METABOLIC FUNCTIONS

OF THE LUNG

LUNG BIOLOGY IN HEALTH AND DISEASE

Executive Editor: **Claude Lenfant**
Director, Division of Lung Diseases
National Institutes of Health
Bethesda, Maryland

METABOLIC FUNCTIONS OF THE LUNG

Edited by

Y.S. Bakhle

Institute of Basic Medical Sciences
Royal College of Surgeons of England
London, England

John R. Vane

Wellcome Research Laboratories
Langley Court
Beckenham, Kent, England

MARCEL DEKKER, INC.   New York and Basel

Library of Congress Cataloging in Publication Data
Main entry under title:

Metabolic functions of the lung.

    (Lung biology in health and disease ; v. 4)
    Includes bibliographical references and indexes.
    1. Lungs. 2. Metabolism. 3. Pulmonary circula-
tion. I. Bakhle, Y. S. II. Vane, John R. III. Title.
RC756.L83 vol. 4 [QP121] 616.2'4'008s [612'.22]
ISBN 0-8247-6383-1   76-41467

MARCEL DEKKER, INC.
270 Madison Avenue, New York, New York 10016

Current printing (last digit):
10 9 8 7 6 5 4 3 2 1

PRINTED IN THE UNITED STATES OF AMERICA

CONTRIBUTORS

Valerie A. Alabaster,* B. Pharm., Ph. D.   Department of Pharmacology, Institute of Basic Medical Sciences, Royal College of Surgeons of England, London, England

Marshall W. Anderson, Ph.D., M.S., B.S.   Head, Pharmacokinetic Section, Biometry Branch, National Institute of Environmental Health Sciences, Research Triangle Park, North Carolina

Y.S. Bakhle, M.A., D.Phil.   Senior Lecturer in Pharmacology, Department of Pharmacology, Institute of Basic Medical Sciences, Royal College of Surgeons of England, London, England

David M. Conning, M.D., B.S.   Deputy Director, Central Toxicology Laboratory, Imperial Chemical Industries Ltd., Alderley Park, Macclesfield, Cheshire, England

Thomas E. Eling, Ph.D., M.S., B.S.   Head, Pharmacokinetic Section, Pharmacology Branch, National Institute of Environmental Health Sciences, Research Triangle Park, North Carolina

John E. Etherton,† M.I.Biol.   Central Toxicology Laboratory, Imperial Chemical Industries, Ltd., Alderley Park, Macclesfield, Cheshire, England

Sergio H. Ferreira, M.S.   Associate Professor, Department of Pharmacology, Faculdade de Medicina de Ribeirão Preto, Ribeirão Preto, Est São Paulo, Brazil

Present affiliation
    *Consultant Pharmacologist, Medicinal Biology, Pfizer Ltd., Sandwich, Kent, England
    †Fitzwilliam College, Cambridge, England

iii

Roderick J. Flower, B.Sc., Ph.D.   Department of Pharmacology, Wellcome Foundation Ltd., Wellcome Research Laboratories, Langley Court, Beckenham, Kent, England

C. Norman Gillis, Ph.D.   Professor, Departments of Anesthesiology and Pharmacology, Yale University School of Medicine, New Haven, Connecticut

Nicholas M. Greene, M.D.   Professor of Anesthesiology, Department of Anesthesiology, Yale University School of Medicine, New Haven, Connecticut

Clyde Griffin Huggins, Ph.D.   Professor, Biochemistry and Associate Dean, Academic Affairs, College of Medicine, University of South Alabama, Mobile, Alabama

Gesina L. Longnecker,* Ph.D.   Instructor, Department of Pharmacology, College of Medicine, University of South Alabama, Mobile, Alabama

Richard M. Philpot, Ph.D., B.S.   Research Chemist, Pharmacology Branch, National Institute of Environmental Health Sciences, Research Triangle Park, North Carolina

Priscilla J. Piper, B.Sc., Ph.D.   Lecturer in Pharmacology, Department of Pharmacology, Institute of Basic Medical Sciences, Royal College of Surgeons of England, London, England

James W. Ryan, M.D., D.Phil.   Senior Scientist, Papanicolaou Cancer Research Institute and Associate Professor of Medicine, University of Miami, Miami, Florida

Una S. Ryan, Ph.D.   Senior Scientist, Papanicolaou Cancer Research Institute and Assistant Professor of Medicine, University of Miami, Miami, Florida

Sami I. Said, M.D.   Professor, Department of Internal Medicine and Pharmacology, University of Texas Southwestern Medical School and Veterans Administration Hospital, Dallas, Texas

John R. Vane, D.Sc., F.R.S.   Research Director, Wellcome Foundation Ltd., Wellcome Research Laboratories, Langley Court, Beckenham, Kent, England

Present affiliation
    *Assistant Professor, Department of Pharmacology, University of South Alabama College of Medicine, Mobile, Alabama

FOREWORD

I would be hard put to say whether the expansion of research on the lung and on respiratory disease is a precursor or a result of increasing public awareness of the importance of pulmonary illness. Whatever the case, we have undoubtedly witnessed both phenomena within a relatively short period of time, and with them a rather sobering realization of the limitations in both scientific and general public knowledge of lung disease. New concerns about the impact of environmental and occupational hazards on lung function—impacts that may only manifest themselves in frank disease after decades of seemingly innocuous exposure—serve to remind us all that society pays a heavy price when knowledge lags behind action, and moreover that society looks to science for solutions.

This series of monographs is, therefore, most timely and important. The substantial increase in the number and variety of scientific reports on respiratory and pulmonary topics makes it all the more critical that work in this field be subjected to thorough and comprehensive review as a service to the scientist and the physician who find it virtually impossible to "keep up," let alone to assimilate and evaluate a rapidly growing body of knowledge in an area of human health that is of mounting importance.

Chronic and acute lung diseases are among the major causes of disability and death in all age groups. From a public health standpoint, prevention of these diseases is a goal that amply justifies an increased commitment of research resources. For it is clear that the most effective paths toward prevention will emerge out of disciplined study in many fields, from the physiology and biochemistry of the respiratory system to the pathology and therapy of respiratory disorders.

I feel sure that this series of publications will continue to make a substantial contribution to the science and practice of medicine and to the hopes we have for more effective concepts and·methods of preventing a major segment of human disease.

Theodore Cooper, M.D.
Assistant Secretary for Health
Department of Health, Education,
and Welfare

PREFACE

It is now well established that the pulmonary circulation has another function apart from that associated with the exchange of gases. This is a pharmacokinetic one, in which the cells and enzyme systems of the pulmonary vascular bed change the biological activity of a variety of substances presented to them via the pulmonary circulation.

Our own contribution to this field started some ten years ago with a study of the metabolic fate of several vasoactive amines, peptides, and prostaglandins. For this, we used a dynamic bioassay system, the blood-bathed organ technique, which allows a continuous and immediate estimation of the inactivation (or activation) of any musculotropic substance in the few seconds that it takes to cross a particular vascular bed. At that time, there were already a few scattered reports in the literature showing that some substances, like 5-hydroxytryptamine, were inactivated on passage through the lungs. It was, however, the concentrated effort by my colleagues in the Department of Pharmacology at The Royal College of Surgeons of England that allowed some general principles to be proposed and also provided the stimulus for much of the work described in this book.

We developed the concept that inactivation or removal of vasoactive substances from the venous blood was an important cleansing function of the lungs, protecting the arterial circulation from the potent and sometimes deleterious effects of these substances. Thus, we showed that not only 5-hydroxytryptamine but also bradykinin, noradrenaline, prostaglandins E_1, E_2, and $F_{2\alpha}$ were all inactivated or removed whereas some substances, often very closely related, were allowed free passage through the pulmonary circulation. These included adrenaline, angiotensin II, oxytocin, and vasopressin.

Fundamental developments in this field are discussed in detail in the chapters by Alabaster; Ferreira and Bakhle; Flower; and Philpot, Anderson, and Eling. It is now apparent that uptake processes, storage, and enzymic degradation all play a part in the inactivation processes for these substances.

The removal of some substances but not of others led to the idea that vasoactive hormones could be classified either as *local* or as *circulating*, depending upon whether they were removed by the lungs. A local hormone would be released at or near the target cells, have its effect, and be inactivated before reaching the arterial circulation. Any of the local hormone that escaped immediate inactivation and spilled over into the venous blood would either be inactivated within a few seconds in the blood itself or, if it reached the lungs, by the pulmonary circulation. A circulating hormone would be released into the venous blood and then distributed through the arterial circulation, without loss of activity on passage through the lungs.

The other side of the story began with the work of Ng and Vane which showed that rapid conversion of angiotensin I to the much more active angiotensin II was not in the bloodstream, as previously supposed, but in the pulmonary circulation. Since then, there has been abundant confirmation that the pulmonary vascular bed is an important site of conversion of angiotensin I to angiotensin II, and the lung is a rich source of the peptidase involved (converting enzyme), as can be seen from the chapter by Longenecker and Huggins.

Gillis and Greene present the clinical implications of the laboratory research, diluting the enthusiasms of the bench with the cold water of practical therapeutic considerations.

An essential part of these investigations of lung pharmacokinetics has been the localization of the metabolic processes described. With over 40 different cell types to choose from, this is an unenviable task but the chapters by Ryan and Ryan and by Etherton and Conning summarize two different and successful approaches to this task.

The activation of angiotensin I by conversion to angiotensin II in the pulmonary circulation forced us to look on the lungs as a potential "endocrine" organ which could contribute vasoactive hormones to the circulation, as well as removing them. In this context, I stressed the analogy between the respiratory and metabolic functions of the lung. Just as by the physical processes of diffusion and filtration the lung removes carbon dioxide, emboli, and cellular debris from the blood, so by biochemical processes it removes 5-hydroxytryptamine, bradykinin, and prostaglandins. Just as the respiratory function of the lung adds oxygen, so the metabolic functions can add angiotensin II and, after specific types of stimulation, histamine, prostaglandins, rabbit aorta contracting substance (RCS, now known as Thromboxane A_2), and perhaps other spasmogens. These aspects are covered in the chapters by Piper and by Said.

It is always pleasing to see a new field develop and grow, particularly if one is fortunate enough to contribute at an early stage to its development and growth. All the authors of this book are recognized internationally as authorities on the subjects which they present, and I commend the reader to this work.

John R. Vane

INTRODUCTION

Although it was as far back as the mid 1920s that the first publications appeared indicating an active metabolic function of the lung [E.H. Starling and E.B. Verney, 1925 (5-hydroxytryptamine); H.H. Dale, 1929 (histamine); A.F. Charles and D.A. Scott, 1933 (heparin)], it was not until the 1960s that the importance and tremendous significance of this function was adequately recognized. At that time Vane and his colleagues began to report their elegant experiments clearly demonstrating the role of the lung in handling biochemical substances. Since then many investigators worldwide have pursued new and fascinating avenues of research to attain a better understanding of this aspect of lung function.

Although the metabolic activities that occur in the lung are not unique, they do have a unique role because the lung acts as a "gate" to the blood and hence has an impact on the circulatory system of the entire body.

Various disciplines—biochemistry, physiology, pharmacology, morphology, and clinical medicine—have contributed to the solution of some aspects of this problem, but many questions remain unanswered.

This monograph addresses the question of the role of the lung in the handling of bioactive substances. It is written by distinguished scientists from many disciplines and from three continents. Its breadth is testimony to the complexity of the subject. However, through the dynamic leadership of Drs. Bakhle and Vane, what seemed to be an almost impossible task has been accomplished. This volume is a tribute to its editors and its authors, and it is an asset to the series of monographs on Lung Biology in Health and Disease.

Claude Lenfant
Bethesda, Maryland

CONTENTS

Contents *xv*

METABOLIC FUNCTIONS
OF THE LUNG

Part I

METABOLISM OF BLOODBORNE SUBSTRATES

1

Inactivation of Endogenous Amines in the Lungs

VALERIE A. ALABASTER

Institute of Basic Medical Sciences
Royal College of Surgeons of England
London, England

I. Introduction

It has long been known that the lungs are capable of removing vasoactive substances from the blood. In 1925 Starling and Verney found it impossible to maintain adequate circulation with defibrinated blood through an isolated kidney without including the lungs in the perfusion circuit because a potent vasoconstrictor substance was present in the blood. The vasoconstrictor substance in serum was later identified as 5-hydroxytryptamine (Rapport et al. 1948a,b). However, only within the last 7 years has the ability of the lungs to remove certain hormones from the blood been investigated in any detail and become recognized as an important pulmonary function that can be altered in certain disease states and influenced by drug treatment (Vane 1969, Bakhle and Vane 1974, Gillis et al. 1974).

The biogenic amines, noradrenaline, adrenaline, dopamine, 5-hydroxytryptamine (5-HT), histamine, and acetylcholine, all have marked excitatory or inhibitory actions on a variety of organs and physiologic functions, through an action on smooth muscle and on glandular and neuronal tissues. The concentration of circulating amines can increase as a result of various stimuli or physiologic response: catecholamines, for example, are released into the venous circulation from the adrenal medulla and postganglionic sympathetic nerve endings in response to sympathetic stimulation; 5-hydroxytryptamine can be released from platelets during aggregation and from the gut. The removal of circulating amines by uptake into organs depends both on the magnitude of uptake per unit weight of tissue and on the fraction of cardiac output received by that organ. The lungs, which, in contrast to all other organs, receive the total venous return, are in an ideal position to regulate the concentration of amines in venous blood before they reach the arterial circulation where the biogenic amines can have such a profound effect. Before discussing the metabolic or pharmacokinetic function of lungs with respect to the biogenic amines, I would like to review briefly the methods used to investigate the fate of a drug in the lungs, since it is important to recognize the limitations involved and relevance of the results obtained when comparing experimental data and when attempting to extrapolate the results to the physiologic state.

A variety of techniques and preparations have been used to investigate the fate of drugs in the lung and pulmonary circulation, including distribution studies in the whole animal, measurement of inactivation of drugs by homogenized lung preparations, and measurement of the disappearance of drug from the pulmonary circulation in vivo or in isolated perfused lungs. Distribution studies, where the drug concentration in lung tissue is determined at varying times after administration, do not reflect the ability of the lung to remove drug in one circulation, since the lapse of time allows redistribution to take place. Similarly studies in homogenized or minced lung tissue do not necessarily reflect the metabolizing activity of the pulmonary circulation, since homogenization of tissue can expose enzyme systems not normally accessible to the drug on passage through the pulmonary circulation.

Removal of a drug in one circulation through the lungs in vivo is measured by injecting the drug intravenously or into the right heart and determining the amount surviving passage through the pulmonary circulation by either serial sampling of arterial blood and estimation of the drug chemically or biologically, or by continuous bioassay using the blood-bathed organ technique (Vane 1964, 1969). In these experiments, as in isolated lung preparations, the quantitative determination of removal of an amine will depend on whether the drug is measured in the lung effluent at fixed time intervals or by assaying peak biologic activity. In addition, results obtained will depend on whether the amine is administered as a single bolus injection where a high concentration is attained for a short time, possibly temporarily overwhelming an uptake system, or as an infusion and removal assessed under steady state conditions. For example, the pulmonary circulation of dogs in vivo removed only 33% of 5-HT injected into the pulmonary artery (Davis and Wang 1965), whereas up to 98% of intravenously infused 5-HT was inactivated (Thomas and Vane 1967).

Some measure of the extent to which vasoactive amines are removed from the pulmonary circulation can also be obtained by comparing systemic blood pressure responses, produced by intravenous administration, to responses produced by intra-arterial administration of the amine. The blood pressure responses can, however, be affected by other factors since biogenic amines can induce circulatory and respiratory reflex changes and can release spasmogens from the lung (Alabaster and Bakhle 1970b, Bakhle and Smith 1972).

Isolated lungs perfused through the pulmonary artery offer, perhaps, the best method for investigating the properties of the pulmonary uptake and metabolism systems for biogenic amines, since external factors can be varied and controlled to a greater extent than in whole animal experiments and a lower concentration of amine can be used. The concentration used is an important factor when the amine under study can cause marked changes in pulmonary blood flow and when studying an uptake system that can be saturated. This is illustrated clearly in the results of Boileau and associates (1972a) where lung removal of noradrenaline in the anesthetized dog decreased from 54% to 5% as the infusion concentration increased from 0.2 to 3 μg/kg/ min. In studies of pulmonary uptake in isolated perfused lungs, biogenic amines are administered via the pulmonary artery and measurements are made of either the amount of biogenic amine retained by the lung or the amount of amine surviving passage through the lung. Quantitative assessment of pulmonary removal of biogenic amines will obviously vary according to the method used, especially if the amine is rapidly metabolized in lung tissue.

The term *amine uptake* refers strictly to the transfer of an amine across a cell membrane, and the true rate of uptake cannot be measured unless the amine is retained in the tissue without significant leakage or enzyme inactivation. Since pulmonary metabolism of certain biogenic amines involves both an uptake and enzyme inactivation process, the term *pulmonary removal* is used in this chapter to describe the reduction in biologic activity or concentration of amine during passage through the lungs.

II. Noradrenaline

The first demonstration that the lungs could remove noradrenaline was made by Eiseman and associates (1964). These investigators found that isolated lungs of the dog, perfused with blood in a recirculating system, removed 96%

of administered noradrenaline over a 30-min period, as opposed to 51% inactivation in blood alone during this same time period. The lungs of many species have since been shown to remove noradrenaline. Approximately 20% to 35% of injected noradrenaline was removed on passage through the pulmonary circulation in anesthetized cats and dogs when removal was estimated by the blood-bathed organ technique (Ginn and Vane 1968); similar results were obtained in cats, dogs, rabbits, and rats by the systemic pressor response method (Boileau et al. 1972a). Noradrenaline was removed to a comparable degree from the pulmonary circulation of man, as estimated either by radiochemical analysis of pulmonary arterial and left atrial blood (Gillis et al. 1972) or by the systemic pressor response technique (Boileau et al. 1972a).

Pulmonary removal of noradrenaline has been studied in isolated lung preparations by measuring both uptake of noradrenaline into lung tissue (Hughes et al. 1969, Nicholas et al. 1974) and the amount of noradrenaline surviving passage through the pulmonary circulation (Gillis and Iwasawa 1972, Alabaster and Bakhle 1973). Radioactivity derived from infusions of $[^3H]$ noradrenaline through rat isolated lungs was concentrated in lung tissue by a saturable uptake process (Hughes et al. 1969). Uptake of noradrenaline was approximately 30% when the lungs were perfused with low concentrations of amine (3×10^{-8} M, 5 ng/ml), although uptake decreased significantly at concentrations above 6×10^{-7} M (100 ng/ml). Nicholas et al. (1974) confirmed that uptake of noradrenaline in rat lungs obeyed saturation kinetics, the process tending to saturate at perfusion concentrations of 6 to 8×10^{-7} M. Removal was slightly higher when assessed by measuring the amount of noradrenaline surviving passage through the pulmonary circulation, but similar evidence of saturation was obtained. The biologic activity of infusions of noradrenaline (2 to 50 ng/ml) was reduced by 35% to 40% in rat isolated lungs (Alabaster and Bakhle 1973), but removal decreased as infusion concentrations increased to 6×10^{-7} M (100 ng/ml). Noradrenaline removal in rabbit isolated lungs (Gillis and Iwasawa 1972) varied between 35% to 50% at infusion concentrations of 6×10^{-7} M, but declined significantly when the concentration was increased to 6×10^{-6} M (1 μg/ml). In these experiments the noradrenaline surviving passage through the lungs was measured fluorometrically.

In rat isolated lungs only 19% of the radioactivity concentrated by the tissue after a 5-min infusion of $[^3H]$ noradrenaline (3×10^{-8} M) was unchanged noradrenaline, the greater proportion being associated with O-methylated and deaminated metabolites (Hughes et al. 1969). Inhibition of either catechol-O-methyltransferase or monoamine oxidase reduced metabolite formation and increased the lung accumulation of unchanged $[^3H]$ noradrenaline. Although the loss of tritium was faster from untreated lungs than from lungs treated with enzyme inhibitors (Hughes et al. 1969), the total amount of noradrenaline removed from the perfusion fluid was unaffected by enzyme inhibitors (Iwasawa and Gillis 1974), implying that the rate-limiting step in lung removal of noradrenaline was the uptake of amine rather than its metabolism.

Studies in isolated lungs from rats and rabbits suggest that the pulmonary uptake system for noradrenaline requires energy, but this may be supplied by oxidation of noncarbohydrate substrates since perfusion of lungs with a glucose-free medium did not affect pulmonary removal of noradrenaline (Iwasawa et al. 1973, Nicholas et al. 1974). The uptake is however sensitive to temperature. Noradrenaline uptake (at 1.5×10^{-6} M) was inhibited by 81% when the temperature of perfusion was lowered from 35° to 6°C in rabbit isolated lungs (Iwasawa et al. 1973). In contrast to that occurring at 35°C, amine uptake at 6°C was probably passive and dependent on physical factors alone. Perfusion at 4°C also inhibited noradrenaline removal by approximately 85% in rat isolated lungs (Nicholas et al. 1974). There is direct evidence for the participation of sodium ions, since uptake was inhibited by decreasing the sodium concentration of the perfusion fluid in rat lungs (Nicholas et al. 1974). Uptake is also inhibited by ouabain, but a high concentration of ouabain (10^{-3} M) was required to inhibit noradrenaline uptake in rat lungs (Nicholas et al. 1974). In rabbit lungs ouabain at 10^{-4} M, produced only a 33% inhibition of uptake (Iwasawa et al. 1973). Consequently, it is not known if inhibition of uptake by ouabain is a result of inhibition of a sodium-linked transport of amine, as reported in other cellular systems (Tissari et al. 1969, Bogdanski and Brodie 1969) or through some other action.

Pharmacologic analysis of noradrenaline uptake in isolated lungs has shown it to be inhibited by cocaine (Hughes et al. 1969, Alabaster and Bakhle 1973, Iwasawa and Gillis 1974) and tricyclic antidepressants (Iwasawa and Gillis 1974, Nicholas et al. 1974).

In contrast to this wide agreement, reports on the effects of other uptake inhibitors vary (Table 1). Phenoxybenzamine, at 10^{-5} M, inhibited the uptake of 1.5×10^{-6} M noradrenaline in rabbit lung (Iwasawa and Gillis 1974), but at the same concentration it did not inhibit the removal of lower concentrations of noradrenaline (1 to 6×10^{-8} M) in rat lungs (Alabaster and Bakhle 1973). While it is generally agreed that metaraminol, at 10^{-5} M (Alabaster and Bakhle 1973) or 5×10^{-4} M (Nicholas et al. 1974) has no effect in rat lungs, the investigators cited do not agree about the effect of normetanephrine. As these examples and the data in Table 1 show, many of the divergences could be due to differences in species, in concentrations of substrate and inhibitor, and to other experimental conditions. For instance, in one set of experiments (Nicholas et al. 1974), control uptake was measured in the presence of monoamine oxidase and catechol-*o*-methyltransferase inhibitors, whereas in other experiments control uptake was that occurring in the absence of any drug.

TABLE 1. Comparison of Pulmonary Uptake of Noradrenaline With Other Catecholamine Uptake Systems

Characteristic	Pulmonary uptake[a]	Neuronal uptake (Uptake 1)[a]	Extraneuronal uptake (Uptake 2)[a]
Fate of amine taken up	Metabolized by MAO and COMT [1,12,17,20]	Protected from metabolism by storage in nerve granules [14]	Metabolized by MAO and COMT [5,14,19]
Effects of experimental conditions and drugs			
Low [Na] in perfusion medium	Inhibited [20]	Inhibited [2,10]	Partially inhibited [11]
Cold ($4^\circ - 6^\circ$C)	Inhibited [17,20]	Inhibited [9,13]	Inhibited [8]
Anoxia (N_2 in perfusion medium)	Inhibited [17]		
Ouabain ($10^{-4} - 10^{-3}$ M)	Inhibited [17,20]	Inhibited [10,22]	Not inhibited [6]
Cocaine (10^{-6} M)	Inhibited [1,12]	Inhibited [14]	Not inhibited [14,21]
Tricyclic antidepressants (10^{-5} M)	Inhibited [18,20]	Inhibited [14]	Not inhibited [7,14,21]
Normetanephrine (5×10^{-6} M) (10^{-4} M) (5×10^{-6} M)	Not inhibited [1] Partially inhibited [18] Inhibited [20]	Not inhibited [14] — —	Inhibited [6,14] — —
Metaraminol ($10^{-5} - 5 \times 10^{-4}$ M)	Not inhibited [1,20]	Inhibited [14,19]	Not inhibited [6,14,19]
Phenoxybenzamine (10^{-5} M) (10^{-5} M)	Not inhibited [1] Partially inhibited [18]	Inhibited [19] —	Inhibited [6,19] —
Steroids (10^{-5} M)	Inhibited [16]	Not inhibited [15]	Inhibited [15,21]
Monoamine oxidase inhibitors ($3 - 5 \times 10^{-4}$ M)	Not inhibited [18]	—	—

MAO and COMT inhibitors (10^{-4} M)	Not inhibited [18,20]	—	—
Kinetic constants			
Km (M)	1.4×10^{-6} [12] $1 \quad \times 10^{-6}$ [20] 2.4×10^{-6} [17]	6.6×10^{-7} [14]	2.5×10^{-4} [14]
Vmax (moles $g^{-1}min^{-1}$)	2.2×10^{-9} [12] 2.8×10^{-9} [20] 5.7×10^{-9} [17]	1.4×10^{-6} [14]	$1 \quad \times 10^{-4}$ [14]
Transport of other catecholamines. Order of affinity.	Noradrenaline ≫ adrenaline. No uptake of dopamine or isoprenaline (see text for references).	Dopamine > noradrenaline > adrenaline [3] No uptake of isoprenaline.	Isoprenaline > adrenaline > noradrenaline ≫ dopamine [4,14]

aReferences are in brackets. For full source see References.
b[1] Alabaster and Bakhle 1973; [2] Bogdanski and Brodie 1969; [3] Burgen and Iversen 1965; [4] Callingham and Burgen 1966, [5] Eisenfeld et al. 1967a; [6] Eisenfeld et al. 1967b; [7] Farnebo and Malmfors 1969; [8] Gillespie et al. 1970; [9] Gillis and Paton 1966; [10] Gillis and Paton 1967; [11] Gulati and Sivaramakrishna 1975; [12] Hughes et al. 1969; [13] Iversen 1963; [14] Iversen 1965; [15] Iversen and Salt 1970; [16] Iwasawa and Gillis 1973; [17] Iwasawa et al. 1973; [18] Iwasawa and Gillis 1974; [19] Lightman and Iversen 1969; [20] Nicholas et al. 1974; [21] Salt 1972; [22] Tissari et al. 1969.

Despite these minor differences all results demonstrated that the pulmonary uptake of noradrenaline cannot be identified with either $Uptake_1$ or $Uptake_2$ (Iversen 1965), but that it comprises features of both uptake mechanisms. For instance, pulmonary uptake resembles neuronal uptake of noradrenaline ($Uptake_1$) into rat heart (Iversen 1963, 1965), rat brain synaptosomes (Tissari et al. 1969), and heart slices (Gillis and Paton 1966, 1967, Bogdanski and Brodie 1969) in that uptake is inhibited by cocaine, tricyclic antidepressants, and hypothermia and is dependent on sodium ions. However, metaraminol, which is a specific inhibitor of $Uptake_1$ (Iversen 1965, Lightman and Iversen 1969), had no effect on lung removal of noradrenaline (Alabaster and Bakhle 1973, Nicholas et al. 1974). Furthermore, pulmonary uptake did not show any optical specificity in rats (Nicholas et al. 1974) or rabbits (Iwasawa et al. 1973), whereas neuronal uptake generally favors the naturally-occurring (−) isomer (Iversen 1963, Coyle and Snyder 1969), although there are exceptions (Draskóczy and Trendelenburg 1970, Iversen et al. 1971). Perhaps the strongest evidence against pulmonary uptake being a neuronal uptake is that the amine taken up in lung is rapidly metabolized, whereas that taken up into adrenergic neurones is characteristically protected from enzymic attack. Degeneration of adrenergic neurones is caused by 6-hydroxydopamine, abolishing neuronal uptake, but in lungs from rabbits pretreated with this amine, the uptake of noradrenaline was unchanged (Iwasawa and Gillis 1974).

Autoradiographic studies support pharmacologic data showing that pulmonary removal of noradrenaline is an extraneuronal process. Examination of rat lung tissue by light and electron microscopy after infusions of labeled noradrenaline (3×10^{-8} M) showed that the only sites of intense labeling were capillary endothelial cells, both in untreated and in lungs treated with pargyline (monoamine oxidase inhibitor) and tropolone (catechol-O-methyltransferase inhibitor) (Hughes et al. 1969). In rat lungs treated with iproniazid and tropolone, Nicholas et al. (1974) observed that only 30% of the capillary endothelial cells were labeled but that 90% of the small distended vessels leading into or from the capillary beds were labeled, suggesting a regional specificity in the uptake of $[^3H]$ noradrenaline by the lung vasculature. In addition, some labeling was observed in the walls of the large veins but not in those of the large arteries. Studies by fluorescence microscopy in rabbit lung after perfusion with higher concentrations of noradrenaline (6–30×10^{-6} M) showed noradrenaline fluorescence in capillary endothelial cells and immediate postcapillary venules only when the metabolism of noradrenaline was prevented (Iwasawa et al. 1973).

If, therefore, pulmonary uptake is not neuronal, how does it compare with extraneuronal uptake systems already described? The chief characteristic of extraneuronal uptake in a variety of tissues is rapid metabolism of the amine taken up (Iversen 1965, Eisenfeld et al. 1967a, Avakian and Gillespie

1968, Gillespie et al. 1970). The rat heart has been the most extensively studied tissue in which extraneuronal uptake of noradrenaline was termed Uptake$_2$ to distinguish it from neuronal uptake, Uptake$_1$ (Iversen 1965, Lightman and Iversen 1969). Uptake$_2$ is an amine transport mechanism that differs pharmacologically from Uptake$_1$ in that it is unaffected by cocaine and metaraminol and inhibited by metanephrine and normetanephrine (Iversen 1965). Phenoxybenzamine inhibits both Uptake$_1$ and Uptake$_2$ (Lightman and Iversen 1969). Extraneuronal uptake of noradrenaline, with sensitivity to inhibitors similar to that in heart, has also been described in vascular smooth muscle of the rabbit ear artery (Avakian and Gillespie 1968), human umbilical artery (Gulati and Sivaramakrishna 1975), and cat spleen (Gillespie et al. 1970) as well as in the guinea pig trachea (Foster 1968) and nictitating membrane (Draskóczy and Trendelenburg 1970). Biochemically, Uptake$_2$ has been differentiated from Uptake$_1$ by its higher K_m and V_{max} (Iversen 1971) for noradrenaline. Although pulmonary uptake of noradrenaline resembles extraneuronal uptake processes in other tissues in being followed by rapid metabolism and being unaffected by metaraminol, it is also inhibited by cocaine. More significantly, the K_m and V_{max} values for pulmonary uptake are lower than those for Uptake$_2$, and very comparable with those for Uptake$_1$.

Table 1 summarizes some of the properties of the lung noradrenaline uptake system and compares them with those of neuronal and various extraneuronal uptake processes described in other tissues. So far, the characteristics of pulmonary uptake, Uptake$_3$?, that differentiate it from other uptake processes are high affinity (low K_m) combined with rapid and extensive metabolism. Another characteristic is the almost complete specificity of the uptake, as neither adrenaline nor isoprenaline are taken up in lung (see below). The presence of an inactivating system for noradrenaline in the pulmonary circulation, operative at low physiologic concentrations of noradrenaline, strongly suggests a physiologic role for this system in controlling and limiting levels of noradrenaline that reach the arterial circulation.

III. Adrenaline and Isoprenaline

As early as 1905, Elliot showed that adrenaline did not disappear in the lungs as it did in other vascular beds. This observation was not investigated further until Ginn and Vane (1968) compared the biologic inactivation of catecholamines in the pulmonary circulation and other vascular beds in anesthetized cats and dogs, using the blood-bathed organ technique. Unlike noradrenaline, intravenous infusions of adrenaline passed through the pulmonary circulation without loss of activity. Similarly, pulmonary inactivation of adrenaline was negligible when determined by comparing systemic pressor responses to adrenaline injected into the pulmonary artery with responses produced by injections into the left atrium or ascending aorta in rats, dogs, cats, and man (Boileau et al. 1971)

Rat isolated lungs, perfused with tritiated adrenaline (3×10^{-8} M, 5 ng/ml), accumulated a small amount of radioactivity that was increased by treating the lungs with the enzyme inhibitors pargyline and tropolone (Hughes et al. 1969). The removal process therefore was qualitatively similar to that described for noradrenaline, but the amount of adrenaline taken up was approximately seven times less than the uptake of amine after a similar infusion of noradrenaline. Gillis and Iwasawa (1972) compared the removal of adrenaline and noradrenaline in lungs isolated from rabbits by measuring the concentration of amine in the lung perfusate fluorometrically during a 30-min infusion of either adrenaline or noradrenaline (100 ng/ml) into the pulmonary circulation. Adrenaline removal was calculated to be 13% in contrast to the 39% removal of noradrenaline.

Isoprenaline is another catecholamine not removed significantly in the pulmonary circulation. Infusions of this amine passed through the lungs of anesthetized cats without loss of biologic activity (Ginn and Vane 1968), and there was no evidence of pulmonary inactivation in patients undergoing cardiac catheterization and in anesthetized dogs when systemic depressor responses to intravenous and intraarterial isoprenaline were compared (Boileau et al. 1970).

The fact that both adrenaline and isoprenaline are better substrates than noradrenaline for the extraneuronal Uptake$_2$ process in rat heart (Callingham and Burgen 1966), emphasizes the difference between the extraneuronal catecholamine uptake process in the pulmonary circulation and that described in other tissues.

IV. Dopamine

Dopamine-containing neurones in certain areas of the brain possess a specific high affinity uptake system for dopamine, which differs in drug sensitivity to that described for noradrenaline in other central adrenergic neurones (Hamberger 1967, Coyle and Snyder 1969). Dopamine is also taken up by the neuronal catecholamine uptake process (Uptake$_1$) in rat heart (Peskar et al. 1968) and by mast cells (Eränkö and Jansson 1967). However, there is no evidence that dopamine is taken up or metabolized in the pulmonary circulation. Thus, in rats and man, depressor responses to dopamine injected via the left atrium and pulmonary artery were similar (Boileau et al. 1972b). More direct evidence of the lack of pulmonary uptake was obtained by these workers, using chemical measurements of pre- and postpulmonary plasma levels of dopamine during its constant intravenous infusion into anesthetized dogs.

There was no significant difference between the mean pulmonary arterial and mean aortic level of dopamine.

In lungs isolated from the rat very little tritium accumulated after an infusion of [³H] dopamine into the pulmonary artery, compared with the amount accumulated after infusing [³H] noradrenaline (Nicholas et al. 1974). The lung perfusate was not analyzed, so this result could be explained either by a lower rate of uptake of dopamine or its more rapid metabolism compared with noradrenaline. The latter possibility seems unlikely in view of results obtained from experiments in vivo.

Dopamine is present in low concentration in lung tissue of the cat, dog, rabbit, mouse, guinea pig, and man, while in ruminants the concentration is very much higher (Euler and Lishajko 1957, Aviado and Sadavongvivad 1970). It would be interesting to know if the fate of dopamine in the pulmonary circulation of ruminants differs from that in other species.

V. 5-Hydroxytryptamine

The 5-hydroxytryptamine (5-HT) content of lung tissue is relatively low, varying from 0.5 to 0.7 $\mu g/g$ depending on the species (Weissbach et al. 1957, Sadavongvivad 1970). It is formed from 5-hydroxytryptophan by decarboxylation and, as the required decarboxylase is present in lung (Sadavongvivad 1970), 5-HT could be synthesized in the lungs in situ. Distribution studies in mice (Axelrod and Inscoe 1963), in rats, and in guinea pigs (Sadavongvivad 1970) indicate that the lungs can also store exogenously administered 5-HT. However, these studies do not necessarily reflect the properties of the pulmonary circulation, since platelets, which take up 5-HT (Stacey 1961), can become trapped and lodged in lung capillaries (Aviado and Sadavongvivad 1970), and could contribute to the amount of 5-HT in lung.

Studies in anesthetized animals (Davis and Wang 1965, Thomas and Vane 1967) and in isolated blood-perfused lung preparations (Gaddum et al. 1953) have shown that there is an efficient removal process for 5-HT in the pulmonary circulation. Up to 98% of an infusion of 5-HT was removed in a single passage through the pulmonary circulation in anesthetized dogs (Thomas and Vane 1967). However, it was not clear from these experiments, whether the 5-HT removed from the pulmonary circulation was stored or inactivated by lung tissue. Since removal of 5-HT in the pulmonary circulation of anesthetized dogs was not affected by monoamine oxidase inhibitors (Thomas and Vane 1967, Davis and Wang 1965), it was assumed that lung removal of 5-HT did not involve inactivation by monoamine oxidase. However, extracts of lung tissue could inactivate 5-HT (Rapport et al. 1948c), and in isolated, blood-perfused lungs of the dog, 5-HT added to the recirculating blood was metabolized to 5-hydroxyindoleacetic acid within 60 min (Eiseman et al. 1964). The fate of 5-HT in the pulmonary circulation has been further investigated in isolated lungs perfused with physiologic salt solution by two methods: (a) measuring, by bioassay or chemical analysis, the amount of 5-HT surviving passage through the lungs (Alabaster and Bakhle 1970a, Alabaster 1971, Gruby et al. 1971, Gillis and Iwasawa 1972) and (b) measuring the retention of infused 5-HT in lung tissue (Junod 1972).

Tritiated 5-HT was infused through isolated lungs of rats, dogs, and guinea pigs and pulmonary removal assessed by analyzing both the biologic activity and radioactivity of the lung perfusate (Alabaster and Bakhle 1970a, Alabaster 1971). Biologic activity was reduced by 90% to 94% on a single passage through lungs of rats and dogs. Radioactivity measurements confirmed this degree of inactivation since, after a 4-min infusion of [^{3}H] 5-HT through the lungs, 10% of the radioactivity appeared in the perfusate as unchanged 5-HT within 5 min, and the rest of the radioactivity was recovered over the next 40 to 60 min. Chromatographic analysis of the lung perfusate revealed only one metabolite, which corresponded with 5-hydroxyindoleacetic acid. The pulmonary removal process was less efficient in the guinea pig, since 75% of an infusion of 5-HT was removed. Similar results were obtained by Gruby et al. (1971): 50% of an infusion of 5-HT was removed on a single passage through guinea pig lungs, and chromatographic analysis of the perfusate after recycling labeled 5-HT through the lungs for 30 min revealed almost total conversion to 5-hydroxyindoleacetic acid. Studies involving analysis of lung tissue after infusions into the pulmonary circulation have also demonstrated the efficient removal of 5-HT. In rat lungs approximately 60% of a 3-min infusion of [^{14}C] 5-HT was taken up: metabolism was rapid since only 4% to 8% of the radioactivity was accounted for as unchanged 5-HT (Junod 1972).

Experiments in isolated lungs of rabbit and rat indicate that pulmonary uptake of 5-HT is a saturable process (Alabaster 1971, Junod 1972, Iwasawa et al. 1973). In rat lungs 90% to 94% of the biologic activity of an infusion of 5-HT (1 to 100 ng/ml, 0.6 to 55 $\times$ 10^{-9} M) was removed, but the degree of removal decreased as the concentration of 5-HT infused was increased up to 2 μg/ml; 1.1 $\times$ 10^{-6} M. This reduced inactivation at high concentrations was not due to the pulmonary vasoconstrictor effects of 5-HT leading to reduced efficiency of lung perfusion, since methysergide, which antagonized the 5-HT induced increases in pulmonary artery perfusion pressure, had no effect on the amount of 5-HT removed (Alabaster 1971). Similarly, the removal of 5-HT was found to decrease with concentrations of infused 5-HT over 1 μg/ml in the rat (Junod 1972) and over 500 ng/ml in the rabbit (Iwasawa et al. 1973).

Although 5-HT taken up by the lung is rapidly metabolized, enzymic inactivation does not appear to be the rate-limiting step in the removal process. In the presence of the monoamine oxidase inhibitors, iproniazid or mebanazine, the initial removal of 5-HT in isolated lungs of the rat was little affected although metabolism of 5-HT was markedly reduced, and unchanged 5-HT was detected both biologically and by chromatographic analysis in the lung perfusate for up to 40 min after the infusion period (Alabaster and Bakhle 1970a). Figure 1 shows the effect of mebanazine on 5-HT removal in lungs isolated from dogs, where the biologic activity of lung perfusate was measured by using two rat stomach-strip preparations superfused in series. The biologic activity of an infusion of 5-HT was reduced by 95.5% on passing through untreated lungs. In the presence of mebanazine, a similar amount of 5-HT was removed, as measured by the peak height of contraction of the assay tissues, but the contractions were prolonged in duration, indicating that 5-HT was slowly being washed from the lungs after the end of the infusion (Alabaster 1971). In Junod's experiments (1972), the metabolism of 5-HT in rat lung

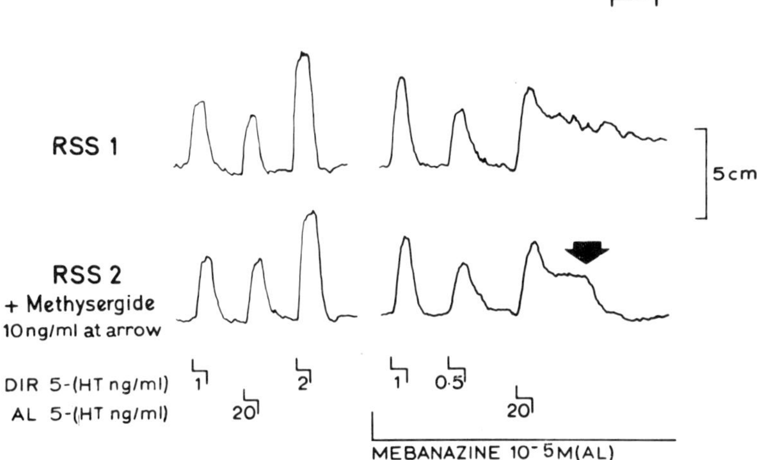

FIGURE 1 Effect of mebanazine on 5-HT removal in dog isolated lung. Record shows contractions of two rat stomach strips (RSS 1 and RSS 2) superfused in series with effluent from lobe of dog lung perfused with Krebs solution. Infusions of 5-HT given either directly to assay tissues (DIR) or into cannula in pulmonary artery (AL). First panel shows removal of 5-HT in untreated lung was 95.5%. Second panel shows that when mebanazine was infused through the lungs as indicated, 96% 5-HT was removed, as measured by the height of contraction of both stomach strips, but contractions were prolonged in duration. Methysergide infused over bottom strip, as shown at arrow, abolished contraction of this tissue showing that prolonged contraction was due to 5-HT (Alabaster and Bakhle, unpublished data).

tissue was almost completely prevented by pretreatment with iproniazid, but uptake of 5-HT from the pulmonary circulation was the same as that under control conditions. Similarly, no inhibition of 5-HT uptake was produced in rabbit lungs treated with pargyline (Gillis and Iwasawa 1972) or in guinea pig lungs treated with nialamide (Gruby et al. 1971).

Pulmonary uptake of 5-HT appears to be an energy-requiring process, since the removal is very dependent on temperature. In rat lungs, lowering the temperature of the perfusing fluid from $37°$ to $4°C$ produced an 86% inhibition of 5-HT removal (Alabaster 1971). Cooling the lung did not damage the removal process since the inhibition could be reversed by warming. The inhibitory effect of hypothermia and its reversibility, on the removal of 5-HT in lungs isolated from rats, is shown in Figure 2. In the same tissue, Junor (1972) also found that uptake of $[^{14}C]$ 5-HT was inhibited by approximately 86% during perfusion at $4°C$. Proportionally more of the radioactivity accumulated by the lung was present as unchanged 5-HT than under control conditions, indicating that metabolism was also reduced by hypothermia. Similarly, in lungs isolated from rabbits, 5-HT removal was reversibly inhibited by 54% to 64% during perfusion at $6°C$ (Iwasawa et al. 1973), while in guinea pig lungs, perfusion at $5°C$ completely prevented pulmonary removal of 5-HT (Gruby et al. 1971).

A sodium carrier system is probably involved in the transport of 5-HT across a cellular membrane in the pulmonary circulation, since lung removal of 5-HT was inhibited by a lowered sodium concentration in the perfusing fluid (Junod 1972). Ouabain (10^{-5} M) had no effect on 5-HT removal in rat lungs (Alabaster 1971), but higher concentrations (10^{-3} M) did have some effect (Junod 1972), which may reflect the insensitivity of $Na^+–K^+$ activated ATPase of rat tissues to cardiac glycosides (Repke et al. 1965). In rabbit lungs ouabain (10^{-4} M) reduced 5-HT uptake by about 33%. Uptake of 5-HT was strongly inhibited by cocaine and tricyclic antidepressant drugs (Alabaster and Bakhle 1970a, Alabaster 1971, Junod 1972, Alabaster and Bakhle 1973, Iwasawa and Gillis 1974). Cocaine, for example, infused through rabbit lungs at a concentration of 10^{-5} M reduced 5-HT removal by 60% (Iwasawa and Gillis 1974). The uptake of 5-HT in lung, therefore, closely resembles that of noradrenaline, since both are inhibited by these drugs. However, noradrenaline and 5-HT are probably taken up at different sites, since noradrenaline in concentrations of up to sixfold molar excess had no effect on pulmonary uptake of 5-HT (10^{-7} M) in lungs isolated from rats (Alabaster and Bakhle 1973) and further increases in concentrations of noradrenaline to 10^{-5} M only reduced 5-HT uptake by 10% in rabbit isolated lungs (Iwasawa and Gillis 1974). Partial inhibition of noradrenaline uptake by 5-HT (2×10^{-7} M $-$ 10^{-5} M) was found in rat lungs by Nicholas et al. (1974), but these results were obtained in the presence of the enzyme inhibitors tropolone and iproniazid.

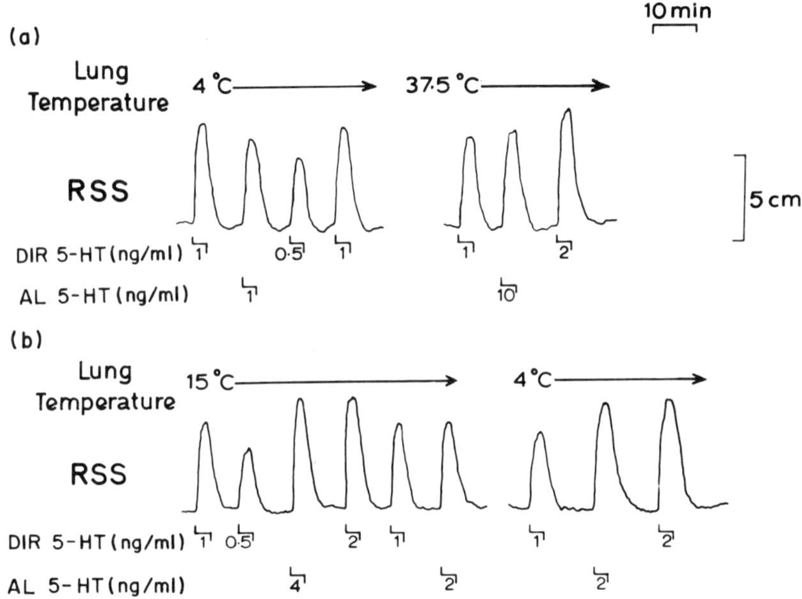

FIGURE 2   Effect of temperature on 5-HT removal in rat isolated lungs. Contractions of rat stomach strip superfused with effluent from lung perfused with Krebs solution, to infusions of 5-HT directly to tissue (DIR) or into pulmonary artery cannula (AL). Temperature of Krebs solution entering lungs varied, but effluent was, in all cases, warmed to 37°C before passing over assay tissues. (a) When lungs perfused with Krebs at 4°C, lung removal of 5-HT was 24%, but on warming the Krebs to 37.5°C, lung removal of 5-HT increased to 90%. (b) Similar experiment in which lung removal of 5-HT at 15°C (panel 1) was compared with lung removal at 4°C (panel 2). At 15°C, lung removal of 5-HT was 50%, but when the Krebs perfusing lung was cooled to 4°C, all 5-HT infused came through lung unchanged (Alabaster and Bakhle, unpublished data).

The pulmonary uptake sites for noradrenaline and 5-HT can be separated pharmacologically. In rabbit lungs, phenoxybenzamine inhibited removal of both 5-HT and noradrenaline at 1.5×10^{-6} M. A high concentration of 5-HT (10^{-5} M) infused together with phenoxybenzamine protected the lung from the inhibitory effect of phenoxybenzamine on 5-HT removal, but it did not prevent the inhibitory effect on noradrenaline removal (Iwasawa and Gillis 1974).

In the lungs the process responsible for uptake and metabolism of 5-HT shows some structural specificity. 5-Hydroxy-*a*-methyltryptamine (*a*-methyl 5-HT) is equipotent with 5-HT as a spasmogen (rat stomach strip preparation) but is not a substrate for monoamine oxidase (Blaschko et al. 1937, Vane

1960). This 5-HT analog had less affinity for the pulmonary uptake site, since the rat lung removed 60% of an infusion of a-methyl 5-HT (4 ng/ml), as measured by the peak contraction height of the assay tissues, compared with 92% removal of a similar infusion of 5-HT. However, since no enzymic inactivation took place, unchanged a-methyl 5-HT slowly reappeared in the lung perfusate for 40 to 60 min after the infusion was stopped (Alabaster 1971). The results of one experiment comparing lung removal of a-methyl 5-HT and 5-HT are shown in Figure 3. Tryptamine is a substrate for monoamine oxidase, but it is not so rapidly oxidized as 5-HT by tissue preparations (Blaschko and Philpot 1953, Hope and Smith 1960). The biologic activity of infusions of tryptamine (1 to 4 ng/ml) was reduced by 65% on passage through lungs isolated from rats. This degree of removal was less than that of equiactive (spasmogenic activity) concentrations of 5-HT (10–50 ng/ml), but similar to that of equimolar concentrations of 5-HT (Alabaster 1971). These results confirm that the important step in the pulmonary removal of 5-HT and other tryptamines is not enzymic inactivation but the initial uptake process.

The properties and sensitivity to drugs of the pulmonary removal process for 5-HT are summarized in Table 2. The platelets take up 5-HT by a process that is temperature and sodium dependent and is inhibited by ouabain, cocaine, and tricyclic antidepressants (Stacey 1961, Todrick and Tait 1969, Pletscher et al. 1967, Sneddon 1969). Similar uptake processes have been described for 5-HT in mast cells (Furano and Green 1964), serotonin and adrenergic neurones in the brain (Tissari et al. 1969, Shaskan and Snyder 1970) and of the vas deferens of rats (Thoa et al. 1969) and cats, and the cat iris (Snipes et al. 1968). However, unlike pulmonary uptake of 5-HT, which is followed by

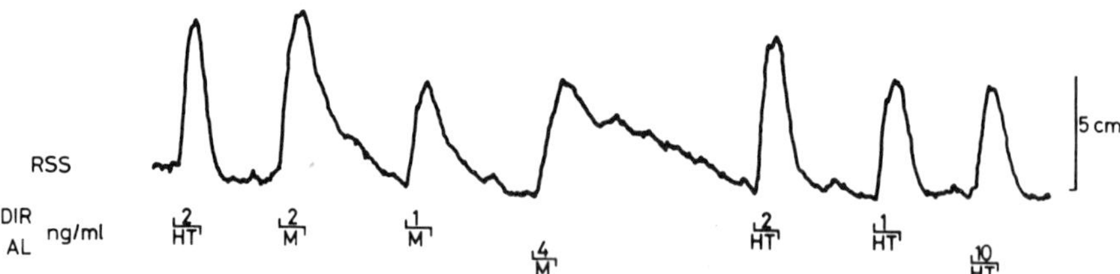

FIGURE 3   Removal of a-methyl 5-hydroxytryptamine by rat isolated lung. Record shows contractions of rat stomach strip (RSS) superfused with effluent from rat lung perfused with Krebs solution to infusions of a-methyl 5-hydroxytryptamine (M) and 5-HT (HT) directly (DIR) or into pulmonary artery cannula (AL). The lung removed 67% of infusion of M compared with 90% of infusion of 5-HT. Note prolonged contraction in response to AL infusion of a-M-5-HT (Alabaster and Bakhle, unpublished data).

TABLE 2   Comparison of Pulmonary Uptake Processes for 5-Hydroxytryptamine and Noradrenaline

Characteristic	5-Hydroxytryptamine[a]	Noradrenaline[b]
Fate of amine taken up	Metabolized [2,3,6]	Metabolized
Effect of experimental conditions and drugs		
Cold $(4°-6°C)$	Inhibited [1,3,4,6]	Inhibited
Sodium-free perfusion medium	Inhibited [6]	Inhibited
Glucose-free perfusion medium	Not inhibited [6]	—
Anoxia (N_2 in perfusion and ventilation)	Inhibited [6,4]	Inhibited
Ouabain $(10^{-5} - 10^{-4}$ M)	Not inhibited [1,6]	Inhibited
$(10^{-3}$ M)	Inhibited [6]	
Cocaine $(10^{-6} - 10^{-4}$ M)	Inhibited [1,5,6]	Inhibited
Tricyclic antidepressants $(5 \times 10^{-6} - 10^{-4}$ M)	Inhibited [2,5,6]	Inhibited
Normetanephrine (5×10^{-6} M)	Not inhibited [2]	Not inhibited
$(10^{-4}$ M)	Inhibited [5]	Inhibited
Metaraminol (10^{-6} M)	Not inhibited [2]	Not inhibited
Phenoxybenzamine (10^{-5} M)	Inhibited [5]	Inhibited
Monoamine oxidase inhibitors $(10^{-5} - 3 \times 10^{-4}$ M)	Not inhibited [1,2,3,5]	Not inhibited
Reserpine, acute	Not inhibited [2]	—
pretreatment	Not inhibited [1,6]	—
Kinetic constants		
K_m (M)	5.2×10^{-6} [4] 5.9×10^{-6} [6]	$1 - 2.4 \times 10^{-6}$
V_{max} (mol g^{-1} min^{-1})	12.8×10^{-9} [4] 19.0×10^{-9} [6]	$2.2 - 5.7 \times 10^{-9}$
Alternative substrates[c]		
Noradrenaline (6×10^{-7} M)	Not inhibited [2]	—
$(10^{-4}$ M)	Inhibited [6]	—
Tryptamine (10^{-5} M)	Inhibited [6]	—

[a] [1] Alabaster 1971; [2] Alabaster and Bakhle 1970; [3] Gruby et al. 1971; [4] Iwasawa et al. 1973; [5] Iwasawa and Gillis 1974; [6] Junod 1972.
[b] For references see Table 1.
[c] Alternative substrates as judged by their ability to inhibit 5-HT uptake.

rapid enzymic inactivation, 5-HT taken up into platelets, mast cells, and neurones is bound and stored in intracellular membrane-bound granules (Green 1962). The accumulated 5-HT in platelets (Pletscher et al. 1967) and vas deferens (Thoa et al. 1969) is oxidized slowly, but the degree of metabolism is very small. Reserpine, which interferes with the binding of amines within membrane-bound granules, inhibited the accumulation of 5-HT in sympathetic nerves of the vas deferens of guinea pigs (Thoa et al. 1969) and in platelets (Hughes and Brodie 1959) but had no effect on lung removal of 5-HT (Alabaster and Bakhle 1970a, Alabaster 1971, Junod 1972).

Thus pulmonary removal of 5-HT is unlike 5-HT uptake described in other tissues and more closely resembles pulmonary uptake of noradrenaline in its characteristics (Tables 1 and 2). Although there is little evidence that 5-HT and noradrenaline share a common uptake site, uptake sites for both amines are probably located in endothelial cells of the pulmonary vasculature. In autoradiographic studies of rat lungs after perfusion with [^{3}H] 5-HT, light microscopy revealed that most of the label was concentrated in alveolar cells (Cross et al. 1974). In the presence of the monoamine oxidase inhibitor mebanazine, additional labeling was seen in arteriolar endothelial cells. This site of uptake revealed in the presence of mebanazine, may represent a site at which the 5-HT taken up is normally metabolized rapidly and lost quickly from the lung. No label was present in vascular smooth muscle cells or mast cells. Similar results were obtained in rat lungs perfused with [^{3}H] 5-HT in the presence of iproniazid and examined by electron microscopy, where over 90% of the label was in capillary endothelial cells (Strum and Junod 1972). In rabbit lungs also, fluorescence microscopy showed intense 5-HT fluorescence within capillary endothelial cells when amine metabolism was prevented (Iwasawa et al. 1973).

Monoamine oxidase appears to be the only enzyme responsible for the metabolism of 5-HT removed from the pulmonary circulation of rats, guinea pigs, and dogs, since only one metabolite, corresponding to 5-hydroxyindoleacetic acid, was detected in lung perfusate after 5-HT was infused through isolated lungs (Alabaster 1971, Gruby et al. 1971). Treating the lungs with monoamine oxidase inhibitors can almost totally inhibit enzyme inactivation. Whereas 72% to 96% of the 5-HT taken up by rat lungs was metabolized under control conditions, after treatment with iproniazid, unchanged 5-HT accounted for more than 95% of the radioactivity in lung tissue and for 93% to 100% of the radioactivity recovered in the perfusate (Junod 1972). An enzyme that methylates 5-HT has been isolated from rabbit lungs (Axelrod 1962), but monoamine oxidase is probably the most important enzyme involved in pulmonary inactivation of 5-HT in this species also, since pargyline produced a fourfold increase in the 5-HT measured fluorometrically in rabbit lungs after perfusion (Gillis and Iwasawa 1972). Recent evidence suggests that more than one type of monoamine oxidase is involved in pulmonary inactivation of amines. Phenylethylamine, a substrate for monoamine oxidase-B, was removed and metabolized in lungs isolated from rats (Bakhle and Youdim 1975) and rabbits (Gillis et al. 1975), metabolism being prevented by a specific monoamine oxidase-B inhibitor. In contrast, metabolism of 5-HT was preferentially inhibited by a specific monoamine oxidase-A inhibitor.

VI. Histamine

Histamine was not removed by the pulmonary circulation in anesthetized dogs since the biologic activity of blood sampled from the femoral artery was the same whether histamine was infused into the superior vena cava or into the base of the ascending aorta or left ventricle (Ferreira et al. 1973). In anesthetized rats and dogs, the degree of inactivation assessed by comparing depressor responses to intravenous and intraarterial histamine was also negligible or very small (Boileau et al. 1970).

In blood-perfused, isolated lungs from dogs (Steggeda et al. 1935, Eiseman et al. 1964) and cats (Lilja and Lindell 1961) histamine was not removed in the pulmonary circulation. For example, there was no loss of histamine attributable to the lung when histamine (2 to 10 mg) was recirculated for 60 min through dog isolated lungs (Eiseman et al. 1964). Further experiments in isolated lungs of the rat, perfused with Krebs solution, have shown that the biologic activity of an infusion of histamine was reduced by only 5% to 10% in a single passage through the pulmonary circulation (Alabaster 1971). This is shown in Figure 4, where the biologic activity of lung perfusate was measured by passing the perfusate over two cat terminal ileum preparations in series. Contractions of the ileum preparations to histamine, infused at 20 ng/ml through the lungs, were equal to 19 ng/ml of histamine infused directly to the assay tissues, representing a removal of 5%. Mepyramine infused over the lower terminal ileum antagonized its responses to histamine, indicating that contractions of the other tissue were due to histamine and not to other substances released by histamine from the lung.

Although histamine was not removed in the pulmonary circulation in whole lungs, this amine was readily inactivated by lung slices or by chopped or homogenized lung preparations from man (Lilja et al. 1960), cat (Brown et al. 1959, Lilja and Lindell 1961), rabbit (Thithapandha 1972), and guinea pig and rat (Bennett 1965). The main metabolite formed was species dependent and reflected the types of histamine-metabolizing enzymes in the lung of each species (Schayer 1959, Schayer and Reilly 1974) and their concentrations in the lung. Guinea pig and cat lung contain a high concentration of imidazole-N-methyltransferase (Brown et al. 1959, Schayer and Reilly 1974), while the rat lung contains a much higher concentration of diamine oxidase than do lungs of the guinea pig, dog, or man (Valette et al. 1956). The lack of histamine inactivation in whole lung could be due, therefore, to the absence of a transport mechanism for histamine in the pulmonary circulation. The fact that chopped lung did not inactivate histamine as readily as did homogenates of lung (Bennett 1965) indicated that there were barriers to the free diffusion of histamine to sites of inactivation in lung tissue.

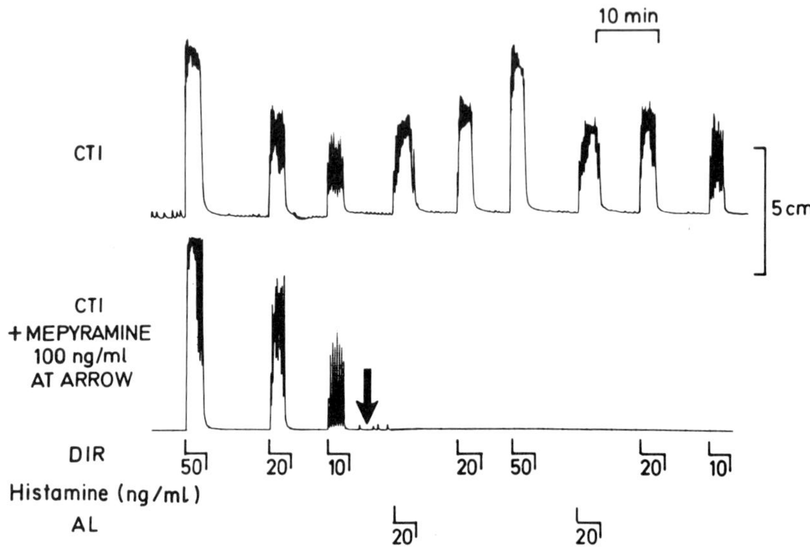

FIGURE 4 Lack of removal of histamine in rat isolated lungs. Record
shows contractions of two cat terminal ileums (CTI) superfused in series with
effluent from rat lungs perfused with Krebs solution. Histamine was infused
either directly to assay tissues (DIR) or into pulmonary arterial cannula (AL).
Only 5% to 10% of histamine infusion was removed by rat lung. Mepyramine
infused over lower tissue, as shown at arrow, antagonized responses to histamine given (AL), showing that contractions were in fact due to histamine and
not to other substances released from the lung (Alabaster and Bakhle, unpublished data).

The lung has the capacity to synthesize histamine, since histidine decarboxylase is present in lung tissue (Schayer 1956). Histamine is present in
lungs of most species, the amount being generally related to the population of
mast cells (Riley and West 1953, Parratt and West 1957). These cells can take
up and store histamine (Furano and Green 1964), but uptake is a slow process
and not likely to contribute to the removal of exogenous histamine during a
single passage through the pulmonary circulation. However, the uptake of
histamine by mast cells could contribute to its eventual distribution after exogenous administration to the whole animal. In distribution studies in rats and
mice, histamine was found in the lung 5 min and 1 hr after intravenous injection, but lung histamine content was normal at 2 to 3 hr (Snyder et al. 1964,
Halpern et al. 1959, Rose and Browne 1938). However, Furano and Green
(1964) found small quantities of $[^{14}C]$histamine present in lungs 24 hr after
an intravenous injection of the radioactive amine in the rat. In addition, histamine uptake by leukocytes and red cells (Lindell and Viske 1961) and by

platelets in some species (Weissbach et al. 1958), which then become trapped or lodged in lung capillaries, may contribute to the increased concentration of histamine in lungs after intravenous injection.

VII. Acetylcholine

Acetylcholinesterases and pseudocholinesterases are present in variable amounts in lung tissue of different species. In cat lung, for example, acetylcholinesterase is the predominant cholinesterase in smooth muscle of bronchioles, but both types of enzyme are present in endothelial and muscle cells of the pulmonary vasculature (Koelle 1950).

The contribution of lung enzymes to the metabolism of acetylcholine in transit through the pulmonary circulation can only be assessed in the absence of blood cholinesterases. The experiments by Eiseman et al. (1964) utilized dog isolated lung perfused with a Ringers-dextran solution until the effluent was free of blood. The perfusion was then changed to a closed system, ie., with recirculation of effluent, and acetylcholine added to the perfusate reservoir. Within one circulation time (4 min), only 12% of the original acetylcholine load could be detected.

Recently, however, experiments with guinea pig and rat lungs have shown more than 90% of acetylcholine or acetylthiocholine could be recovered unchanged either on single or repeated passage through the pulmonary circulation (Bakhle and Martin, unpublished observations). Acetylcholine was measured by bioassay and by radiochemical assay ([^{3}H]acetylcholine) and the hydrolysis of acetylthiocholine was measured spectrophotometrically (Ellman et al. 1961). The difference between these two sets of experiments has not yet been explained. It is, however, not due to a lack of cholinesterase activity in the lung, as guinea pig and rat lung homogenates inactivated acetylcholine and hydrolyzed acetylthiocholine (Ellman et al. 1961). There may be differences in the transport of acetylcholine in the different species or else in the location of the cholinesterases in the lung.

The absence of an inactivating system operating on acetylcholine in the pulmonary circulation is perhaps not surprizing since the action of acetylcholine is usually terminated by hydrolysis close to its site of release from nerve endings. Furthermore, any acetylcholine escaping into the circulation is rapidly inactivated by plasma and erythrocyte cholinesterases. Consequently, it is extremely unlikely that acetylcholine would, under normal circumstances, be present in the blood perfusing the pulmonary circulation. However, the pharmacokinetics of more stable quaternary esters, such as succinylcholine and methacholine, could be seriously influenced by the presence of a pulmonary inactivating system for choline esters.

VIII. Physiologic Consequences of Amine Removal

The physiologic significance of the pulmonary metabolic function has not yet been fully assessed. Vane (1969) suggested that the lung differentiates between local hormones whose actions are restricted at or near the site of release, and circulating hormones, which pass through the pulmonary circulation unchanged. The pulmonary circulation, due to its position, blood supply, and large surface area of cells comprising the alveolar capillaries, is certainly well-fitted to monitor and control levels of circulating hormones, and consequently influence the cardiovascular and other responses produced by hormones reaching the arterial circulation. Thus potentiation of the cardiovascular effects of noradrenaline produced by some drugs eg., cocaine, tricyclic antidepressants, some steroids, and certain antihypertensive drugs, may be due to inhibition of pulmonary removal of noradrenaline in addition to interference with uptake and storage in peripheral tissues.

Noradrenaline and 5-HT are removed in the pulmonary circulation in man (Gillis et al. 1972). Assuming that the properties of the removal systems in man are similar to those found in experimental animals, we would expect the pulmonary circulation to provide a similar control of the blood levels of these amines in man. Defects in this metabolic function of the lung could prove to be implicated in some clinical conditions. For example, as suggested by Gruby et al. (1971), failure to clear the venous plasma of free 5-HT would affect aggregation of platelets and increase the tendency to formation of venous thrombosis. Some steroids, for example estradiol and corticosterone, inhibit lung removal of noradrenaline (Iwasawa and Gillis 1973) and probably 5-HT also, since pulmonary removal processes for both amines show a similar sensitivity to drugs. It is possible that increased levels of circulating 5-HT could contribute to the increased risk of thrombosis during oral contraceptive and other steroid therapy. The anesthetics, halothane and nitrous oxide, inhibit pulmonary removal of noradrenaline in the rabbit isolated lung (Naito and Gillis 1973) and halothane abolished pulmonary inactivation of noradrenaline in anesthetized dogs (Bakhle and Block 1976). In man this effect could have clinical significance by permitting higher concentrations of vasoactive amines to reach the arterial circulation. This may be especially important in surgery involving hypothermia when pulmonary removal mechanisms would be expected to be markedly depressed.

The concentration of circulating noradrenaline and 5-HT is low under normal conditions, but in certain disease states the concentration can rise to high levels, for example, up to 4 μg/ml noradrenaline in phaeochromocytoma (Etsten and Shimosato 1965) and to 1 to 3 μg/ml 5-HT in carcinoid syndrome (Stacey 1966, Goble et al. 1955), concentrations which would be expected to saturate pulmonary removal mechanisms. Indirect evidence indicates that pulmonary inactivation of 5-HT is functioning in carcinoid syndrome, since these patients develop cardiac lesions and fibrosis predominantly on the right side of the heart (Goble et al. 1955, Sjoerdsma et al. 1957). However, it is now recognized that the metabolic function of the lung can be altered in some pathologic and disease states. Thus the removal process for 5-HT can be reduced in patients with certain cardiac disorders (Davis 1968), and recently it was shown that in patients with pulmonary hypertension secondary to valvular disease significantly more 5-HT and noradrenaline was removed from the pulmonary circulation than in patients with normal pulmonary artery pressures (Gillis et al. 1974). Pulmonary removal of noradrenaline and 5-HT was also markedly increased immediately after total cardiopulmonary bypass, an effect that was not correlated with changes in pulmonary blood flow or volume (Gillis et al. 1972, 1974). One possibility is that pulmonary removal processes may be influenced by changes in the concentration of circulating endogenous amines or peptides and consequently the metabolic function of the lung may be directly related to many other physiologic functions and control mechanisms. Clearly a great deal remains to be learned about the properties and physiologic and pharmacologic significance of the pulmonary removal of amines.

References

Alabaster, V. A. (1971). The Metabolism of Vasoactive Substances by the lung. Ph.D. Thesis, University of London.

Alabaster, V. A. and Bakhle, Y. S. (1970a). Removal of 5-hydroxytryptamine in the pulmonary circulation of rat isolated lungs. *Br. J. Pharmacol.,* **40**:468–482.

Alabaster, V. A. and Bakhle, Y. S. (1970b). The release of biologically active substances from isolated lungs by 5-hydroxytryptamine and tryptamine. *Br. J. Pharmacol.,* **40**:582P–583P.

Alabaster, V. A. and Bakhle, Y. S. (1973). The removal of noradrenaline in the pulmonary circulation of rat isolated lungs. *Br. J. Pharmacol.,* **47**:325–331.

Avakian, O. M. and Gillespie, J. J. (1968). Uptake of noradrenaline by adrenergic nerves, smooth muscle and connective tissue in isolated perfused arteries, and its correlation with the vasoconstrictor response. *Br. J. Pharmacol. Chemother.* **32**:168–184.

Aviado, D. M. and Sadavongvivad, C. (1970). Pharmacological significance of biogenic amines in the lungs: noradrenaline and dopamine. *Br. J. Pharmacol.* **38**:374–385.

Axelrod, J. (1962). The enzymatic N-methylation of serotonin and other amines. *J. Pharmacol. Exp. Ther.,* **138**:28–33.

Axelrod, J. and Inscoe, J. K. (1963). The uptake and binding of circulating serotonin and the effect of drugs. *J. Pharmacol. Exp. Ther.,* **141**:161–165.

Bakhle, Y. S. and Block, A. J. (1976). Effects of halothane on pulmonary inactivation of noradrenaline and prostaglandin E$_2$ in anesthetized dogs. *Clin. Sci. Molec. Med.*, **50**:87–90.

Bakhle, Y. S. and Smith, T. W. (1972). Release of spasmogenic substances induced by vasoactive amines from isolated lungs. *Br. J. Pharmacol.*, **46**: 543P–544P.

Bakhle, Y. S. and Vane, J. R. (1974). Pharmacokinetic function of the pulmonary circulation. *Physiol. Rev.*, **54**:1007–1045.

Bakhle, Y. S. and Youdim, M. B. H. (1975). Inactivation of phenylethylamine and 5-hydroxytryptamine in rat isolated lungs: evidence for monoamine oxidase A and B in lung. *J. Physiol. (Lond.)*, **248**:23–25P.

Bennett, A. (1965). The metabolism of histamine by guinea pig and rat lung in vitro. *Br. J. Pharmacol. Chemother.*, **24**:147–155.

Blaschko, H. and Philpot, F. J. (1953). Enzymic oxidation of tryptamine derivatives. *J. Physiol. (Lond.)*, **122**:403–408.

Blaschko, H., Richter, D. and Schlossman, H. (1937). The oxidation of adrenaline and other amines. *Biochem. J.*, **31**:2187–2196.

Bogdanski, D. F. and Brodie, B. B. (1969). The effects of inorganic ions on the storage and uptake of H^3-norepinephrine by rat heart slices. *J. Pharmacol. Exp. Ther.*, **165**:181–189.

Boileau, J. C., Campeau, L., and Biron, P. (1970). Pulmonary fate of histamine, isoproterenol, physalaemin and substance P. *Can. J. Physiol. Pharmacol.*, **48**:681–684.

Boileau, J. C., Campeau, L., and Biron, P. (1971). Comparative fate of intravenous epinephrine. *Rev. Can. Biol.*, **30**:281–286.

Boileau, J. C., Campeau, L., and Biron, P. (1972a). Pulmonary fate of intravenous noradrenaline. *Rev. Can. Biol.*, **31**:185–192.

Boileau, J. C., Crexells, C., and Biron, P. (1972b). Free pulmonary passage of dopamine. *Rev. Can. Biol.*, **31**:69–72.

Brown, D. D., Tomchick, R., and Axelrod, J. (1959). The distribution and properties of a histamine methylating enzyme. *J. Biol. Chem.*, **234**:2948–2950.

Burgen, A. S. V. and Iversen, L. L. (1965). The inhibition of noradrenaline uptake by sympathomimetic amines in the rat isolated heart. *Br. J. Pharmacol.*, **25**:34–49.

Callingham, B. A. and Burgen, A. S. V. (1966). The uptake of isoprenaline and noradrenaline by the perfused rat heart. *Molec. Pharmacol.*, **2**:37–42.

Coyle, J. T. and Snyder, S. H. (1969). Catecholamine uptake by symptosomes in homogenates of rat brain: stereospecificity in different areas. *J. Pharmacol. Exp. Ther.*, **170**:221–231.

Cross, S. A. M., Alabaster, V. A., Bakhle, Y. S., and Vane, J. R. (1974). Sites of uptake of ^{3}H-5-hydroxytryptamine in rat isolated lung. *Histochemistry*, **39**:83–91.

Davis, R. B. (1968). Discussion of the role of 5-hydroxytryptamine in the carcinoid syndrome. In S. Garrattini, P. A. Shore, E. Costa, and M. Sandler (eds.): *Advances in Pharmacology*, vol. 6B. Academic Press, New York, pp. 146–149.

Davis, R. B. and Wang, Y. (1965). Rapid pulmonary removal of 5-hydroxytryptamine in the intact dog. *Proc. Soc. Exp. Biol. Med.*, **118**:799–800.

Draskóczy, P. R. and Trendelenburg, U. (1970). Intraneuronal and extraneuronal accumulation of sympathomimetic amines in the isolated nictitating membrane of the cat. *J. Pharmacol. Exp. Ther.*, **174**:290–306.

Eiseman, B., Bryant, L., and Waltuch, T. (1964). Metabolism of vasomotor agents by the isolated perfused lung. *J. Thorac. Cardiovasc. Surg.*, **48**: 798–806.

Eisenfeld, A. J., Azelrod, J., and Krakoff, L. (1967a). Inhibition of the extraneuronal accumulation and metabolism of noradrenaline by adrenergic blocking agents. *J. Pharmacol. Exp. Ther.*, **156**:107–113.

Eisenfeld, A. J., Landsberg, L., and Axelrod, J. (1967b). Effect of drugs on the accumulation and metabolism of extraneuronal noradrenaline in rat heart. *J. Pharmacol. Exp. Ther.*, **158**:378–385.

Elliot, T. R. (1905). The action of adrenaline. *J. Physiol (Lond.)*, **32**:401–467.

Ellman, G. E., Courtney, K. D., Andres, V., and Featherstone, R. M. (1961). A new and rapid colorimetric determination of acetylcholinesterase activity. *Biochem. Pharmacol.*, **7**:88–95.

Eränkö, O. and Jansson, S. E. (1967). Uptake of monoamines by mouse peritoneal mast cells in vitro. *Acta Physiol. Scand.*, **70**:449–450.

Etsten, B. E. and Shimosato, S. (1965). Halothane anesthesia and catecholamine levels in a patient with phaeochromocytoma. *Anesthesiology*, **26**: 688–691.

Euler, U. S. von and Lishajko, F. (1957). Dopamine in mammalian lung and spleen. *Acta Physiol. Pharmacol. Neerl.*, **6**:295–303.

Farnebo, L. O. and Malmfors, T. (1969). Histochemical studies on the uptake of noradrenaline and a-methylnoradrenaline in the perfused rat heart. *Eur. J. Pharmacol.*, **5**:313–320.

Ferreira, S. H., Ng, K. K. and Vane, J. R. (1973). The continuous bioassay of the release and disappearance of histamine in the circulation. *Br. J. Pharmacol.*, **49**:543–553.

Foster, R. W. (1968). A correlation between inhibition of the uptake of ^{3}H from $\pm^3$H-noradrenaline and potentiation of the responses to (−)noradrenaline in the guinea pig isolated trachea. *Br. J. Pharmacol. Chemother.*, **33**:357–367.

Furano, A. V. and Green, J. P. (1964). Uptake of biogenic amines by mast cells of the rat. *J. Physiol. (Lond.)*, **170**:263–271.

Gaddum, J. H., Hebb, C. O., Silver, A., and Swan, A. A. B. (1953). 5-hydroxytryptamine. Pharmacological action and destruction in perfused lungs. *Q. J. Exp. Physiol.*, **38**:255–262.

Gillespie, J. S., Hamilton, D. M. H., and Hosie, R. J. A. (1970). The extraneuronal uptake and localization of noradrenaline in the cat spleen and the effect on this of some drugs, of cold and of denervation. *J. Physiol. (Lond.)*, **206**:563–590.

Gillis, C. N., Cronau, L. H., Greene, N. M. and Hammond, G. L. (1974). Removal of 5-hydroxytryptamine and norepinephrine from the pulmonary vascular space of man: influence of cardiopulmonary bypass and pulmonary arterial pressure on these processes. *Surgery,* **76**:608–616.

Gillis, C. N., Greene, N. M., Cronau, L. H., and Hammond, G. L. (1972). Pulmonary extraction of 5-hydroxytryptamine and norepinephrine before and after cardiopulmonary bypass in man. *Circ. Res.,* **30**:666–674.

Gillis, C. N. and Iwasawa, Y. (1972). Technique for measurement of noradrenaline and 5-hydroxytryptamine uptake by rabbit lung. *J. Appl. Physiol.,* **33**:404–408.

Gillis, C. N. and Paton, D. M. (1966). Effects of hypothermia and anoxia on retention of noradrenaline by the cat perfused heart. *Br. J. Pharmacol.,* **26**: 426–434.

Gillis, C. N. and Paton, D. M. (1967). Cationic dependence of sympathetic transmitter retention by slices of rat ventricles. *Br. J. Pharmacol.,* **29**:309–318.

Gillis, C. N., Roth, J. A., and Baker, J. R. (1975). Evidence for different forms of monoamine oxidase in perfused rabbit lung. *Chest,* **67**:26–28S.

Ginn, R. and Vane, J. R. (1968). Disappearance of catecholamines from the pulmonary circulation. *Nature (Lond.),* **219**:740–742.

Goble, A. J., Hay, D. R., and Sandler, M. (1955). 5-hydroxytryptamine metabolism in acquired heart disease associated with argentaffin carcinoma. *Lancet,* **2**:1016–1017.

Green, J. P. (1962). Binding of some biogenic amines in tissues. In S. Grattini and P. A. Shore (eds.): *Advances in Pharmacology,* Academic Press, London, pp. 349–422.

Gruby, L. A., Rowland, C., Varley, B. Q., and Wyllie, J. H. (1971). The fate of 5-hydroxytryptamine in the lungs. *Br. J. Surg.,* **58**:525–532.

Gulati, O. D. and Sivaramakrishna, N. (1975). Kinetics and some characteristics of uptake of noradrenaline by the human umbilical artery. *Br. J. Pharmacol.,* **53**:152–154.

Halpern, B. N., Neveu, T., and Wilson, C. W. M. (1959). The distribution and fate of radioactive histamine in the rat. *J. Physiol. (Lond.),* **147**:437–449.

Hamberger, B. (1967). Reserpine resistant uptake of catecholamines in isolated tissues of the rat. *Acta Physiol. Scand.,* **71**: Suppl. 295, 1–200.

Hope, D. B. and Smith, A. D. (1960). Distribution and activity of monoamine oxidase in mouse tissues. *Biochem. J.,* **74**:101–107.

Hughes, F. B. and Brodie, B. B. (1959). The mechanism of serotonin and catecholamine uptake by platelets. *J. Pharmacol. Exp. Ther.,* **127**:96–102.

Hughes, J., Gillis, C. N., and Bloom, F. E. (1969). The uptake and disposition of dl-noradrenaline in perfused rat lung. *J. Pharmacol. Exp. Ther.,* **169**:237–248.

Iversen, L. L. (1963). The uptake of noradrenaline by the isolated perfused rat heart. *Br. J. Pharmacol.,* **21**:523–537.

Iversen, L. L. (1965). The uptake of catecholamines at high perfusion concentrations in the rat isolated heart: a novel catecholamine uptake process. *Br. J. Pharmacol.,* **25**:18–33.

Iversen, L. L. (1971). Role of transmitter uptake mechanisms in synaptic neurotransmission. *Br. J. Pharmacol.,* **41**:571–591.

Iversen, L. L., Jarrott, B., and Simmonds, M. A. (1971). Differences in the uptake, storage and metabolism of (+)- and (−)-noradrenaline. *Br. J. Pharmacol.*, **43**:845–855.

Iversen, L. L. and Salt, P. J. (1970). Inhibition of catecholamine Uptake$_2$ by steroids in the isolated rat heart. *Br. J. Pharmacol.*, **40**:528–530.

Iwasawa, Y. and Gillis, C. N. (1973). Effect of steroid and other hormone on lung removal of noradrenaline. *Eur. J. Pharmacol.*, **22**:367–370.

Iwasawa, Y. and Gillis, C. N. (1974). Pharmacological analysis of norepinephrine and 5-hydroxytryptamine removal from the pulmonary circulation: differentiation of uptake sites for each amine. *J. Pharmacol. Exp. Ther.*, **188**:386–393.

Iwasawa, Y., Gillis, C. N., and Aghajanian, G. (1973). Hypothermic inhibition of 5-hydroxytryptamine and noradrenaline uptake by lung: cellular location of amines after uptake. *J. Pharmacol. Exp. Ther.*, **186**:489–507.

Junod, A. F. (1972). Uptake, metabolism and efflux of ^{14}C-5-hydroxytryptamine in isolated perfused rat lungs. *J. Pharmacol. Exp. Ther.*, **183**:341–355.

Koelle, G. B. (1950). The histochemical differentiation of types of cholinesterases and their localizations in tissues of the cat. *J. Pharmacol. Exp. Ther.*, **100**:158–179.

Lightman, S. L. and Iversen, L. L. (1969). The role of Uptake$_2$ in the extraneuronal metabolism of catecholamines in the isolated rat heart. *Br. J. Pharmacol.*, **37**:638–649.

Lilja, B. and Lindell, S. E. (1961). Metabolism of ^{14}C-histamine in heart-lung-liver preparation of cats. *Br. J. Pharmacol. Chemother.*, **16**:203–208.

Lilja, B., Lindell, S. E., and Saldeen, T. (1960). Formation and destruction of ^{14}C-histamine in human lung tissue in vitro. *J. Allergy*, **31**:492–496.

Lindell, S. E. and Viske, K. (1961). A note on the distribution of ^{14}C-histamine added to blood. *Br. J. Pharmacol., Chemother.*, **17**:131–136.

Naito, H. and Gillis, C. N. (1973). Effects of halothane and nitrous oxide on removal of noradrenaline from the pulmonary circulation. *Anaesthesiology*, **39**:575–580.

Nicholas, T. E., Strum, J. M., Angelo, L. S., and Junod, A. F. (1974). Site and mechanism of uptake of ^{3}H-l-norepinephrine by isolated perfused rat lungs. *Circ. Res.*, **35**:670–680.

Parratt, J. R. and West, G. B. (1957). 5-hydroxytryptamine and tissue mast cells. *J. Physiol. (Lond.)*, **137**:169–178.

Peskar, B., Hellman, G., and Hertting, G. (1968). Kinetik der Aufnahme und der Transformation von 7-^{3}H-Dopamin im isoliert perfundierten Rattenherzen. *Arch. Exp. Pathol. Pharmakol.*, **260**:186–187.

Pletscher, A., Burkard, W. P., Tranzer, J. P., and Gey, K. F. (1967). Two sites of 5-hydroxytryptamine uptake in blood platelets. *Life Sci.*, **6**:273–280.

Rapport, M. M., Greene, A. A., and Page, I. H. (1948a). Crystalline serotonin. *Science,* **108**:329–330.

Rapport, M. M., Greene, A. A., and Page, I. H. (1948b). Serum vasoconstrictor (serotonin). *J. Biol. Chem.*, **176**:1243–1251.

Rapport, M. M., Greene, A. A., and Page, I. H. (1948c). Enzymatic inactivation of serum vasoconstrictor. *Proc. Soc. Exp. Biol. Med.,* **68**:582.

Repke, K., Est, M., and Portius, H. J. (1965). Ueber die Ursache der Speciesunterschiede in der Digitalisempfindlichkeit. *Biochem. Pharmacol.,* **14**:1785–1802.

Riley, J. F. and West, G. B. (1953). The presence of histamine in tissue mast cells. *J. Physiol. (Lond.),* **120**:528–533.

Rose, B. and Browne, J. S. L. (1938). The distribution and rate of disappearance of intravenously injected histamine in the rat. *Am. J. Physiol.,* **124**:412–420.

Sadavongvivad, C. (1970). Pharmacological significance of biogenic amines in the lungs: 5-hydroxytryptamine. *Br. J. Pharmacol.,* **38**:353–365.

Salt, P. J. (1972). Inhibition of noradrenaline Uptake$_2$ in the isolated rat heart by steroids, clonidine and methoxylated phenylethylamines. *Eur. J. Pharmacol.,* **20**:329–340.

Schayer, R. W. (1956). The metabolism of histamine in various species. *Br. J. Pharmacol. Chemother.,* **11**:472–473.

Schayer, R. W. (1959). Catabolism of physiological quantities of histamine in vivo. *Physiol. Rev.,* **39**:116–126.

Schayer, R. W. and Reilly, M. A. (1974). Histamine catabolism in guinea pigs, rats and mice. *Eur. J. Pharmacol.,* **25**:101–107.

Shaskan, E. G. and Snyder, S. H. (1970). Kinetics of serotonin accumulation into slices from rat brain: relationship to catecholamine uptake. *J. Pharmacol. Exp. Ther.,* **175**:404–418.

Sjoerdsma, A., Weissbach, H., Terry, L. T., and Udenfriend, S. (1957). Further observations on patients with malignant carcinoid. *Am. J. Med.,* **23**:5–7.

Sneddon, J. M. (1969). Sodium dependent accumulation of 5-hydroxytryptamine by rat blood platelets. *Br. J. Pharmacol.,* **37**:680–688.

Snipes, R. L., Thoenen, H., and Tranzer, J. P. (1968). Fine structure localization of exogenous 5-hydroxytryptamine in vesicles of adrenergic nerve terminals. *Experientia (Basel),* **24**:1024–1027.

Snyder, S. H., Axelrod, J., and Bauer, H. (1964). The fate of C^{14}-histamine in animal tissues. *J. Pharmacol. Exp. Ther.,* **144**:373–379.

Stacey, R. S. (1961). Uptake of 5-hydroxytryptamine by platelets. *Br. J. Pharmacol. Chemother.,* **16**:284–295.

Stacey, R. S. (1966). Clinical aspects of cerebral and extracerebral 5-hydroxytryptamine. In V. Erspamer (ed.): *Handbook of Experimental Pharmacology: 5-Hydroxytryptamine and Related Indolealkylamines.* Springer-Verlag, Berlin, p. 760.

Starling, E. H. and Verney, E. B. (1925). The secretion of urine as studied on the isolated kidney. *Proc. R. Soc. B.,* **97**:321–363.

Steggeda, F. R., Essex, H. E., and Mann, F. C. (1935). The inactivation of histamine in perfused organs. *Am. J. Physiol.,* **112**:70–73.

Strum, J. M. and Junod, A. F. (1972). Radioautographic demonstration of 5-hydroxytryptamine-^{3}H uptake by pulmonary endothelial cells. *J. Cell Biol.,* **54**:456–467.

Thithapandha, A. (1972). Substrate specificity and heterogeneity of N-methyl-transferases. *Biochem. Biophys. Res. Comm.*, **47**:301–308.

Thoa, N. B., Eccleston, D., and Axelrod, J. (1969). The accumulation of C^{14}-serotonin in the guinea pig vas deferens. *J. Pharmacol. Exp. Ther.*, **169**: 68–73.

Thomas, D. P. and Vane, J. R. (1967). 5-hydroxytryptamine in the circulation of the dog. *Nature (Lond.)*, **216**:335–338.

Tissari, A. H., Schönhöfer, P. S., Bogdanski, D. F., and Brodie, B. B. (1969). Mechanism of biogenic amine transport. II: Relationship between sodium and the mechanism of ouabain blockade of the accumulation of serotonin and noradrenaline by synaptosomes. *Molec. Pharmacol.*, **5**:593–604.

Todrick, A. and Tait, C. (1969). The inhibition of human platelet 5-hydroxy-tryptamine uptake by tricyclic antidepressive drugs. *J. Pharm. Pharmacol.*, **21**:751–762.

Valette, G., Cohen, Y., and Burkuerd, W. (1956). Répartition de l'histamine dans differents organes de certain animaux. *Pharm. Acta Helv.*, **31**:382–390.

Vane, J. R. (1960). The actions of sympathomimetic amines on tryptamine receptors. In J. R. Vane, G. E. W. Wolstenholme, and M. O'Connor (eds.): *Adrenergic Mechanisms.* Churchill, London, pp. 356–372.

Vane, J. R. (1964). The use of isolated organs for detecting active substances in the circulating blood. *Br. J. Pharmacol. Chemother.*, **23**:360–373.

Vane, J. R. (1969). The release and fate of vasoactive hormones in the circulation. *Br. J. Pharmacol.*, **35**:209–242.

Weissbach, H., Bogdanski, D. F., and Udenfriend, S. (1958). Binding of serotonin and other amines by blood platelets. *Arch. Biochem.*, **73**:492–499.

Weissbach, H., Waalkes, T. P., and Udenfriend, S. (1957). Presence of serotonin in lung and its implication in the anaphylactic reaction. *Science*, **125**:235–236.

2

Inactivation of Bradykinin
and Related Peptides in the Lung

SERGIO H. FERREIRA

Faculdade de Medicina de Ribeirão Preto
Ribeirão, Est São Paulo, Brazil

Y. S. BAKHLE

Institute of Basic Medical Sciences
Royal College of Surgeons of England
London, England

I. Introduction

In this chapter we shall review the inactivation of bradykinin and related peptides (a) during passage through the pulmonary circulation in vivo, (b) in perfused lung preparations and (c) by enzyme preparations from lung homogenates. In each of these sections experimental evidence will be examined relating to the suggestion that lung kininase and lung angiotensin I-converting enzyme activities result from the action of a single enzyme, a dipeptidylcarboxypeptidase (Ng and Vane 1968). Most of the recent work on lung kininase has concentrated on this suggestion, and these investigations have been greatly advanced by the discovery of potent kininase and converting enzyme inhibitors in snake venoms (Ferreira 1965, Kato and Suzuki 1971).

Also an hypothesis will be proposed to explain what determines which enzymic activity, of all those present in lung homogenates, is exhibited by the whole perfused tissue in vitro or in vivo. Finally, attempts will be made to assess the relevance of pulmonary kininase activity to some physiologic and pathologic situations.

II. Inactivation In Vivo

The rapid destruction of bradykinin by blood was noted by Rocha e Silva et al.(1949). Indeed, even if tissues did not participate in the removal of bradykinin from the circulation, its destruction by blood alone would result in a half-life shorter than two circulation times. Despite this high background inactivation by blood, there were soon indications that, in vivo, bradykininase activity could also be attributed to tissues, particularly the kidneys (Bumpus et al. 1964, Trautschold et al. 1966). Furthermore, a venous-arterial difference in kinin concentration had been suggested, although this suggestion had not been pursued (Sicuteri et al. 1963, Oates et al. 1964).

In 1967 the kininase activity associated with several discrete vascular beds, e.g., hind legs, liver, head, renal, and pulmonary, was systematically examined by Ferreira and Vane (1967a). They used the blood-bathed organ technique (Vane 1964), which permitted measurement of small amounts of kinin (1 to 5 ng/ml) in the circulating blood without laborious extraction procedures (Ferreira and Vane 1967b). By comparing the concentration of bradykinin in femoral arterial blood following infusions either into the right ventricle or into the aorta just distal to the aortic valve, they showed that about 80% of infused bradykinin disappeared during passage through the lung and heart chambers of the cat. This degree of inactivation was greatly in excess of that seen in other vascular beds and of that expected from the known activity of blood kininases during the time of transit through the pulmonary circulation. Only 50% inactivation of bradykinin took place during a 17-sec (one circulation time) incubation with cat's blood in an extracorporeal circuit at 37°C.

The conclusion that the lungs were important in controlling levels of circulating kinins was at variance with the then current belief that blood and kidneys played major roles in the inactivation of kinins. Involvement of the kidneys in kinin metabolism was based on the finding that this organ concentrated most of the radioactivity derived from labeled bradykinin injected into the animal (Bumpus et al. 1964). However, it is now known that the lung hydrolyzes bradykinin without retaining its fragments (Ryan et al. 1970) and that the accumulation of radioactivity in the kidney probably represents the accumulation, perhaps prior to excretion, of fragments of bradykinin rather than a major site of its inactivation. It is interesting to reflect here that the metabolic properties of organs are generally deduced from the results first obtained in vitro and to point out that the importance of the lungs in the removal of circulating kinins was first established by experiments performed in vivo.

The almost complete pulmonary removal of bradykinin has since been confirmed in vivo in rats, dogs, and sheep. Some of these further observations were made by matching the hypotensive effect of kinins administered into the jugular vein with the effects of kinins administered into the ascending aorta, the systemic pressure response technique of Biron (1968). In the rat the pulmonary inactivation of bradykinin varies between 75% and 98% (Biron 1968, Roblero et al. 1973) and in dogs it is 82% (Ferreira and Vane 1967b). Bradykinin is also probably inactivated in the lungs of man for it was one-sixth as active as histamine when given intravenously but more potent than histamine when administered intraarterially (Fox et al. 1961). Inactivation in the lung now seems a more likely explanation of this result than inactivation by blood, as suggested by the authors. Study of the pulmonary inactivation of bradykinin in sheep has led to the suggestion that the inactivation of bradykinin is a pulmonary function that develops late in fetal life (Friedli et al. 1973). These authors observed a high degree of inactivation in mature ewes (93%), which was greater than that in newborn lambs (68%), fetal lambs at term (46%), and preterm fetuses (0%). These results however conflict with those of Hébert et al. (1972) who found the same degree of inactivation (68%) in ewes, newborn lambs, and fetuses. Both groups used the systemic pressure response technique, and the only apparent difference was that the former group used infusions and the latter used injections of bradykinin.

It is appropriate here to make a few remarks with regard to the systemic pressure response technique. This technique is based on the well-established hypotensive effective of intravenously administered bradykinin. However, bradykinin infused through isolated guinea pig lungs caused the release of prostaglandin-like substances (Vargaftig and Dao Hai 1972). Thus there is always the possibility that an intravenous injection of kinin would release an endogenous substance that adds to the effect of bradykinin on blood pressure. This certainly seems to be the case in the rabbit where the depressor effect of bradykinin, given intravenously, was more sustained than that of bradykinin given into the aorta (Vane and Ferreira 1975). This prolonged effect of bradykinin is curtailed in this species after treatment with a prostaglandin synthesis inhibitor. Whether such interactions occur in other species is not known, but the readiness with which lungs of all species release prostaglandin-like substances (Bakhle and Vane 1974) does emphasize the possible source of error in results obtained by this technique. Furthermore, when injections rather than infusions are made, a removal of about 10% can probably be attributed to dilution by blood during pulmonary transit. To this dilution effect there should be added inactivation by blood during this time, giving a total minimal removal of about 30%. Finally, the lowering of blood pressure itself activates a number of homeostatic reflexes, the rapidity and efficacy of which may influence the final magnitude of the depressor response measured. Advantages of the blood-bathed organ technique are that small amounts of bradykinin, less than those lowering systemic blood pressure, can be detected and by a careful choice of assay tissues, the release of other substances can be assessed.

Other hypotensive, kinin-like peptides (Fig. 1) have different degrees of susceptibility to the pulmonary inactivation process in vivo. Thus, Lys-bradykinin and Met-Lys-bradykinin are inactivated, whereas d-Pro[7]-bradykinin, physalaemin, eledoisin, polistes kinin, and substance P are all essentially resistant to pulmonary inactivation (Roblero et al. 1973, Boileau et al. 1970). The substrate specificity of this inactivation process will be discussed later.

Several substances have been shown to potentiate the effects of bradykinin in vivo, and perhaps the most interesting derive from bradykinin-potentiating factor (BPF, Fig. 2), a mixture of peptides extracted from the venom of *Bothrops jararaca* (Ferreira 1965). The inhibition of pulmonary inactivation by this factor in vivo was demonstrated directly by the sixfold increase in the amount of bradykinin surviving pulmonary transit in dogs and cats treated with BPF (Ferreira and Vane 1967b). Since then, the peptides responsible for the pharmacologic activity of BPF have been isolated, characterized, and synthesized (Ferreira et al. 1970a, Ondetti et al. 1971). Only two of the *Bothrops* peptides, the pentapeptide BPP 5a and the nonapeptide BPP 9a (Fig. 2) have been extensively studied. The normal disappearance of bradykinin (98%) during a single passage through the rat lung in vivo could be reduced to a minimum of 30% with increasing doses of the pentapeptide (Stewart et al. 1971).

Bradykinin	H-Arg-Pro-Pro-Gly-Phe-Ser-Pro-Phe-Arg-OH
Lys-bradykinin	H-Lys-Arg-Pro-Pro-Gly-Phe-Ser-Pro-Phe-Arg-OH
Met-Lys-bradykinin	H-Met-Lys-Arg-Pro-Pro-Gly-Phe-Ser-Pro-Phe-Arg-OH
Lys-Lys-bradykinin	H-Lys-Lys-Arg-Pro-Pro-Gly-Phe-Ser-Pro-Phe-Arg-OHOSO$_3$H
Phyllokinin	H-Arg-Pro-Pro-Gly-Phe-Ser-Pro-Phe-Arg-Ile-Tyr-OH
Polistes kinin	Pca-Thr-Asn-Lys-Lys-Lys-Leu-Arg-Gly-Arg-Pro-Pro-Gly-Phe-Ser-Pro-Phe-Arg-OH
Substance P	H-Arg-Pro-Lys-Pro-Gln-Gln-Phe-Phe-Gly-Leu-Met-NH$_2$
Eledoisin	Pca-Pro-Ser-Lys-Asp-Ala-Phe-Ile-Gly-Leu-Met-NH$_2$
Physalaemin	Pca-Ala-Asp-Pro-Asn-Lys-Phe-Tyr-Gly-Leu-Met-NH$_2$

FIGURE 1   Bradykinin and other hypotensive peptides.

Bothrops jararaca

BPP 5a; SQ20475   Pca-Lys-Trp-Ala-Pro

BPP 9a; SQ20881   Pca-Trp-Pro-Arg-Pro-Gln-Ile-Pro-Pro

Decapeptide SQ20859   Pca-Ser-Trp-Pro-Gly-Pro-Asn-Ile-Pro-Pro

Decapeptide SQ20858   Pca-Asn-Trp-Pro-His-Pro-Gln-Ile-Pro-Pro

Agkistrodon halys blomhoffii

Potentiator C   Pca-Gly-Leu-Pro-Pro-Gly-Pro-Pro-Ile-Pro-Pro

         E   Pca-Lys-Trp-Asp-Pro-Pro-Pro-Val-Ser-Pro-Pro

FIGURE 2   Peptides isolated from snake venom. (Purification, structure, synthesis: from Ferreira et al. 1970a, Kato and Suzuki 1971, Ondetti et al. 1971.)

The nonapeptide, besides being more potent, has longer lasting effects than the pentapeptide (Greene et al. 1972, Engel et al. 1972). It should be pointed out that although many of the snake venom peptides have bradykinin-potentiating properties on smooth muscle (Ferreira et al. 1970b), comparatively few (Table 1) have been tested as inhibitors of bradykinin inactivation in any system, and efficacy as a bradykinin potentiator does not necessarily parallel potency as a bradykininase inhibitor.

Inhibitors of plasma kininase, like 2:3-dimercaptopropanol (BAL) and 2-mercaptoethanol (2-ME) (Ferreira and Rocha e Silva 1962, Erdös and Wohler 1963), are well-established potentiators of the hypotensive effect of an intravenous injections of bradykinin. However, more direct evidence of the inhibition of pulmonary inactivation came later. Thus, 2-ME exerted a greater potentiation when bradykinin was given intravenously than when it was given intraarterially, indicating an inhibition of pulmonary inactivation of kinin in rats (Stewart and Roblero 1967, Scholz and Biron 1969). Stewart and Freer (1973) found that an intravenous infusion of 2-ME completely inhibited destruction of bradykinin by rat lungs. The suggestion, by Ng and Vane (1968), that the same enzyme was responsible for pulmonary inactivation of bradykinin and the conversion of angiotensin I was supported by the fact that BPF and the synthetic peptides BPP 5a and BPP 9a inhibit both processes in vivo (Engel et al. 1972). However, refuting this idea is the finding that 2-ME inhibits the inactivation of bradykinin by lung but has no effect on the conversion of angiotensin I by dog and rat lungs in vivo (Scholz and Biron 1969, Stewart and Freer 1973) and that potentiation of bradykinin occurs with much smaller doses of the *Bothrops* nonapeptide than those necessary to inhibit the pressor effects of angiotensin I (Engel et al. 1972). The latter effect

TABLE 1 Inhibition of Pulmonary Bradykininase

Inhibitor	In vivo[a]	Perfused lung[a]	Homogenates[a,b]
2:3-Dimercaptopropanol	−	+ [1]	+ [2]
2-Mercaptoethanol	+ [12,13,14]	+ [1,11]	0 [2]
n-Ethyl maleimide	−	+ [1]	0 [2]
EDTA	−	0 [1]	+ [2,4]
Peptides			
Alternative substrates			
Insulin	−	−	+ [7]
B-chain of insulin	−	−	+ [7]
Angiotensin I	−	−	+ [2]
Hydrolysis products			
Phe-Arg	−	−	+ [9]
Arg-Pro-Pro	−	−	+ [9]
Angiotensin II	−	−	0 [2]
Venom peptides			
BPF	+ [6]	+ [1,11]	+ [3]
BPP 5a; SQ 20475	+ [5]	+ [1]	+ [2]
BPP 9a; SQ 20881	+ [5]	+ [1]	+ [2,4,7,8]
Decapeptide:SQ20858	+ [5]	−	+ [2]
Decapeptide:SQ20859	−	+ [1]	−
Potentiator C	−	−	+ [2,7]
Potentiator E	−	−	+ [2]

[a]References in brackets: [1] Alabaster and Bakhle (1972a), [2] Alabaster and Bakhle (1973), [3] Bakhle (1968), [4] Dorer et al. (1974), [5] Engel et al. (1972), [6] Ferreira and Vane (1967), [7] Igic et al. (1973), [8] Nakajima et al. (1973), [9] Oshima and Erdös (1974), [10] Ryan et al. (1968), [11] Ryan et al. (1970), [12] Scholz and Biron (1969), [13] Stewart and Freer (1973), [14] Stewart and Roblero (1967).
[b]Refers to all preparations of bradykininases from homogenized lung and includes the highly purified dipeptidylcarboxypeptidase.

could be due to either a higher affinity of the enzyme for bradykinin (see Dorer et al. 1974) or to the participation of mechanisms other than the inhibition of enzymic degradation (Camargo and Ferreira 1971).

III. Inactivation in Isolated Lungs

Bradykinin inactivation in the pulmonary circulation was originally explained in terms of a highly active bradykininase in the lung (Ferreira and Vane 1967a). An alternative location of the bradykininase could have been in the heart. A more complicated alternative would be to suggest that bradykininase activity in blood (Erdös et al. 1963) was increased temporarily as it passed through the pulmonary circulation, perhaps due to some particular gas concentration gradient. To distinguish between these two alternatives, isolated lungs perfused with a nonblood fluid, generally Krebs solution (sometimes supplemented with dextran), have been used. These preparations eliminated the contribution of blood bradykininases and minimized those of bradykininase in the heart chambers.

The inactivation of bradykinin in isolated lungs from rat, guinea pig, and dog was extensive, varying from 75% to 99.9% (Ryan et al. 1968, 1970, Pojda and Vane 1971, Alabaster and Bakhle 1972a, Levine et al. 1973). The 84% to 96% inactivation of bradykinin by dog lung perfused with blood drops to 75% when perfused with Locke's solution (Levine et al. 1973). Thus, during passage through the lung, about 10% to 20% of the disappearance can be attributed to blood kininases. Using a mock isolated lung, Levine et al. (1973) demonstrated that plasma kininases can account for 25% of the bradykinin destroyed through the pulmonary circulation. These values agree with our estimate of a maximum of 30% inactivation, which could be due to blood during passage through the lungs (Ferreira and Vane 1967a).

The results obtained with isolated perfused lungs clearly showed that the tissue had enough bradykininase activity to account for the inactivation observed in vivo. However, little was known of the nature of the bradykinin inactivating system. Was there uptake and storage of the peptide in lung cells as though it were a catecholamine? Was there uptake followed by enzymic breakdown? Was there enzymic breakdown without uptake? The experiments of Ryan et al. (1970) showed that the third possibility was most likely. They infused radioactive bradykinin through isolated rat lungs perfused with Locke-Ringer solution and found that 98% of the radioactivity entering the lungs emerged in the effluent within 10 min of the end of the infusion. Thus, no radioactivity was retained by the lung, as would be expected by a storage mechanism. Furthermore, none of the radioactivity emerged as bradykinin, but as a mixture of di- and tetrapeptide fragments. The radioactivity emerged from the lungs in the same time as did blue dextran infused via the pulmonary arterial cannula. Blue dextran is a polysaccharide of molecular weight about 2,000,000, and it is confined to the vascular space.

These are two crucial findings. First the presence of several small fragments of bradykinin demonstrate several points of cleavage in the molecule. The significance of this is that the cleavage of any one peptide bond in bradykinin will result in biologic inactivation (Suzuki et al. 1969), and we are therefore faced with the problem of deciding which bond is cleaved at the fastest rate and thus which kininase is rate-determining for the inactivation process in lung. We shall return to this question later on. Second, the finding that radioactivity has the same transit time as dextran demonstrates clearly that the substrate, bradykinin, does not have to leave the vascular space to be hydrolyzed. Thus the enzymic activities must be located in free communication with the vascular space, for instance, on the surface of endothelial cells, or be released into the vascular space. The latter possibility is unlikely, as the effluent fluid from the lung had no significant bradykininase activity (Ryan et al. 1970).

In the isolated lung a variety of compounds have been investigated as inhibitors of the inactivation of bradykinin. Inactivation was prevented by BAL, although another sulfhydryl compound, 2-ME, did not prevent inactivation (Alabaster and Bakhle 1972a,b), or the metabolism of bradykinin (Ryan et al. 1968, 1970) in isolated lungs despite its ability to potentiate the effects of bradykinin in vivo (Erdös and Yang 1966, Scholz and Biron 1969).

Several peptide inhibitors of the kininase of isolated lung have been described (see Table). In rat isolated lung the crude BPF mixture altered the metabolism of infused bradykinin, especially at the COOH terminal (Ryan et al. 1970). In rat and guinea pig lungs, BPF, some of its constituent peptides, and some of the potentiating peptides from *Agkistrodon halys blomhoffii* venom all inhibited the inactivation of bradykinin (Alabaster and Bakhle 1972b, 1973). Igic et al. (1972), using, as substrate, the tetrapeptide corresponding to the COOH terminal of bradykinin, found that besides the nonapeptide from *Bothrops jararaca,* a much larger peptide, the B-chain of insulin, prevented hydrolysis of this substrate. The latter inhibitor was an alternative substrate for the dipeptidylcarboxypeptidase that attacks bradykinin.

The presence of more than one enzymic component in the pulmonary inactivation process in isolated lungs was reemphasized by some recent experiments with rat and guinea pig isolated lungs in which we used the *Bothrops* nonapeptide as an inhibitor of bradykininase (Bakhle 1976). Whereas, the nonapeptide depressed bradykinin inactivation in isolated guinea pig lungs from 90% to 42%, in rat lungs the same concentration of nonapeptide only depressed inactivation from 97% to 91%. This suggested that there was proportionately less of the nonapeptide-sensitive bradykininases in rat lungs than in guinea pig lungs. The suggestion was supported by the study of the inactivation of a bradykinin analog, 7β-homo-Pro-bradykinin, which is not a substrate for the purified converting enzyme from rabbit lung (Ondetti and Engel 1975). Its inactivation in guinea pig lungs was only 58% compared with 89% in rat lungs, and the inactivation in either species was not inhibited by the nonapeptide. These results show that there are nonapeptide-sensitive and nonapeptide resistant bradykininases, both contributing to overall pulmonary inactivation and, furthermore, that the proportion of these kininases may well vary markedly between different species. The latter point must be taken into consideration when the results obtained by different workers are compared. On the other hand, the relative ineffectiveness of the nonapeptide in isolated rat lung, when compared with its effectiveness in vivo (100% inhibition of bradykinin inactivation, Stewart and Freer 1973), may indicate that kininases not usually accessible in vivo are operating in the isolated preparation (see below).

IV. Inactivation by Cell-free Extracts and Purified Enzymes from Lungs

Most of our detailed knowledge of lung kininases in vitro, since the work of Nobili (1965), has come, paradoxically, from angiotensin I converting enzyme, although homogenates of dog lung have been scanned for kininase activity (Alabaster and Bakhle 1973). There was significant activity in the high-speed supernatant fraction (80,000 $\times$ g), but most of the bradykininase from dog (Alabaster and Bakhle 1973) and rabbit (Sander and Huggins 1971) lungs was associated with a light particulate material corresponding to the microsomal fraction. There was evidence for at least two bradykininases in this particulate fraction (Alabaster and Bakhle 1973). Igic et al. (1972) purified, from pig lungs, a peptidase very similar to a bradykininase found in kidney some years earlier (Erdös and Yang 1967). Like that from kidney, this lung enzyme removed the COOH terminal dipeptide unit from bradykinin. Apart from bradykinin and its COOH terminal tetrapeptide, the lung dipeptidylcarboxypeptidase also hydrolyzed angiotensin I to angiotensin II and attacked several other natural and synthetic peptides. Dorer et al. (1974) purified, from the same source (pig lung), a peptidase they characterized in terms of its converting enzyme activity. This enzyme also hydrolyzed bradykinin, removing at least four amino acid residues from the COOH terminal in dipeptide units. Another homogenous peptidase has been purified from rabbit lung by following its converting enzyme activity and it also was capable of hydrolyzing the four COOH terminal residues from bradykinin dipeptide units. Chemical analysis of this peptide preparation showed it to be a glycoprotein with galactose, *N*-acetylglucosamine, and mannose as the major sugar residues (Soffer et al. 1974). The purification of these enzymes has necessitated the development of nonbiologic assay methods, and there are now many and various synthetic peptide substrates designed for spectrophotometric assays. However, what is lacking is information on the action of these purified enzymes, on bradykinin analogs, and on related kinins, and it is hoped that a study of this point will soon be undertaken.

The crude particulate bradykininase (Sander and Huggins 1971, Alabaster and Bakhle 1973) and the highly purified dipeptidylcarboxypeptidases of lung, described above, have several important characteristics in common. They hydrolyze bradykinin and convert angiotensin I to angiotensin II; they are inhibited by chelating agents such as EDTA and BAL, by snake venom peptides, and by alternative substrates (see Table); they have a divalent cation requirement, usually for cobalt and manganese (Alabaster and Bakhle 1972b, Igic et al. 1972). It is therefore possible to attribute most of the bradykininase activity in these crude particulate fractions to the activity of lung dipeptidylcarboxypeptidase.

As mentioned earlier, much of our knowledge of lung dipeptidylcarboxypeptidase stemmed from the investigation of lung angiotensin I converting enzyme, and there is now no doubt that one enzyme catalyzes both the inactivation of bradykinin and the conversion of angiotensin I to angiotensin II, as suggested originally by Ng and Vane in 1968. Although it is most likely that the substrate and inhibitor specificities described for the angiotensin I hydrolyzing activity of dipeptidylcarboxypeptidase will also apply to the bradykinin hydrolyzing activity of this enzyme, we must point out that less work has actually been carried out on the bradykininase activity of dipeptidylcarboxypeptidase. Now that highly purified dipeptidylcarboxypeptidase from lung is available, a systematic investigation of its bradykinin hydrolyzing activity in terms of cation and anion dependence, substrates, and inhibitors is long overdue.

One very interesting property of the dipeptidylcarboxypeptidase is its requirement for chloride ions. When Skeggs et al. (1954) first described converting enzyme, one of its characteristics was its absolute requirement for halide ions, usually chloride, for activity. This dependence on chloride ions is still shown by the purified dipeptidylcarboxypeptidase with regard to the hydrolysis of angiotensin I, but hydrolysis of bradykinin has been found in different preparations to be less dependent (Igic et al. 1972) or totally independent (Sander et al. 1971, Alabaster and Bakhle 1972b) on chloride. Recently, Dorer et al. (1974) found that their lung dipeptidylcarboxypeptidase required chloride for bradykinin hydrolysis as well as for angiotensin I hydrolysis, though the optimum concentration for bradykinin was ten times less than that for angiotensin I. Furthermore, at the optima, the Km for bradykinin was almost ten times less than that for angiotensin I.

These findings have gone some way towards settling the question of chloride dependence, but other questions of equal importance remain. Is there a chloride-requirement binding site in the enzyme that angiotensin I needs to utilize but bradykinin does not? Which of the many synthetic peptide substrates also need chloride ion? Is it possible, from their structures, to pick out the amino acid residue(s) involved with the chloride-dependent site? Angiotensin I inhibited bradykinin inactivation equally in high (170 mM) and low (15 mM) chloride concentrations (Alabaster and Bakhle 1973) and this was interpreted in terms of two modes of binding for angiotensin I. In high chloride, the binding is in the correct orientation for hydrolysis but in low chloride, the binding, although still occurring, is in the incorrect orientation, thus preventing hydrolysis (abortive binding). Are there any other inhibitors whose efficacy is chloride dependent? Can inhibitors change in relative potency, i.e., towards converting enzyme or bradykininase, with changes in chloride concentration? We have now the opportunity and the techniques to tackle these questions, which may have physiologic as well as biochemical implications.

V.   Which Kininases Are Active in Lung?

The dipeptidylcarboxypeptidase is the only well-characterized bradykininase from lung. The others, perhaps an aminopeptidase and an endopeptidase, remain to be investigated. We can, however, speculate on the types of kininases active in the isolated lung on the basis of the fragments of bradykinin identified in lung effluent (Ryan et al. 1970).

In Figure 3 all the positions of cleavage of bradykinin are shown. We can reasonably expect the dipeptidylcarboxypeptidase activity, already discussed, to act successively at positions 1, 3 and, perhaps, 5 (see, however,

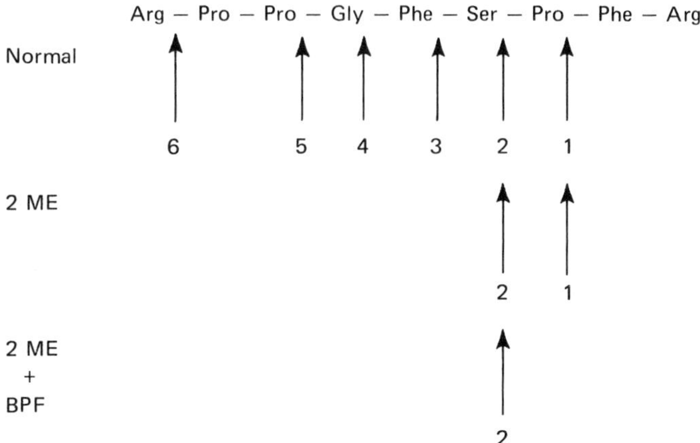

FIGURE 3   Points of hydrolysis in bradykinin during passage through isolated rat lungs (data from Ryan et al. 1970).

Soffer et al. 1974). An aminopeptidase could act at position 6 with the possibility of the carboxypeptidase activity known to be present in lung (Barrett and Sambhi 1971), acting on the pentapeptide fragment 1–5, at position 4. What is particularly interesting is that in the presence of 2-ME, a new cleavage point is disclosed at position 2 and the hydrolyses at positions 3, 4, 5, and 6 are all suppressed. Only the first step of the dipeptidylcarboxypeptidase action at position 1 is still present, suggesting that bradykinin is a better substrate than the heptapeptide (1–7) for this enzyme. Certainly the cleavage of Ser-Pro from the heptapeptide is slower than that of Phe-Arg from bradykinin (Dorer et al. 1974). The hydrolysis at the Ser^6-Pro^7 bond, i.e., in position 2, is resistant to inhibition by both 2-ME and BPF and discloses the actions of an endopeptidase capable of acting on the complete molecule.

This endopeptidase must cleave bradykinin more slowly than the dipeptidylcarboxypeptidase, since there is an increase in biologic activity surviving transit through the lung in the presence of BPF. The relative rate of the aminopeptidase activity is difficult to estimate, but it must be less than that of the dipeptidylcarboxypeptidase, as the inactivation of bradykinin is not altered when the aminopeptidase activity is suppressed by 2-ME. The effect of the *Bothrops* peptides on aminopeptidase activity is not known. Carboxypeptidase *N*, which hydrolyzes the COOH terminal arginine from bradykinin, is not inhibited by the nonapeptide (Igic et al. 1972) and this carboxypeptidase has been recently identified in homogenates of lung (Petakova et al. 1972) although there is, as yet, no evidence of its action in perfused lung (see however, Barrett and Sambhi 1971) or in the pulmonary circulation in vivo.

It seems, therefore, that under normal circumstances in perfused lung the fastest kininase is the dipeptidylcarboxypeptidase, and it is the rate-determining step in the inactivation of bradykinin. However, there is an endopeptidase that is perhaps half as fast and can take over much of the inactivation in the presence of the *Bothrops* peptidase inhibitors. This may be one of the enzymic activities that we suggested earlier were present in perfused lung but not in vivo.

Earlier in this review we referred to the fate of several peptides related to bradykinin, both in vivo and in isolated perfused lungs. What can we deduce from these results to help us decide which of the enzymes present in lung plays a crucial role in the inactivation?

The presence of lung metabolizing enzymes in lung homogenates is not a guarantee that they will act on their substrates in the pulmonary circulation. For instance, the lung contains at least two enzymes capable of inactivating histamine, and lung homogenates readily inactivate histamine (Bennett 1965) but histamine is unaffected by passage through the pulmonary vascular bed in vitro and in vivo (Boileau et al. 1970, Ferreira et al. 1973, Bakhle and Vane

1974). Another more apposite example is that of angiotensin II which, in spite of angiotensinase activity in lung homogenates, passes through the pulmonary circulation unchanged. Eledoisin, a kinin-like hypotensive peptide, provided in our early work another example of this divergence between in vitro and in vivo conditions. This peptide, though resistant to plasma kininases, is easily metabolized by lung homogenates (Nobili 1965), but it passed unchanged through the pulmonary vascular bed in vivo (Ferreira and Vane 1967a).

VI. Substrate Specificity of Inactivation Mechanisms

Although we do not know a great deal about the biologic activity of fragments of peptides other than bradykinin, it is noticeable that three hypotensive peptides resistant to pulmonary inactivation (eledoisin, physalaemin, and substance P) have COOH terminal amide groups. This correlation may be extended to oxytocin, vasopressin, gastrin, and cholecystokinin, all of which are COOH terminal amides and are not inactivated by passage through the pulmonary circulation (for references see Bakhle and Vane 1974). The terminal amide makes such peptides resistant to attack by dipeptidylcarboxypeptidase, and the simplest deduction is that resistance to dipeptidylcarboxypeptidase correlates with resistance to pulmonary inactivation. Since the activity of fragments of other hypotensive peptides is not known, the contribution of the BPF-resistant endopeptidase, postulated earlier, to the inactivation process cannot be estimated. However, the Ser-Pro bond, which it cleaves in bradykinin, does not occur in any other resistant peptide apart from *Polistes* kinin and Lys-Lys-bradykinin.

If we take as a working hypothesis that the determinant of pulmonary inactivation is susceptibility primarily to dipeptidylcarboxypeptidase, and secondarily to the Ser-Pro endopeptidase, how can we explain the results obtained with peptides possessing a free COOH terminal? The NH_2 terminal homologs of bradykinin, kallidin, and Met-Lys-bradykinin, would be equivalent to bradykinin and would be as susceptible to dipeptidylcarboxypeptidase. Phyllokinin has the COOH terminal sulfonic acid, and the negative charge associated with this group may well make it resistant to dipeptidylcarboxypeptidase, since COOH terminal dibasic amino acids confer protection against dipeptidylcarboxypeptidase action (Elisseeva et al. 1971). Here it could be postulated that the observed inactivation is due to the Ser-Pro endopeptidases, as phyllokinin is structurally equivalent to bradykinin with a COOH terminal extension. The D-amino acid analog, D-Pro[7]-bradykinin, is not inactivated because the Pro[7] residue is involved both in the action of the dipeptidylcarboxypeptidase cleaving at Pro[7]-Phe[8] and in the action of the Ser[6]-Pro[7] endopeptidase.

The real difficulty arises with *Polistes* kinin and Lys-Lys-bradykinin. These peptides have the complete sequence of bradykinin at the COOH terminal, with more residues attached at the NH_2 terminal. They should therefore be susceptible to both the dipeptidylcarboxypeptidase and the endopeptidase, but they are totally resistant to inactivation in the perfused lung. We can only surmise that their NH_2 terminal additions somehow prevent their binding to the enzyme. This could be tested by measuring their ability to inhibit the hydrolysis of, eg., bradykinin either by perfused lungs or by purified enzymes, as substrates for dipeptidylcarboxypeptidase compete for binding (Sander et al. 1971).

What is needed is a detailed structural and pharmacologic analysis of the peptide fragments emerging from the lung. The fragments of bradykinin are known to be virtually inactive on isolated intestinal or uterine smooth muscle and as systemic vasodepressors. Nevertheless, these fragments may have other bradykinin-like activities, eg., increase of capillary permeability, contraction of bronchial smooth muscle, mediation of inflammation, ability to cause pain, and we cannot yet afford to disregard these possibilities.

Earlier it was suggested that bradykininase activities other than the dipeptidylcarboxypeptidase do not act on bradykinin passing through the pulmonary circulation in vivo. It is now suggested further that the detection of other kininases in isolated lungs perfused with salt solutions may be due to an increased permeability of, say, the endothelial cells to the peptide substrate. Our hypothesis would be that in vivo and in isolated lungs the dipeptidylcarboxypeptidase is easily accessible to the substrate, being located on the luminal surface of the endothelial cells. All other kininases would be intracellular and accessible only when the permeability of the endothelial cells is increased, for instance in isolated lungs.

Indirect support for this hypothesis comes from the findings that a preparation of endothelial cell membranes will convert angiotensin I to angiotensin II but that the other fragments of angiotensin I present in the effluent from isolated lungs are not formed by this membrane preparation (Ryan et al. 1972). The authors suggest that peptidases other than dipeptidylcarboxypeptidase might have been inhibited by the lead nitrate used in the preparation of the membrane fractions, but an alternative explanation is that the membranes contain only dipeptidylcarboxypeptidase and that the other peptidases are intracellular. A direct consequence of our hypothesis is that fragments of bradykinin, other than the COOH terminal dipeptide, would be delayed in transit relative to the blue dextran marker used by Ryan et al. (1970). Experiments with radioactive substrate showing that all radioactivity passed through the lung in the same time as blue dextran, were carried out with 8-([^{3}H]Phe)-bradykinin, and thus the radioactive label would be associated with the COOH terminal dipeptide. Experiments with 2-($[^{14}C]$Pro)-bradykinin would enable the transit time of other fragments to be measured.

Another test of the hypothesis would be to analyze the fragments in arterial blood after the passage of radioactive bradykinin, labeled in the Pro^2 position, through the pulmonary circulation in vivo. We know that the dipeptidylcarboxypeptidase acts in vivo on angiotensin I and therefore can assume its action on bradykinin, but we would not need to show the absence of other peptidase activity.

VII. Systemic Effects of the Pulmonary Kininase Activity

Finally, let us consider the contribution made by the pulmonary inactivation system to the effects of circulating kinins in the body.

Earlier it was pointed out that even without the participation of tissues in the degradation of bradykinin, its half-life in the circulation would be very short, less than two circulation times, as a result of blood kininases. However, bradykinin does have potent systemic effects once it reaches the arterial side of the circulation. Thus, the pulmonary circulation, by attenuating the activity of circulating kinins during their transit from the venous to the arterial side, acts as a filter for the kinins formed in peripheral tissues. This has led to the proposal that kinins, like prostaglandins and 5-hydroxytryptamine, should be regarded as local hormones (Ferreira and Vane 1967c, Vane 1969).

If the inactivation of kinins in the pulmonary circulation is an important mechanism for controlling the amount of kinins in arterial blood, is there significance in the low level of kininase in fetal and neonatal lungs? Bradykinin has been implicated in the closing of the ductus arteriosus and other circulatory changes that occur at birth (Melmon et al. 1968). These changes take some hours to complete, and during such time it would clearly be of advantage to have low pulmonary inactivation, thus maintaining high arterial levels of kinin without the continuous consumption of large amounts of kininogen. The involvement of bradykinin in these circulatory changes might be assessed using venom peptides; these inhibitors may, for instance, shorten the time taken for the ductus arteriosus to close. Conversely, delay in closing might be due to abnormally high, i.e., adult levels of kininase activity in the pulmonary circulation. Clearly, there are many fascinating and important questions to be answered in this area.

The aspects of pulmonary peptidases related to angiotensin have recently attracted more attention, and since it seems that converting enzyme is also a bradykininase, it is relevant to discuss these results here. The peptides from

Bothrops jararaca have been used to prevent hypertension induced by infusion of angiotensin I in animals and man and also to prevent the hypertension consequent on increased renin secretion in animals (Krieger et al. 1971, Miller et al. 1972, Engel et al. 1973, Collier et al. 1973, Muirhead et al. 1974) and in man (Gavras et al. 1974). Attempts to correlate hypertensive states with increases in angiotensin I-converting enzyme activity in lungs have not yet been successful. However, the possibility of variations in lung bradykininase activity correlating with hypertensive or hypotensive states cannot be ignored and merits investigation. Recently, the *Bothrops* nonapeptide has been shown to increase survival of dogs with irreversible hemorrhagic shock (Errington and Rocha e Silva 1974) and to modify the acute changes in blood pressure following endotoxin or hemorrhagic shock (Erdös et al. 1974). These findings could have considerable clinical importance even though it is not clear yet whether the beneficial effects were due to less vasoconstriction consequent on inhibition of the conversion of angiotensin I or to more vasodilatation consequent on the inhibition of the destruction of bradykinin.

The mechanism by which changes in enzyme activity may be brought about could be either chemical, i.e., changes in synthesis rates of enzyme or changes in activity due to changed levels of cofactors; or physical, altered permeability allowing substrates access to intracellular enzymes, altered membrane configurations changing accessibility or activity of membrane-bound enzymes.

Enough is now known about the normal functioning of the pulmonary inactivating system for kinins; it is time to start inquiring into the functioning of this system in abnormal situations.

VIII.   Summary

The pulmonary circulation in vivo and in isolated lungs inactivates about 80% of bradykinin passing through it. This inactivation is chiefly and, perhaps entirely, due in vivo to the action of a dipeptidylcarboxypeptidase located in free communication with the vascular space, probably on the plasma membrane of the endothelial cells. This enzyme is inhibited by peptides from snake venom, also capable of potentiating some of the actions of bradykinin itself. Additional kinin-hydrolyzing enzymes are active in isolated perfused lungs, possibly because the permeability of the endothelial cells to substrates is increased. Homogenates of lung contain several kinin-inactivating enzymes, including the dipeptidylcarboxypeptidase, which has been purified and also shown to be capable of converting angiotensin I to angiotensin II. Despite the numerous kininases present in lung tissue, the dipeptidylcarboxypeptidase activity appears to be the rate-determining step in the pulmonary inactivation of bradykinin and other hypotensive peptides.

Although there is still a need for work on the basic mechanism of pulmonary inactivation of kinins, it is now possible to test critically the contribution of this inactivating system to many physiologic and pathologic problems.

References

Alabaster, V. A. and Bakhle, Y. S. (1972a). The inactivation of bradykinin in the pulmonary circulation of isolated lungs. *Br. J. Pharmacol.*, **45**:299–309.

Alabaster, V. A. and Bakhle, Y. S. (1972b). Converting enzyme and bradykininase in the lung. *Circ. Res.*, **30** and **31**, Suppl. 2:72–81.

Alabaster, V. A. and Bakhle, Y. S. (1973). The bradykininase activities of extracts of dog lung. *Br. J. Pharmacol.*, **47**:799–807.

Bakhle, Y. S. (1976). The nature of the bradykinin inactivating system in isolated lungs. *Br. J. Pharmacol.*, **56**:349–350P.

Bakhle, Y. S. and Vane, J. R. (1974). Pharmacokinetic function of the pulmonary circulation. *Physiol. Rev.*, **54**:1007–1045.

Barrett, J. D. and Sambhi, M. P. (1971). Pulmonary activation and degradation of angiotensin I, a dual enzyme system. *Res. Commun. Chem. Pathol. Pharmacol.*, **2**:128–145.

Bennett, A. (1965). The metabolism of histamine by guinea pig and rat lung in vitro. *Br. J. Pharmacol.*, **24**:147–155.

Biron, P. (1968). Pulmonary extraction of bradykinin and eledoisin. *Rev. Can. Biol.*, **27**:75–76.

Boileau, J. C., Campeau, L., and Biron, P. (1970). Pulmonary fate of histamine, isoproterenol, physalaemin and substance P. *Can. J. Physiol. Pharmacol.*, **48**:681–684.

Bumpus, F. M., Smeby, R. R., Page, I. H., and Khairallah, P. A. (1964). Distribution and metabolic fate of angiotensin II and various derivatives. *Can. Med. Assoc. J.*, **90**:190–193.

Camargo, A. and Ferreira, S. H. (1971). Action of bradykinin potentiating factor (BPF) and dimercaptol (BAL) on the responses to bradykinin of isolated preparations of rat intestines. *Br. J. Pharmacol.*, **42**:305–307.

Collier, J. G., Robinson, B. F., and Vane, J. R. (1973). Reduction of the pressor effects of angiotensin I in man by synthetic nonapeptide (BPP$_{9a}$ or SQ 2088a) which inhibits converting enzyme. Lancet, **1**:72–74.

Dorer, F. E., Kahn, J. R., Lentz, K. E., Levine, M., and Skeggs, L. T. (1974). Hydrolysis of bradykinin by angiotensin-converting enzyme. *Circ. Res.*, **34**:824–827.

Elisseeva, Y. E., Orekhovich, V. N., Pavlikhina, L. V., and Alexeenko, L. P. (1971). Carboxycathepsin – a key regulatory component of two physiological systems involved in regulation of blood pressure. *Clin. Chem. Acta*, **31**:413–419.

Engel, S. L., Schaeffer, T. R., Gold, B. I., and Rubin, B. (1972). Inhibition of pressor effects of angiotensin I and augmentation of depressor effects of bradykinin by synthetic peptides. *Proc. Soc. Exp. Biol. Med.,* **140**:240–244.

Engel, S. L., Schaeffer, T. R., Waugh, M. H., and Rubin, B. (1973). Effects of the nonapeptide SQ 20881 on blood pressure of rats with experimental renovascular hypertension. *Proc. Soc. Exp. Biol. Med.,* **143**:483–487.

Erdös, E. G., Massion, W. H., Downs, D. R., and Gecse, A. (1974). Effect of the inhibition of angiotensin I converting enzyme in endotoxin and hemorrhagic shock. *Proc. Soc. Exp. Biol. Med.,* **145**:948–951.

Erdös, E. G., Renfrew, A. G., Sloane, E. M., and Wohler, J. R. (1963). Enzymatic studies on bradykinin and similar peptides. *Ann. N.Y. Acad. Sci.,* **104**:222–235.

Erdös, E. G. and Wohler, J. R. (1963). Inhibition in vivo of the enzymatic inactivation of bradykinin and kallidin. *Biochem. Pharmacol.,* **12**:1193–1199.

Erdös, E. G. and Yang, H. Y. (1966). Inactivation and potentiation of the effects of bradykinin. In E. G. Erdös, N. Back, and F. Sicuteri (eds.): *Hypotensive Peptides.* Springer-Verlag, New York, pp. 235–251.

Erdös, E. G. and Yang, H. Y. (1967). An enzyme in microsomal fraction of kidney that inactivates bradykinin. *Life Sci.,* **6**:569–574.

Errington, M. L. and Rocha e Silva, M., Jr. (1974). On the role of vasopressin and angiotensin in the development of irreversible haemorrhagic shock. *J. Physiol.,* **242**:119–141.

Ferreira, S. H. (1965). A bradykinin-potentiating factor (BPF) present in the venom of *Bothrops jararaca. Br. J. Pharmacol.,* **24**:163–169.

Ferreira, S. H., Bartelt, D. C., and Greene, L. J. (1970a). Isolation of bradykinin potentiating peptides from *Bothrops jararaca* venom. *Biochemistry,* **9**:2583–2593.

Ferreira, S. H., Greene, L. J., Alabaster, V. A., Bakhle, Y. S., and Vane, J. R. (1970b). Activity of various fractions of bradykinin potentiating factor against angiotensin I converting enzyme. *Nature,* **225**:379–380.

Ferreira, S. H., Ng. K. K. F., and Vane, J. R. (1973). The continuous bioassay of the release and disappearance of histamine in the circulation. *Br. J. Pharmacol.,* **49**:543–553.

Ferreira, S. H. and Rocha e Silva, M. (1962). Potentiation of bradykinin by dimercaptopropanol (BAL) and of other inhibitors of its destroying enzyme in plasma. *Biochem. Pharmacol.,* **11**:1123–1128.

Ferreira, S. H. and Vane, J. R. (1967a). The disappearance of bradykinin and eledoisin in the circulation and vascular beds of the cat. *Br. J. Pharmacol. Chemother.,* **30**:417–424.

Ferreira, S. H. and Vane, J. R. (1967b). The detection and estimation of bradykinin in the circulating blood. *Br. J. Pharmacol. Chemother.,* **29**:367–377.

Ferreira, S. H. and Vane, J. R. (1967c). Half-lives of peptides and amines in the circulation. *Nature,* **215**:1237–1240.

Fox, R. H., Goldsmith, R., Kidd, D. J., and Lewis, G. P. (1961). Bradykinin as a vasodilator in man. *J. Physiol. (Lond.),* **157**:589–602.

Friedli, B., Kent, G., and Olley, P. M. (1973). Inactivation of bradykinin in the pulmonary vascular bed of newborn and fetal lambs. *Circ. Res.*, **33**:421–427.

Gavras, H., Brunner, H. R., Laragh, J. H., Sealey, J. E., Gavras, I., and Vukovich, R. A. (1974). An angiotensin converting enzyme inhibitor to identify and treat vasoconstrictor and volume factors in hypertensive patients. *N. Engl. J. Med.*, **291**:817–821.

Greene, L. J., Camargo, A. C. M., Krieger, E. M., Stewart, J. M., and Ferreira, S. H. (1972). Inhibition of the conversion of angiotensin I to II and potentiation of bradykinin by small peptides present in *Bothrops jararaca* venom. *Circ. Res.*, **30** and **31**:Suppl. 2:62–71.

Hébert, F., Fouron, J. C., Boileau, J.-C. and Biron, P. (1972). Pulmonary fate of vasoactive peptides in fetal, newborn and adult sheep. *Am. J. Physiol.*, **225**:20–23.

Igic, R., Erdös, E. G., Yeh, H. S. J., Sorrells, K., and Nakajima, T. (1972). Angiotensin I converting enzyme of the lung. *Circ. Res.*, **30** and **31**:Suppl. 2: 51–61.

Kato, H. and Suzuki, T. (1971). Bradykinin-potentiating peptides from venom of *A. halys blomhoffii*. Isolation of five bradykinin potentiators and the amino acid sequence of two of them, potentiators B and C. *Biochemistry*, **10**:972–980.

Krieger, E. M., Salgado, H. C., Assan, C. J., Greene, L. J., and Ferreira, S. H. (1971). Potential screening test for detection of overactivity of renin-angiotensin system. Lancet, **1**:269–271.

Levine, B. W., Talamo, R. C., and Kazemi, H. (1973). Action and metabolism of bradykinin in dog lung. *J. Appl. Physiol.*, **34**:821–826.

Melmon, K. L., Cline, M. J., Hughes, T., and Nies, A. S. (1968). Kinins: possible mediators of neonatal circulatory changes in man. *J. Clin. Invest.*, **47**: 1279–1302.

Miller, E. D. Jr., Samuels, A. I., Haber, I., and Barger, A. C. (1972). Inhibition of angiotensin conversion in experimental renovascular hypertension. *Science*, **117**:1108–1109.

Muirhead, E. E., Brooks, B., and Arora, K. K. (1974). Prevention of malignant hypertension by the synthetic peptide SQ 20881. *Lab. Invest.*, **30**:129–135.

Nakajima, T., Oshima, G., Yeh, H. S. J., Igic, R., and Erdös, E. G. (1973). Purification of the angiotensin I-converting enzyme of the lung. *Biochem. Biophys. Acta*, **315**:430–438.

Ng, K. K. F. and Vane, J. R. (1968). Fate of angiotensin I in the circulation. *Nature*, **218**:144–150.

Nobili, M. B. (1965). Sulla inattivazione della eledoisina e della physalaemin da parte del sangue totale e di omogenati tissutali di alcuni vertebrati. *Arch. Int. Pharmacodyn.*, **158**:187–201.

Oates, J. A., Melmon, K., Sjoerdsma, A., Gillespie, L., and Mason, D. T. (1964). Release of a kinin peptide in the carcinoid syndrome. Lancet, **1**:514–517.

Ondetti, M. A. and Engel, S. L. (1975). Bradykinin analogs containing β-homo-amino acids. *J. Med. Chem.*, **18**:761–763.

Ondetti, M. A., Williams, N. J., Sabo, E. F., Pluscec, J., Weaver, E. R., and Kocy, O. (1971). Angiotensin converting enzyme inhibitors from the venom of *Bothrops jararaca*. Isolation, elucidation of structure and synthesis. *Biochemistry*, **10**:4033–4039.

Oshima, G. and Erdös, E. G. (1974). Inhibition of the angiotensin I converting enzyme of the lung by a peptide fragment of bradykinin. *Experientia*, **30**: 733–734.

Petakova, M., Simonianova, E., and Rybak, M. (1972). Carboxypeptidases N (Kininases I) in rat serum lungs, liver and spleen and the inactivation of kinins (bradykinin). *Physiol. Bohemoslov.*, **21**:287–293.

Pojda, S. M. and Vane, J. R. (1971). Inhibitory effects of aprotinin on kallikrein and kininases in dog's blood. *Br. J. Pharmacol.*, **42**:558–568.

Roblero, J., Ryan, J., and Stewart, J. M. (1973). Assay of kinins by their effects on blood pressure. *Res. Commun. Chem. Pathol. Pharmacol.*, **6**:207–212.

Rocha e Silva, M., Beraldo, W. T., and Rosenfeld, G. (1949). Bradykinin: hypotensive and smooth muscle stimulating factor released from plasma globulin by snake venom and by trypsin. *Am. J. Physiol.*, **156**:261–273.

Ryan, J. W., Roblero, J., and Stewart, J. M. (1968). Inactivation of bradykinin in the pulmonary circulation. *Biochem. J.*, **110**:795–797.

Ryan, J. W., Roblero, J., and Stewart, J. M. (1970). Inactivation of bradykinin in rat lung. *Adv. Exp. Med. Biol.*, **8**:263–271.

Ryan, J. W., Smith, U., and Niemeyer, R. S. (1972). Angiotensin I: metabolism by plasma membrane of lung. *Science*, **176**:64–66.

Sander, G. E. and Huggins, C. G. (1971). Subcellular localization of angiotensin I converting enzyme in rabbit lung. *Nature, New Biol.*, **230**:27–29.

Sander, G. E., West, D. W., and Huggins, C. G. (1971). Peptide inhibitors of pulmonary angiotensin I converting enzyme. *Biochem. Biophys. Acta*, **242**: 662–667.

Scholz, W. H. and Biron, P. (1969). Non-identity between pulmonary bradykininase and converting enzyme activity. *Rev. Can. Biol.*, **28**:197–200.

Sicuteri, F., Fanciullacci, M., and Anselmi, B. (1963). Bradykinin release and metabolism in man. *Int. Arch. Allergy*, **22**:77–84.

Skeggs, L. T., Marsh, W. H., Kahn, J. R., and Shumway, N. P. (1954). The existence of two forms of hypertensin. *J. Exp. Med.*, **99**:275–282.

Soffer, R. L., Reza, R., and Caldwell, P. R. B. (1974). Angiotensin-converting enzyme from rabbit pulmonary particles. *Proc. Natl. Acad. Sci.*, **71**:1720–1724.

Stewart, J. M., Ferreira, S. H., and Greene, L. J. (1971). Bradykinin potentiating peptide PCA-Lys-Trp-Ala-Pro. An inhibitor of the pulmonary inactivation of bradykinin and conversion of angiotensin I to II. *Biochem. Pharmacol.*, **20**:1557–1567.

Stewart, J. M. and Freer, R. J. (1973). Inhibitors of the pulmonary destruction of bradykinin in the rat. In H. Peeters (ed.): *Protides of the Biological Fluids*. 20th Colloquium, Pergamon Press, Oxford and New York, pp. 331–333.

Stewart, J. M. and Roblero, J. (1967). Studies on the pulmonary inactivation of bradykinin. In O. Ludescher (ed.): Vasoactive Polypeptides and Inhibitors of Proteolytic Enzyme. K. K. Bayer-Yakuhin, Tokyo, pp. 52–55.

Suzuki, K., Abiko, T., Endo, N., Kameyama, T., Sasaki, K., and Nabeshima, J. (1969). Biologically active synthetic fragments of bradykinin. *Jap. J. Pharmacol.*, **19**:325–327.

Trautschold, I., Fritz, H., and Werle, E. (1966). Kininogenases, kininases and their inhibitors. In E. G. Erdös, N. Back, and F. Sicuteri (eds.): *Hypotensive Peptides*. Springer Verlag, New York, pp. 221–232.

Vane, J. R. (1964). The use of isolated organs for detecting active substances in the circulating blood. *Br. J. Pharmacol.*, **23**:360–373.

Vane, J. R. (1969). The release and fate of vasoactive hormones in the circulation. *Br. J. Pharmacol.*, **35**:209–242.

Vane, J. R. and Ferreira, S. H. (1976). Interactions between bradykinin and prostaglandins. In *Chemistry and Biology of the Kallikrein-Kinin System in Health and Disease*. Fogarty International Center Proceedings, vol. 27, in press.

Vargaftig, B. B. and Dao Hai, N. (1972). Selective inhibition by mepacrine of the release of rabbit aorta contracting substance evoked by the administration of bradykinin. *J. Pharm. Pharmacol.*, **24**:159–161.

3

Biochemistry of the Pulmonary Angiotensin-Converting Enzyme

GESINA L. LONGENECKER and
CLYDE G. HUGGINS

University of South Alabama, College of Medicine
Mobile, Alabama

I. Introduction

The biochemistry, physiology, and pharmacology of the angiotensins and the angiotensin-converting enzyme have been reviewed extensively in recent years (Sander and Huggins 1972, Lubran 1973, Page and Bumpus 1974, Oparil and Haber 1974, Erdos 1975 and Soffer 1976). The angiotensins were variously named in earlier literature, e.g., angiotonin, by Page and Helmer (1940), and hypertensin, by Braun-Menendez et al. (1940), with the term angiotensin adopted in 1958 by Braun-Menendez and Page. There are two forms of angiotensin, referred to as angiotensin I and angiotensin II. Angiotensin II is the physiologically active form. The description of angiotensin I converting enzyme (Skeggs et al. 1954), which is responsible for the production of angiotensin II (Fig. 1) initiated an intensive investigation regarding the biochemical

Supported in part by Grant No. 5 RO1 HL 15384-03, from the National Heart and Lung Institute, National Institutes of Health.

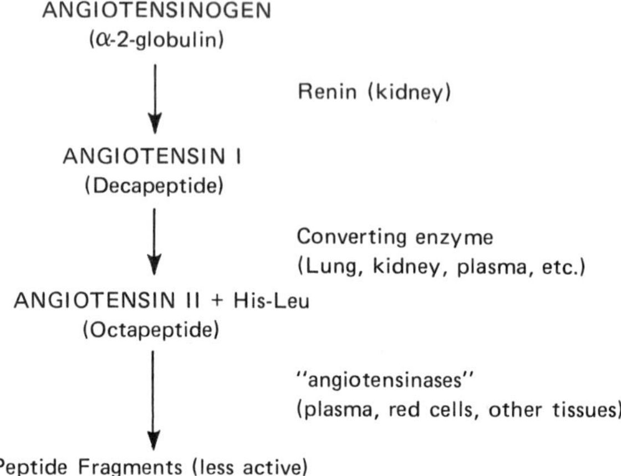

FIGURE 1   The metabolism of angiotensin.

and physiologic role of the enzyme. The term *converting enzyme* was applied by Skeggs to the enzyme isolated from horse plasma, but more specifically it was applied to the *function* of conversion. Other terms have been proposed, e.g., kininase II and dipeptidyl hydrolase (DH) (Yang et al. 1971), although *converting enzyme* is the usual term used. Since its original description, converting enzyme activity has been found in several tissues of various species (Cushman and Cheung 1971b, Roth et al. 1969).

The presence of converting enzyme activity in lung is a relatively recent finding (Ng and Vane 1967, Huggins and Thampi 1968). These early reports on the presence of converting enzyme in lung have resulted in a remarkable quantity of published data on the properties of this enzyme and more recently on the role of the lung in regulatory processes in general (Fishman and Pietra 1974, Bakhle and Vane 1974, Junod and de Haller 1975). Interest in non-respiratory lung functions has resulted from recognition of the facts that almost all blood is ultimately *seen* by the microcirculation of lung and that lung is an important and highly selective organ of metabolism (Vane 1968, 1969, Marshall 1973, Gillis 1973). It is the purpose of this chapter to examine an increasingly important aspect of lung biochemistry, i.e., the metabolism of the angiotensins.

The biochemistry and cellular and subcellular distribution of pulmonary angiotensin converting enzyme will be described in detail. The regulatory role of the lungs in terminating angiotensin activity will also be considered.

II. Biochemistry of the
Renin-Angiotensin System

A brief consideration of the biochemistry of the renin-angiotensin system may serve to make clear subsequent descriptions. Renin, an enzyme present in the juxtaglomerular apparatus of the kidney, acts on angiotensinogen (or renin substrate), which moves electrophoretically with α_2-globulin, to form a decapeptide, angiotensin I (Fig. 1). The amino acid sequence of this decapeptide is remarkably constant from species to species, varying in the substitution of a single amino acid at position 5. Bovine angiotensin has Val in position 5 (Elliott and Peart 1956), while horse and human have Ile (Lentz et al. 1956, Arakawa et al. 1957). The decapeptide, angiotensin I, is, in turn, acted on by converting enzyme, which splits off the dipeptide His-Leu at the carboxyl terminus (thus converting enzyme is a dipeptidylcarboxypeptidase) to form the octapeptide angiotensin II. Angiotensin II is one of the most potent pressor substances known. The pressor effect is due to the action of angiotensin II on receptors in smooth muscle, resulting in contraction and vasoconstriction. Smooth muscle from sources other than vasculature is responsive to angiotensin as well (uterus: Luduena 1940, colon: Regoli and Vane 1964). Angiotensin II usually gives a much greater response (10 to 50 times) than angiotensin I, but this is not true for all tissues (e.g., guinea pig ileum: Collins 1948, Picarelli et al. 1954). Prevention of the formation, and thus pharmacologic activity, of endogenous angiotensin II may be accomplished by inhibitors of converting

H$_2$N-Asp-Arg-Val-Tyr-Ile-His-Pro-Phe-His-Leu-COOH

ANGIOTENSIN I

H$_2$N-Asp-Arg-Val-Tyr-Ile-His-Pro-Phe-COOH

ANGIOTENSIN II

H$_2$N-Arg-Pro-Pro-Gly-Phe-Ser-Pro-Phe-Arg-COOH

BRADYKININ

PCA-Lys-Trp-Ala-Pro

BPP-Pentapeptide SQ 20475

PCA-Trp-Pro-Arg-Pro-Gln-Ile-Pro-Pro-COOH

BPP-Nonapeptide SQ 20881

FIGURE 2 Amino acid sequences of some active peptides.

enzyme activity (Sander and Huggins 1972, Page and Bumpus 1974), but the most effective are the peptides isolated from *Bothrops jararaca* venom (Ferreira 1965, Ferreira et al. 1970, Sander et al. 1971). Pharmacologic or physiologic activity of angiotensin II is terminated by the action of the *angiotensinases,* a group of enzymes with wide tissue distribution and a large number of sites of cleavage in the peptide molecule (Sander and Huggins 1972, Ledingham and Leary 1976). The terminal Pro-Phe bond is the usual, but not exclusive, site of cleavage. Structures of angiotensin I and II, bradykinin, and two peptide inhibitors of converting enzyme are given in Figure 2.

III.   Methods of Assay of Converting Enzyme

A.   Bioassay

Some tissues are much more sensitive to angiotensin II than to angiotensin I. This specific and differential sensitivity to the angiotensins is the basis for many bioassay systems. Helmer (1957) described the use of spirally cut strips of rabbit aorta, which is much more responsive to angiotensin II than to angiotensin I. The response of the aorta is so specific to angiotensin II, in fact, that mixtures of both angiotensins may be used in the assay without interference from angiotensin I. Angiotensin I can be measured indirectly, using the rabbit aorta after conversion in vitro to angiotensin II by exposure to a converting enzyme preparation from, e.g., lung. Obviously the same system can be used to quantitate converting enzyme by the rate of conversion of angiotensin I to II. Up to 40 μg/ml of angiotensin I, converted to angiotensin II may be accurately determined with this bioassay system (Huggins et al. 1970). Rat uterus is also more responsive to angiotensin II, with responses being 10 to 40 times greater than for an equivalent amount of angiotensin I (Bumpus et al. 1961). Substrate concentration for assay with this tissue is about 200 ng/ml of angiotensin I (Bakhle 1974). The rat colon assay gives a differential of angiotensin II to I of about 20 to 1 (Regoli and Vane 1964, Ng and Vane 1967). A complete tabulation of various tissues used for bioassay, together with a comparison of the amounts of substrate that can be measured has been made by Bakhle (1974). A discussion of other aspects of bioassay is given by Khairallah and Smeby (1974) and by Boucher and Genest (1974).

For many years bioassay was the principal system used, requiring a large investment in time. Despite the fact that it is sensitive (within the physiologic range), response by bioassay provides only indirect evidence of conversion. Specificity has been refined in bioassay by the use of several sensitive organs in series (e.g., Bakhle et al. 1969). Addition of organs (tissues) responsive to other, possibly interfering, vasoactive or contraction-inducing materials (catecholamines, prostaglandins, histamine, etc.), allows correction of responses to account for these agents (e.g., Jakschik et al. 1974, Turker et al. 1974). Despite these refinements, however, bioassay is still subject to the same criticism, i.e., it is indirect, and the above refinements actually add to the time required for the assay. These consideration have stimulated two important advances: (a) coupling chemical identification techniques (substrate or products) with bioassay and (b) preparing synthetic substrates for converting enzyme, allowing spectrophotometric analysis.

B. Radiometric Assay

In an effort to avoid some of the difficulties associated with bioassay for quantitative determinations of angiotensin II, Huggins and Thampi (1968) devised a system for separating His-Leu from angiotensin I and angiotensin II on Biogel P_2, with subsequent colorimetric assay of His-Leu by the ninhydrin reaction. This procedure proved to be time consuming and required relatively large amounts of starting material for colorimetry (ninhydrin reaction is effective in the 20 to 2000 μg/ml range). By introducing ^{14}C-labeled Leu into position 10 in angiotensin I, the product His-Leu was made radioactive and could be measured by radiometric techniques. Column chromatography with Biogel P_2 was replaced by a much faster separation process, using silica gel-impregnated glass-fiber paper chromatography. Identification of separated materials was confirmed by bioassay, the only method readily available for angiotensin II at that time. These studies used plasma enzyme, but marked the beginning of biochemical analytic techniques for radiometric measurement of angiotensin I and II, which facilitated later work on pulmonary converting enzyme.

Ryan et al. (1970) and Lee et al. (1971) have used [^{14}C] Leu^{10}-labeled angiotensin I to demonstrate the formation of His-Leu by lung in situ and by lung converting enzyme preparations, respectively. Formation of angiotensin II in these systems was confirmed by bioassay, without direct confirmation by biochemical procedures. Chiu and coworkers (1975) have developed an assay based on use of ^{125}I-Tyr^8-bradykinin which is reported to be both specific and sensitive enough to be used for assay of conversion in cell cultures. This was obviously better than completely inferential evidence, but the development of radioimmunoassay allowed the identification of the active product directly.

C. Radioimmunoassay

The introduction of radioimmunoassay (RIA) has made it possible to assay
minute physiologic quantities of the angiotensins directly. Also, the rapidity
and simplicity of RIA allow large numbers of assays to be undertaken. Either
of the angiotensins is coupled to a carrier (e.g., charcoal: Boyd et al. 1967,
protein: Deodhar 1960) to increase its size and antigenicity. Antibodies are
then produced to these complexes by the usual immunologic techniques (Worobec et al. 1972). The antibodies thus produced are very specific to the initiating hapten, with only slight cross-reactivity (5%, Haber et al 1969) of one to
the other, or to degradation homologs. Interference from degradation products has been minimized by the use of arterial blood samples (Cain et al.
1969). Unreacted angiotensin is separated from antibody-bound angiotensin
by treatment with charcoal or by other techniques (Oparil and Haber 1974).

Menard and Catt (1972) have applied the use of RIA of angiotensin I in
plasma as a measure of renin activity. Converting enzyme has also been quantitated by RIA (Oparil et al. 1970, Fitz et al. 1971). Boyd and Peart (1968)
have measured as little as 30 pg angiotensin II, a very impressive accomplish-
ment. Physiologic concentrations are thus well within the reach of direct
assay by this technique (see Table, Oparil and Haber 1974).

D. Synthetic Substrates: Spectrophotometric and Colorimetric Assay

Cushman and collaborators (1969, 1971a,b) reported that Hip-His-Leu, a protected tripeptide C-terminal analog of angiotensin I, was a substrate for converting enzyme. This permitted the development of a rapid spectrophotometric assay. Properties of the converting enzyme with this substrate (pH
optimum, chloride dependence, inhibitor profiles) agreed with those for
natural substrate, although Hip-His-Leu had a lower affinity for the enzyme.
Synthesis of a small peptide is obviously much simpler than that of a decapeptide. It is also less expensive to produce and easier to characterize and
purify. Moreover, the reaction proceeds rapidly (with a wavelength shift in
absorption paralleling product formation), allowing any reaction to be monitored directly, either by continuous or endpoint determination. Other small
peptides are also substrates for converting enzyme: e.g., Hip-Gly-Gly and its
p-NO$_2$ derivative (Stevens et al. 1972), [^{14}C] dansyl Gly-Gly-Gly (Igic et al.
1972 a,b), etc. Substrate concentration for these in vitro incubations is generally in the millimolar range.

Reaction products have also been quantitated colorimetrically by the
ninhydrin reaction (Dorer et al. 1970), with substrate concentrations for this

method in the millimolar range for synthetic substrates (Hip-His-Leu) and about 2.5×10^{-4} M for the natural substrate, angiotensin I. This substrate concentration of angiotensin I is relatively high compared to bioassay or RIA.

Roth et al. (1969), using the artificial substrates Z-Phe-Ala-His-Leu and Z-Phe-His-Leu (previously shown to be effective for converting enzyme, Piquilloud et al. 1970), devised a fluorimetric assay for the product His-Leu. The reaction mixture is dried, dissolved in a very small volume, applied to paper, and developed. The chromatogram is treated with o-phthaldialdehyde, which condenses with the imidazole portion of His-Leu, and the reaction product is measured fluorimetrically. The substrate concentration for this procedure is approximately the same as for the spectrophotometric assays.

There is a clear advantage in using synthetic artificial substrates because of the speed and number of analyses made possible. This is especially advantageous in the purification of the enzyme or in the isolation and purification of inhibitors, where the large numbers of individual assays necessary would swamp bioassay procedures. However, correlation with bioassay is a necessity in endstage enzyme purification, for example, to assure that the enzyme isolated and quantitated with the aid of these compounds is indeed still capable of acting on the natural substrate and that specific activity for the natural substrate has also increased. This is the only assurance that isolated system work has any bearing on the physiology ultimately intended to be elucidated.

IV. Pulmonary Converting Enzyme

A. Introduction

Historically, plasma, which contains converting enzyme activity, was assumed to be the primary site of production of angiotensin II. A circulating enzyme with easy access to its substrate, angiotensin I, and with direct vascular distribution of the active product, angiotensin II, provided a rational explanation for the rapid pressor action of angiotensin. The ready availability of blood and the ease of working with an already soluble enzyme had a definite influence on the above concept (Bakhle 1974). Several observations complicated the assumption, however. The first was that the angiotensin I pressor effect was essentially equivalent to that of an equal dose of angiotensin II. Additionally, less than 20% conversion from angiotensin I to angiotensin II occurred in blood in vitro during a time period equivalent to one circulation time. The third was that a significant difference in the physiologic and pharmacologic effects was obtained, depending on whether angiotensin I was administered intravenously or intraarterially. Finally, there was greater than an order of magnitude difference (120 sec versus 4 to 8 sec) in the time required for conversion of angiotensin I to II in peripheral blood as compared with passage through the pulmonary circulation (Ng and Vane 1967). These observations, combined with those of Goffinet and Mulrow (1965), who reported that angiotensin II had *free passage* through lungs, led to the conclusion that lung was the primary site of production of angiotensin II and stimulated the intensive research in progress on pulmonary converting enzyme.

B. In Vivo Site of Conversion

Investigations by Hodge and associates (1967) and Ng and Vane (1968), using a blood-bathed rat colon assay, showed that other vascular beds (e.g., head, kidneys, limbs) do not convert angiotensin I to angiotensin II to any significant degree. The early observation (Ng and Vane 1967) that conversion in blood was slow (17% after 30 sec) while conversion in the pulmonary circulation was rapid (40% to 50% in less than 10 sec) was confirmed. This observation was made for both synthetic and endogenously produced angiotensin I. These workers suggested that these results were probably indicative of complete conversion of angiotensin I to II during a single passage through the pulmonary circulation. Angiotensin II passed through the pulmonary circulation unchanged, whereas in other vascular beds, there is up to 60% loss. Ng and Vane questioned whether the conversion in the pulmonary circulation was a result of some extraordinary change in the blood enzyme while present in the lung circulation, or whether the lung itself contained a converting enzyme, i.e., a dipeptidylcarboxypeptidase (carboxydipeptidase). The report that isolated perfused lungs also converted angiotensin I to II (Bakhle et al. 1969) partially answered this question by indicating the presence of a physiologically accessible pulmonary converting enzyme activity. It was also noted that renal effects of angiotensin I (reduction in blood flow and urine output) could occur only after the substrate passed through the pulmonary circulation, thereby questioning the intrarenal-only role for the renin-angiotensin system. In contrast, work by Franklin and associates (1970) has shown a significant degree of renal conversion.

Also, in contrast to the observations of Bakhle et al. (1969) regarding lack of peripheral conversion, Biron and Huggins (1968), using synthetic ^{14}C-labeled angiotensin I (Ileu-5-[^{14}C] Leu-10-angiotensin I), demonstrated, by careful comparison of time delays after aortic injection, that some conversion of angiotensin I to II must occur and be effective *at the site* of action. In their scheme angiotensin I remaining after local conversion would be equally distributed to loss or to conversion on reaching the pulmonary circulation. Thus the pressor response of any system would be the result of angiotensin II from the combined sources. In their studies intraaortic injection of angiotensin I resulted in pressor responses approximately half those seen after intra-jugular injection, suggesting that the greater portion of conversion of physiologic significance does indeed occur in lung.

Aiken and Vane (1970) also examined the possibility of in situ conversion, being concerned with the discrepancy of net inactivation by perfused intact organs other than lung, despite the presence of converting enzyme activity in homogenates of these same organs. They first demonstrated the activity of a peptide inhibitor of converting enzyme (the pentapeptide, BPP_{5a} or SQ 20 475) in their superfused rat colon assay and in arterial strip assays from several species. These arterial strips were responsive to both angiotensin I and II, with the ratio of one to the other a function in degree of the source of the strips. The pentapeptide affected not only the ratio of responses to angiotensin I and II, but also the response to angiotensin I alone. This finding, combined with the fact that the response to angiotensin I took much longer than the response to angiotensin II, led them to suggest local formation of and response to angiotensin II. Quantitative consideration of the untreated and inhibitor-treated angiotensin I-angiotensin II response ratios showed that pulmonary arteries had the highest conversion, suggesting that the locus of converting enzyme was in pulmonary vasculature, perhaps throughout the arterioles. This distribution could account for the rapid conversion seen in lungs. In addition, peripheral vasculature had a relatively higher sensitivity to angiotensin II and essentially no converting enzyme activity, suggesting that some systems respond only to a *delivered* substrate. Because of the small local conversion and the time requirement for it, Aiken and Vane concluded that *intramural* conversion was secondary and that conversion in the lung was the primary and important site.

Osborn and associates (1972) made observations similar to those of Biron and Huggins, in several different species. They concluded that conversion cannot occur only in lung, since this would necessitate a response to angiotensin I some 20 sec later than that to angiotensin II after left ventricular injection, a response they did not get. They further concluded that pulmonary conversion is indeed the most important physiologically and that activation or inactivation by blood is relatively unimportant.

Freer and Stewart (1972, 1975) report that *no* pulmonary conversion of angiotensin from I to II occurs in the rat, even though bradykinin is 95% inactivated. Rats do show a pressor response to both angiotensins I and II, with the response to angiotensin I lessened by treatment with converting-enzyme inhibitors. The conclusion is that in the rat, at least, extrapulmonary conversion is very significant. The work of Oates and Stokes (1974) also indicates a significant extrapulmonary conversion in the rat, but their data indicates a significant degree of pulmonary conversion as well.

C.   Classification of Pulmonary Converting Enzyme

Once it was established that lung indeed did contain angiotensin I converting enzyme activity and that the conditions necessary for enzymic conversion of angiotensin I to II in lung were similar to conditions required for plasma converting enzyme, the next question to be answered was whether the lung enzyme was also a dipeptidylcarboxypeptidase or whether it was an enzyme(s) cleaving first Leu and then His from angiotensin I. Ng and Vane (1970) used an undecapeptide analog of angiotensin I with the terminal sequence His-His-Leu to test the hypothesis that pulmonary converting enzyme is a dipeptidyl-carboxypeptidase. The analog had an activity on their superfused rat colon assays of 0.5% to 0.6% of the angiotensin II response. Stepwise conversion of this analog during pulmonary perfusion could result in the formation of angiotensin II and thus an increase in the biologic activity. However, the analog did not show an increase in activity after perfusion through the lung, suggesting that stepwise conversion to angiotensin II did not occur. Angiotension II, which has the same internal sequence as the analog, is not cleaved at any other position in its structure. It was thus unlikely that other bonds within the analog were split.

Biochemical confirmation of the results of Ng and Vane was achieved by Ryan et al. (1970), using $[^{14}C]$ Leu-10-angiotensin I in an in situ perfused lung preparation. Substrate and products were separated by column fractionation, identified by paper chromatography, and quantitated by radiometric analyses. After a single passage through the lung, radioactivity showed up only as His-Leu fragments: there was no free Leu. This indicated that angiotensin II is formed in a single step conversion. Ryan and associates indicated the presence of a C-terminal fragment of angiotensin I, which was believed to be formed by the action of a lung aminopeptidase. Another active peptide with a molecular weight lower than angiotensin II was also found. It was reported to be a C-terminal heptapeptide formed from angiotensin II. Previous suggestions (e.g., Aiken and Vane 1970) that the endothelial surface of vessels was the most probable location of the converting enzyme was supported 'by the fact that metabolism (conversion) does not require enzymes from any other source, and neither the product nor any of its metabolites are retained (Ryan et al. 1971).

Lee and associates (1971), using a $[^{14}C]$ Leu-10-angiotensin I derivative, demonstrated the formation of His-$[^{14}C]$ Leu by partially purified lung preparations from hog or guinea pig. Although they were able to achieve purification, they felt that the total activity recovered was insufficient to account for the amount of conversion seen in the lung under in vivo conditions. They also had a high amount of His-Leu peptidase activity in their preparations.

Oparil and associates (1971) used RIA to examine conversion of angiotensin I by dog lung. The substrates used were synthetic analogs (L-Leu-angiotensin I, D-Leu-angiotensin I and des-Leu-angiotensin I) with cross-reactivity to angiotensin I and angiotensin II. These investigators proposed that des-Leu angiotensin I would be an adequate substrate for a monocarboxypeptidase, i.e., it would yield angiotensin II (as carboxypeptidase A did), while it would be an inadequate substrate for a dipeptidylcarboxypeptidase, i.e., it would produce an inactive heptapeptide. Neither the lung nor the plasma enzyme converted des-Leu-angiotensin I to II, indicating a common mechanism, i.e., both were dipeptidases. L-Leu-angiotensin I was converted by plasma enzyme, and also gave a pressor response in the dog. D-Leu-angiotensin I was only half as reactive as the L-form in the RIA procedure and it was not converted either by the lung or plasma enzymes, an indication of the importance of the C-terminal structure in conversion.

D. Isolation, Purification, and Properties

The plasma enzyme is both soluble and easily accessible. As a result, its biochemical properties have been well described. Since it has been documented that the properties of the plasma and lung converting enzymes are similar, a summary of plasma enzyme properties is given at this point in order to provide the reader with information against which to compare subsequent information on the pulmonary enzyme.

The pH optimum of the plasma enzyme is buffer dependent, and ranges from 6.5 to 8.0 (phosphate and tris buffers, respectively) (Skeggs et al. 1956). Chloride, or one of the halide ions is required for activity. A relationship between the effects of pH and ionic effects, at least for the synthetic substrate Hip-Gly-Gly, has been demonstrated (Dorer et al. 1976): protonation of the enzyme may occur and chloride activation is biphasic. Bicarbonate ion may substitute for chloride, but cyanide anions are inhibitory (Huggins et al. 1970). Most divalent metal cations have no effect on the enzyme (Ca^{2+}, Mg^{2+}, Co^{2+}, Ba^{2+}, Cu^{2+}; Dorer et al. 1970, Huggins et al. 1970), but some are inhibitory (Hg^{2+} and Pb^{2+}, Huggins et al. 1970). However, the enzyme is a metalloprotein, as evidenced by loss of activity if exposed to chelating agents such as EDTA (Skeggs et al. 1956). Activity can be restored by addition of divalent metal cations, such as Ca^{2+}, Co^{2+}, Mn^{2+}, and Zn^{2+}. The enzyme is inhibited by *p*-chloromercuribenzoate (PCMB), *N*-ethylmaleimide, phenylmethylsulfonyl fluoride (PMSF) (Huggins et al. 1970), dimercaprol (Ryan et al. 1971): sensitivity to these compounds, coupled with sensitivity to Hg^{2+}, indicates that the enzyme may require free sulfhydryl groups (Sander and Huggins 1972). Other inhibitors of plasma converting enzyme include 8-quinolinol, oxalic acid

(Fitz et al. 1971), and angiotensin II (Lee et al. 1971). Erdös (1975) has tabulated some inhibitors of converting enzyme and the conditions in which they are effective.

E. Inhibitors

The hydrolysis of Hip-His-Leu by lung-converting enzyme was inhibited by two analogs of angiotensin I, 8-Ile angiotensin I, and 4-Phe, 8-Tyr angiotensin I, as effectively as by angiotensin I itself (Ki 1 to 4 $\times$ 10^{-6} M). The 8-Ile angiotensin I was also converted in vivo to a potent antagonist of angiotensin II, 8-Ile angiotensin II (Needleman et al. 1972, Khosla et al. 1974, Turker et al. 1974). Angiotensin II is a weak inhibitor of converting enzyme (Cushman and Cheung 1971a) and analogs of angiotensin II, for example, 1-Sar, 8-Ala angiotensin II are also inhibitory (Longenecker, Wiseman, and Huggins 1976). The heptapeptide angiotensin III (des-1-Asp angiotensin II) is also an inhibitor of the converting enzyme. Because of its occurrence in vivo, a regulatory role has been proposed for this compound (Tsai et al. 1975). Caldwell and co-workers (1976b) have developed a converting-enzyme antibody which appears able to inhibit converting-enzyme activity in vivo. The in vivo administration of the antibody has the problem of frequently being fatal, and of causing severe pulmonary pathology even when not fatal; this makes use of exogenous antibody unlikely therapeutically.

Some of the most potent and most specific inhibitors, however, are the peptides isolated from *Bothrops jararaca* venom (Ferreira 1965, Ferreira and Vane 1967, Ferreira et al. 1970). These compounds comprise a series ranging from a pentapeptide to a tridecapeptide (Ondetti et al. 1971, Greene et al. 1972), all with a blocked *N*-terminus in the form of pyrrolidone-carboxylic acid (PCA). The pentapeptide and nonapeptide (Fig. 2) are the most effective naturally occurring inhibitors (in vitro I_{50} 0.05 μg/ml and 1.1 μg/ml, respectively; Cushman et al. 1973, Cheung and Cushman 1973). The nonapeptide is a competitive inhibitor, while the pentapeptide is a mixed competitive, non-competitive inhibitor. The bradykinin fragment Arg-Pro-Pro, which has structural similarity to the venom inhibitors, is also inhibitory (Oshima and Erdos 1974). These peptides are generally referred to as bradykinin potentiating peptides (BPP).

That the BPP are inhibitors of converting enzyme brings up a still ongoing controversy, i.e., whether bradykininase, which terminates the physiologic (pharmacologic) activity of the nonapeptide bradykinin, and the angiotensin converting enzyme are an entity. Many feel that the two enzymes are identical because of the similarity of the action of both enzymes (both are dipeptidases) and the inseparability of one enzyme activity from the other.

Even antibody formed to angiotensin-converting enzyme inhibits bradykininase activity as well (Caldwell et al. 1976b). Others feel that differential requirements for chloride and effects of various inhibitors (Schulz and Biron 1969) indicate clearly that the enzymes are indeed different. For instance, chloride is required for converting enzyme activity, perhaps because of conformational changes (Erdös and Oshima 1974), but not for bradykininase, although there is evidence that the K_m of bradykininase is affected by chloride (Dorer et al. 1974); mercaptoethanol and 8-hydroxyquinoline inhibit bradykininase but not angiotensin converting enzyme, and *Agkistrodon piscivorus piscivorus* venom inhibits converting enzyme much more strongly than it inhibits bradykininase (Sander et al. 1972). In some species, the enzyme activities appear to be physically separated (Freer and Stewart 1975, Overturf et al. 1975). Valid arguments exist on both sides of the question, and until an actual physical or absolute pharmacologic separation does occur, if ever, both cases will continue to be made.

F. Particulate Lung Enzyme

Lung converting enzyme was shown to be a particulate enzyme by Bakhle (1968) shortly after pulmonary conversion was first described by Ng and Vane (1967). Centrifugation of an homogenate of dog lung into three fractions showed that no net converting enzyme activity occurred in either the low-speed (1,000g) supernatant or sediment. Differential centrifugation of the low-speed supernatant yielded two pellets, P_2 (20,000g) and P_3 (105,000g), and a supernatant, S_3 (105,000g).*

Bakhle found that most activity occurred in the P_3 fraction. It is of interest that bradykininase activity was found in the P_3 and S_3 fractions as well. The apparent absence of converting enzyme activity in the S_3 fraction is probably due to the presence of high levels of angiotensinase activity (*destroying enzyme*) in this fraction. Lung extracts thus did have the capability for metabolizing angiotensin II, even though angiotensin II passed through the intact or isolated lung without destruction. This indicated that something must ordinarily prevent destruction of angiotensin II in the in vivo situation. Bakhle suggested that a physical difference in localization of enzyme activities could give this kind of protection, for instance, if the converting enzyme were membrane bound and the destroying enzyme was intracellular or soluble. Further, if a similar variance in the localization of the destroying enzyme occurred in peripheral circulation, it might account for the observed net inactivation there as well.

*Bakhle's nomenclature has been adopted, with modifications as to exact speeds, by most investigators.

Bakhle demonstrated that the properties of the P_3 enzyme were essentially the same as those reported for the plasma converting enzyme with respect to chloride activation, EDTA inhibition, and BPF inhibition. The lung enzyme, like the plasma enzyme, was not inhibited by mercaptoethanol or 8-hydroxy-quinoline, but the associated bradykininase activity was. Subsequent work on the various partially purified enzymes confirmed the particulate nature and the similarities of the lung and plasma converting enzymes (Huggins et al. 1970, Cushman and Cheung 1971a, Cushman et al 1971, Yang et al. 1971, Depierre and Roth 1972).

Huggins et al. (1970) have compared the properties of lung converting enzyme with plasma converting enzyme. The lung enzyme was obtained by ammonium sulfate precipitation, followed by centrifugation at 75,000*g*, and dialysis. The substrate was angiotensin I, with quantitation by bioassay (rabbit aortic strip) for angiotensin II. Huggins and associates reported close similarities between plasma and lung enzymes with respect to a broad pH optimum (buffer dependent), chloride dependence, linear kinetics with increasing enzyme concentration as well as substrate concentration, essential lack of effect of divalent ions except for restoration of activity following EDTA dialysis, and inhibitor profiles. Maximum conversion occurred at 8 min for lung and at 45 min for plasma enzyme. Huggins and associates calculated a conversion rate of 6.1 nmol/min/mg protein for plasma. Lineweaver-Burke calculations revealed an apparent K_m of 5.2×10^{-6} M for lung and 4.7×10^{-5} M for plasma, which they interpreted to indicate that the plasma and lung enzymes are distinct.

Lee and coworkers (1971) obtained partially purified converting enzymes from guinea pig and hog lungs. The sources were the 1.6 to 2.2 M ammonium sulfate fractions from 80,000*g* supernatant fluids. The fractions were further purified on Sephadex G150. Conversion was determined radiometrically, using Asp-1-Ile-5-[^{14}C] Leu-10-angiotensin I as substrate, after reaction products were separated by paper electrophoresis. Lee and associates reported the enzyme to be a globular protein with a molecular weight of 150,000, as calculated from gel filtration (Sephadex G100) and sucrose density gradient data. The enzymes exhibited maximum activity in the pH range 7.2 to 7.8 and were chloride dependent. The maximum conversion rates were 30 and 10 nmol/min/g wet tissue for guinea pig and hog, respectively, which they reported to represent a 200-fold purification. The apparent K_m of the enzymes was 2.0 to 2.6×10^{-5} M.

Yang and associates (1971) have reported the isolation and purification of a converting enzyme from hog lung. Their starting material was the 104,000*g* supernatant from lung homogenates. Subsequent purification was carried out using Sephadex G250. Enzyme assays were carried out with several substrates. Hydrolysis of synthetic substrates was shown by spectroscopic assay and by amino acid analysis in the case of Hip-Gly-Gly, and hydrolysis of angiotensin I was measured by bioassay on rat colon. The partially purified enzyme preparation had a pH maximum between 7.4 to 7.7 and was found to be chloride dependent. Conversion rates reported were: 0.1 μmol/min/mg for Hip-Gly-Gly, 0.04 for Hip-His-Leu, and 0.05 for t-boc-Phe(NO$_2$)-Phe-Gly. It is of interest that no conversion rate was reported for angiotensin I, although the preparation did act on it.

Igic and coworkers (1972a,b) used both the supernatant fluid and the pellet from a 50,000g centrifugation of hog lung homogenates for isolation and purification. The supernatant fraction enzyme was purified by means of Sephadex G200 gel filtration, exchange on DEAE-Sephadex, further filtration on Giogel P300, and finally disc-gel electrophoresis. The enzyme isolated from the pellet was treated with Sephadex G250, Biogel P300, DEAE-Sephadex, and finally disk-gel electrophoresis. These investigators used essentially the same assay systems and synthetic substrates as Yang et al. (1971), with the addition of the substrate [^{14}C] dansyl-Gly-Gly-Gly, which was quantitated after TLC separation. Also, angiotensin I conversion was quantitated not only on rat colon but also by RIA. The final enzyme preparations were chloride dependent and had conversion rates of 29 nmol/hr/mg, using the dansyl substrate and 14 μmol/min/mg for Hip-Gly-Gly (significantly higher than the 0.1 figure reported by Yang et al. (1971) for the same substrate).

Further studies by these investigators permitted purification (Nakajima et al. (1973) from a 50,000g-supernatant fraction of hog lung. Purification was accomplished using Sephadex G200, DEAE-Sephadex, and hydroxyapatite. Assay was either spectrophotometric for the synthetic substrate (Hip-Gly-Gly), or by rat uterus for bradykinin. These investigators made use of the accompanying dipeptide hydrolase activity of converting enzyme and assumed that measurement of it was sufficient. The enzyme obtained was chloride dependent and had a specific activity for Hip-Gly-Gly of 13.8 units/mg. Since one unit = 1 μmol/min, this translates to 13.8 μmol/min/mg, approximately the same as reported by Igic et al. (1972a,b). This activity was reported to represent a 380-fold increase in purity. The preparation was homogeneous on gel electrophoresis, showing a single band corresponding to a molecular weight of 206,000 (this value was confirmed on Sephadex G200). Treatment of the material in the electrophoresis band with detergent and mercaptoethanol produced an additional band, corresponding to a molecular weight of 70,000. This separation into multiple bands was interpreted by these investigators to indicate the presence of three subunits in the intact enzyme molecule.

Supernatant fluids from homogenate of hog lung were also used by Dorer et al. (1972) in isolation and purification of converting enzyme.

Purification was achieved by ammonium sulfate fractionation, exchange on both CM- and DEAE-Sephadex, and treatment with hydroxyapatite and finally by column chromatography on Sephadex G200. The enzyme resulting from the above purification was chloride dependent. It had a pH optimum at 8.4. The specific activity for Hip-Gly-Gly was 10 units/mg, where a unit = 1 μmol hydrolyzed/min, which, incidently, is less than that reported by Igic et al. (1972a,b) and Nakajima et al. (1973), although the reported purification by Dorer was 1500-fold. The purified enzyme preparation gave a single band on disc-gel electrophoresis and a molecular weight of 300,000 on the basis of gel filtration data.

A molecular weight of 450,000 was reported by Fitz et al. (1972) for human lung converting enzyme. The source of the enzyme was an *extract* of human lung, which was purified by treatment with Sephadex G200. Conversion by the enzyme was assayed radiometrically, using [^{3}H] angiotensin I. The reaction products were separated by electrophoresis.

Similar enzyme preparations from human lung have been reported to show differential-converting enzyme and bradykininase activities, based on inhibitor data, with one enzyme preparation having usual converting enzyme activity and *no* bradykininase (Overturf et al. 1975).

Another source of converting enzyme is the *acetone powder* of lung. Cushman and Cheung (1969, 1971a) reported a chloride-dependent hydrolysis of Hip-His-Leu by an extract of acetone powder from rabbit lung. They used a spectrophotometric assay and found the preparation to have a pH optimum in the range of 8.1 to 8.3, with a K_m of 2.6 $\times$ 10^{-3} M. This extract was further purified to yield a homogenous preparation, binding AI more avidly than Hip-His-Leu; K_m of 0.05 $\times$ 10^{-3} M and 2.1 $\times$ 10^{-3} M, respectively (Cushman and Cheung 1972). Stevens et al. (1972) used an acetone powder of calf lung for studies on converting enzyme. The soluble enzyme was purified by exchange on CM- and DEAE-cellulose and by gel filtration on Sephadex G200, with isoelectric focusing as the last step to give a final 700-fold purification. Several synthetic substrates were used with UV spectrophotometric assay. The molecular weight of this calf lung enzyme, calculated from gel filtration data, was 300,000.

These data for converting enzyme obtained from fresh supernatant fractions, and acetone powders of lung demonstrate a large molecular weight range (150,000 to 450,000), even though many of the preparations were reported to be a single constituent. Other properties agree much more closely, e.g., chloride dependence and pH optima. Recent work on converting enzyme from solubilized particulate fractions has also produced data covering a large molecular-weight range. These preparations are also homogeneous on disc-gel electrophoresis. Some explanations for the variability in molecular weight have resulted from these studies, and are considered below.

Lanzillo and Fanburg (1974) combined the pellets sedimenting at 3,000*g* and 54,500*g* from homogenates of rabbit lung and used them as their enzyme source. This material was solubilized by treatment with deoxycholate and was partially purified by exchange on DEAE-cellulose and filtration on Sephadex G200. The substrates used were Hip-His-Leu (spectrophotometric assay) and labeled angiotensin I (separation by paper electrophoresis and radiometric assay). The partially purified enzyme was chloride dependent. They obtained conversion rates of 17.6 μmol/min/mg for Hip-His-Leu and 1.8 for angiotensin I. A 100-fold purification was reported with a molecular weight of 270,000 from gel filtration data.

A similar procedure was used by Soffer et al. (1974). The 700 to 78,000*g* pellet from rabbit lung was treated with the detergent Nonidet P-40* The solubilized enzyme was then further purified by treatment with DEAE-cellulose, hydroxyapatite, Sephadex G200, and glycerol gradient centrifugation. Spectrophotometric (Hip-His-Leu) and radiometric ([^{3}H] Leu-10-angiotensin I) methods were used for measuring activity. Using Hip-His-Leu, they found a conversion rate of 91.1 units/mg (unit = 1 μmol substrate/min), a pH optimum of 8.3, and chloride dependence with a maximum at 300 mM. Using natural substrate, they reported a conversion rate of 2.8 μmol/min/mg, a pH optimum of 7.8, and chloride dependence with a maximum at 30 mM. These investigators reported a purification of 2,800-fold for the natural substrate angiotensin I and only 1,000-fold for the synthetic substrate Hip-His-Leu. Several estimates of molecular weight were obtained; e.g., 300,000 by gel filtration, 136,000 by gradient centrifugation, and 140,000 by disc-gel electrophoresis.

In examining the differences obtained by gel filtration versus glycerol gradient centrifugation for this highly purified rabbit lung enzyme, Soffer and associates noted that the appearance of the stained band on disc-gel electrophoresis suggested the presence of carbohydrate. Gas-liquid chromatography showed that 16% of the enzyme was indeed carbohydrate, with the major portion made up of mannose, galactose, and *N*-acetylglucosamine. (Carbohydrate has also been reported in purified kidney enzyme (Oshima et al. 1974)). That the molecular weights from gradient centrifugation and disc-gel electrophoresis were in agreement (136,000 and 140,000) suggested to Soffer and associates that the enzyme is not composed of subunits, in contrast to the report of Nakajima et al. (1973), who felt that the enzyme contained several subunits.

Das and Soffer (1975) have subsequently reported a molecular weight of 129,000, based on equilibrium sedimentation data for a calcium phosphate gel-affinity chromatography (ricin agglutinin) purified enzyme. They conclude

*Shell Chemicals, Manchester, England.

that higher molecular weight values obtained by gel electrophoresis and filtration occur because the enzyme is a glycoprotein. Their preparation contained 26% sugar residues by weight and 1.2 g atoms zinc/mol (10 nmol/mg protein). The preparation had K_m and V_{max} for Hip-His-Leu of 2.3 mM and 130 μmol/min/mg protein, and for angiotensin I, 0.07 mM and 6.67 μmol/min/mg protein. Further studies with the purified enzymes are needed to resolve the questions relating to molecular weight, number, if any, of subunits, and active site, on which there is little data.

G. Subcellular Localization

The particulate nature of lung converting enzyme and the suggestive evidence that the enzyme must be located on the surface of the endothelial cells of the vascular system of the lung led to examination of the subcellular localization and specific properties of the enzyme. Bakhle (1968) investigated the subcellular distribution of the angiotensin I converting enzyme in dog lung; he found that the enzyme was localized in the P_3 fraction, perhaps a microsomal fraction. Using similar preparation techniques for the enzyme, Sander and Huggins (1971) have studied the distribution of this enzyme in rabbit lung. They reported converting enzyme activity to be localized mainly in the P_2 fraction (100 to 25,000g pellet), rather than in P_3. P_2 contained mitochondrial components as well as plasma membrane. Discontinuous sucrose density gradient fractionation and marker enzyme analysis of the converting enzyme preparation showed localization in the plasma membrane fraction. The observation that activity was associated with membranes seems more compatible with physiologic observations than an association with a specific intracellular components.

Smith and Ryan (1971) pointed out that existing evidence for conversion at the endothelium was only inferential. They also pointed out that observed conditions of conversion would require a specialized structure, with direct and immediate access to circulating blood. They demonstrated, by microscopy and histochemical techniques, that the pinocytotic vesicles of the capillary endothelium can metabolize adenine nucleotides, a function associated previously (Sander and Huggins 1971) with conversion. These vesicles open into the capillary lumen and increase the surface area. Only those vesicles, which were open to the lumen, showed activity, suggesting that they represent a facilitatory interface.

Later, Ryan and associates (1972) perfected a highly effective separation technique for plasma membranes in which the *caveolae intracellulares* or pinocytotic vesicles were reacted with 5-AMP in the presence of lead nitrate, thus allowing a clean separation of plasma membranes from intracellular components by centrifugation. They used labeled angiotensin I as substrate. Activity was measured after the materials were separated by gel chromatography and paper electrophoresis by means of rat colon and blood pressure bioassay. Localization of the enzyme on endothelial membrane surfaces was conclusively demonstrated. Membrane fractions obtained by the above technique converted greater than 90% of labeled angiotensin I to II in 15 sec, with no degradation of angiotensin II even after 60 min. In this same paper Ryan and associates reported that the volume distribution of angiotensin I within the perfused lung was the same as that of blue dextran. In addition, they showed that the transit time for blue dextran and radioactivity from labeled angiotensin I was essenequal. These data suggest and support the hypothesis that angiotensin I is distributed only in the intravascular space. In the intact lung preparations essentially all radioactivity was recovered in the perfusate from rat lung following perfusion with radioactive labeled substrate: only 18% appeared as angiotensin II, with the remainder recovered in di- through tetrapeptide homologs. This may be compared with the data obtained with the isolated membrane preparation already described, where 90% conversion to angiotensin II was reported. Ryan and associates concluded that conversion by the membrane was indeed sufficient to account for the conversion of angiotensin I to II in the intact lung, in contrast to the conclusion of Lee et al. (1971).

Fanburg and Glazier (1973) similarly demonstrated that the volume distribution of radioactively labeled angiotensin I and II in isolated perfused lungs was the same as that of indocyanine green. They recovered approximately 95% of radioactivity as angiotensin I and II, even at very high concentrations of angiotensin I. By adjusting perfusion pressure, they were able to demonstrate that conversion is also a function of vascular surface area and transit time. These results are compatible with other data indicating conversion at the endothelial surface of the lung.

In support of the concept that the endothelial cells are central to the localization of pulmonary converting enzyme is the report of Richardson and Beaulines (1971). They coupled angiotensin II to cytochrome c and to horseradish peroxidase. The complex was active in a mouse pressor assay and could be identified histochemically. They were able to show binding of the angiotensin II complex to endothelial cells during the pressor response.

Ryan and associates (1975, 1976) have used a marker tagged antibody to pig-lung converting enzyme to further document the presence of angiotensin-converting enzyme on endothelial surfaces. They demonstrated the attachment of antibody coupled to either microperoxidase or other cytochrome C derivatives to plasma membranes and caveolae which were open to the cell exterior. Binding to endothelium occurred in pulmonary capillaries and venules, as well as in aorta and pulmonary artery. Caldwell and coworkers

(1976a), using a fluorescein-tagged converting-enzyme antibody, have demonstrated the presence of converting enzyme in the luminal cells of *all* organs examined. They feel this does not detract from the contribution of pulmonary-converting enzyme because of the large volume and rapid delivery of blood to the pulmonary circulation with respect to other areas.

V.   Angiotensinases*

Goffinet and Mulrow (1965) showed that angiotensin II is allowed free passage through rat lung, which implied that angiotensin II was neither sequestered nor metabolized. This observation was supported by Hodge et al. (1967) and by Biron et al. (1967) for α-angiotensin and β-angiotensin (an aminopeptidase resistant analog). Leary and Ledingham (1969) demonstrated that angiotensin II could survive in the pulmonary circulation up to 10-min recirculation. Bakhle et al. (1969) also demonstrated lack of pulmonary inactivation of angiotensin II, except when the lungs were damaged by the development of edema. These findings for lack of inactivation are relatively unusual, since many other compounds are either inactivated (e.g., bradykinin; Ferreira and Vane 1967, Ryan et al. 1968. See also Ferreira and Bakhle, this volume.), or are removed by sequestration (e.g., norepinephrine, 5-HT; Said 1970, Gillis 1973. See also Alabaster, this volume.). Other exceptions do exist, e.g., oxytocin and vasopressin also pass through unchanged (Gilmore and Vane 1970, Stewart 1971). However, the observation that angiotensin II is not metabolized remains unusual in light of the fact that preparations of converting enzymes from lung tissue do have contaminating enzymes capable of destroying angiotensin II (Bakhle 1968). It has been pointed out that differences in localization of these enzymes with respect to exposure of circulating angiotensin II may prevent destructive enzyme action in vivo.

The early observations that angiotensin II was not metabolized during passage through the pulmonary system was based solely on bioassay. These observations must now be modified as a result of more careful investigation utilizing radiometric techniques. Ryan and coworkers (1971) showed that in isolated perfused rat lung 20% of [^{14}C] Leu-10-angiotensin I was converted to angiotensin II, while 50% was converted to large C-terminal fragments by means of an aminopeptidase. In addition, a large amount of the biologically active material was from a compound about one-third the size of angiotensin II. This material would obviously be accounted for as being angiotensin II, if only bioassay had been used.

*An excellent coverage of angiotensinases other than those occuring in lung is given by Leary and Ledingham in the chapter on Catabolism of Angiotensin II in Page and Bumpus 1974.

Oparil and associates (1970) showed that a large quantity of free Leu was liberated when high concentrations of angiotensin I were passed through lung. Subsequent work by Oparil and coworkers (1971) failed to confirm the release of free Leu, but rather found just His-Leu. It should be noted that substrate concentration was only one-tenth that in the earlier work. One possible explanation of these conflicting data has been offered by Barrett and Sambhi (1971), who showed that increasing concentrations of angiotensin I apparently resulted in saturation of pulmonary converting enzyme. Saturation was evidenced by formation of des-Leu-10-angiotensin I. Barrett and Sambhi propose the existence of a dual enzyme system, in which converting enzyme alone acts at low substrate concentration and a second monocarboxypeptidase acts on *excessive amounts* of angiotensin I. The second peptidase would function in a *protective inactivation* process, preventing the formation of excessively high levels of angiotensin II.

The studies of Turker and associates (1971) and Turker (1973) indicate an inactivation of angiotensin II in the pulmonary circulation. Their findings are not simply conversion of angiotensin I to biologically active compounds other than angiotensin II, but actual loss of activity of angiotensin II. These data need supporting chemical studies, since the results were obtained using only bioassay. Pulmonary inactivation (or lack of pulmonary conversion) has also been reported by Freer and Stewart (1972).

The presence of a His-Leu hydrolyzing enzyme in lung converting enzyme preparations has been reported (Lee et al. 1971) and may account for the presence of free Leu in some preparations. The in vivo significance of such enzymes is not known.

Ryan and associates (1972) showed that only 18% of radioactivity from 8-1-[^{14}C]Phe-Ala-angiotensin I was recovered as angiotensin II. The remainder was recovered as tetra- and tripeptides (58%): Pro-Phe-Ala (15%), and Phe-Ala (7%).

An interesting, perhaps related, observation is that purified thromboplastin hydrolyzes not only angiotensin I and II, but several bradykinins, substance P, and the BPP pentapeptide (Simmons et al. 1974). This is an interesting finding because of the localization of thromboplastin in the endothelium, the proposed site of angiotensin conversion. However, dansylation studies showed that all bonds in angiotensin I and II were hydrolyzed. Obviously thromboplastin has a questionable role as a converting enzyme, but it is curious that an enzyme localized identically (or similarly) to converting enzyme and capable of hydrolyzing both angiotensins has no apparent effect in vivo.

On the basis of available data it seems reasonable to conclude that lung possesses enzymes that could hydrolyze the angiotensins. The exact nature and locus of these enzymes, their physiologic functions, and their means of control remain to be elucidated.

VI. Summary

Converting enzyme activity occurs in the lung, and as a result, the lung is a major site of production of angiotensin II, a potent naturally occuring pressor peptide. Pulmonary converting enzyme is qualitatively similar to plasma converting enzyme. Conversion is more rapid in lung, which seems to be the physiologically significant site of conversion. Converting enzyme activity occurs in association with membrane components, and these data, combined with electron microscopic and physiologic data, have led to the conclusion that the enzyme is localized on the surface of pulmonary vascular epithelium. This localization accounts for the rapid conversion rates seen in vivo. Partially purified pulmonary converting enzyme has a molecular weight of about 130,000 and contains carbohydrate; it is chloride dependent. Although the lung is capable of producing large quantities of angiotensin II, no significant metabolic breakdown of angiotensin II seems to occur in lung unless extraordinarily large quantities of substrate are used. Physical separation of enzymes capable of metabolizing angiotensin II from their substrate has been suggested as an explanation for the usual lack of metabolism in the lung.

References

Aiken, J. W. and Vane, J. R. (1970). The renin-angiotensin system: inhibition of converting enzyme in isolated tissues. *Nature (Lond.)*, **228**:30–34.

Arakawa, K., Nakatani, M., Minohara, A., and Nakamura, N. (1957). Isolation and amino acid composition of human angiotensin I. *Biochem. J.*, **104**: 900–906.

Bakhle, Y. S. (1968). Conversion of angiotensin I to angiotensin II by cell-free extracts of dog lung. *Nature (Lond.)*, **220**:919–921.

Bakhle, Y. S. (1974). Converting enzyme in vitro; measurement and properties. In I. H. Page and F. M. Bumpus (eds.): *Angiotensin, Handbook of Experimental Pharmacology*. Springer-Verlag, New York-Heidelberg-Berlin, pp. 41–80.

Bakhle, Y. S., Reynard, A. M., and Vane, J. R. (1969). Metabolism of the angiotensins in isolated perfused tissues. *Nature (Lond.)*, **222**:956–959.

Bakhle, Y. S. and Vane, J. R. (1974). Pharmacokinetic function of the pulmonary circulation. *Physiol. Rev.*, **54**:1007–1045.

Barrett, J. D. and Sambhi, M. P. (1971). Pulmonary activation and degradation of angiotensin I: a dual enzyme system. *Res. Comm. Chem. Pathol. Pharmacol.*, **2**:128–145.

Biron, P. and Huggins, C. G. (1968). Pulmonary activation of synthetic angiotensin I. *Life Sci.*, **7**:965–970.

Biron, P., Meyer, P., and Panisset, J. C. (1967). Removal of angiotensins from the systemic circulation. *Can. J. Physiol. Pharmacol.*, **46**:175–178.

Boucher, R. and Genest, J. (1974). Measurement of renin and of angiotensin. In J. H. Page and F. M. Bumpus (eds.): *Angiotensin, Handbook of Experimental Pharmacology.* Springer-Verlag, New York-Heidelberg-Berlin, pp. 201–210.

Boyd, G. W., Landon, J., and Peart, W. S. (1967). Radioimmunoassay for determining plasma levels of angiotensin II in man. *Lancet,* 2:1002–1005.

Boyd, G. W. and Peart, W. S. (1968). The production of high-titre antibody against free angiotensin II in man. *Lancet,* 2:129–133.

Braun-Menendez, E., Fasciolo, J. C., Leloir, L. F., and Munoz, J. M. (1940). The substance causing renal hypertension. *J. Physiol.,* **98**:283–298.

Braun-Menendez, E. and Page, I. H. (1958). Suggested revision of nomenclature. *Science,* **127**:242.

Bumpus, F. M., Khairallah, P. A., Arakawa, K., Page, I. H., and Smeby, R. R. (1961). The relationship of structure to pressor and oxytocic actions of isoleucine 5 angiotensin octapeptide and various analogs. *Biochim. Biophys. Acta,* **46**:38–44.

Cain, M. D., Catt, K. J., and Coghlan, J. P. (1969). Immuno-reactive fragments of angiotensin II in blood. *Nature (Lond.),* **223**:617–618.

Caldwell, P. R., Seegal, B. C., Hsu, K. C., Das, M., and Soffer, R. L. (1976a). Angiotensin converting enzyme: Vascular endothelial localization. *Science,* **191**:1050–1051.

Caldwell, P. R., Wigger, H. J., Das, M., and Soffer, R. L. (1976b). Angiotensin converting enzyme: Effect of antienzyme antibody in vivo. *FEBS Lett.,* **63**:82–84.

Cheung, H. S. and Cushman, D. W. (1973). Inhibition of homogeneous angiotensin converting enzyme of rabbit lung by synthetic venom peptides of *Bothrops jararaca. Biochim. Biophys. Acta,* **293**:451–463.

Chiu, A. T., Ryan, J. W., Ryan, U. S., and Dorer, F. E. (1975). A sensitive radiochemical assay for angiotensin converting enzyme (kininase II). *Biochem. J.,* **149**:297–300.

Collins, D. A. (1948). Influence of tetraethylammonium on responses of isolated intestine to angiotensin and other substances. *J. Pharmacol. Exp. Ther.,* **94**:242–248.

Cushman, D. W. and Cheung, H. S. (1969). Simple substrate for assay of dog lung angiotensin converting enzyme. *Fed. Proc.,* **28**:799.

Cushman, D. W. and Cheung, H. S. (1971a). Spectrophotometric assay and properties of the angiotensin converting enzyme of rabbit lung. *Biochem. Pharmacol.,* **20**:1637–1648.

Cushman, D. W. and Cheung, H. S. (1971b). Concentrations of angiotensin converting enzyme in tissues of the rat. *Biochim. Biophys. Acta,* **250**:261–265.

Cushman, D. W., Cheung, H. S., and Peterson, A. E. (1971). Properties of the angiotensin converting enzyme of lung. *Chest,* **59**:Suppl., 10S–11S.

Cushman, D. W. and Cheung, H. S. (1972). Studies in vitro of angiotensin converting enzyme of lung and other tissues. In J. Genest and E. Koiw (eds.): *Hypertension.* Springer-Verlag, Berlin-Heidelberg-New York, pp. 532–541.

Cushman, D. W., Pluscec, J., Williams, N. J., Weaver, E. R., Sabo, E. F., Kocy, O., Cheung, H. S., and Ondetti, M. A. (1973). Inhibition of angiotensin converting enzyme by analogs by peptides from *Bothrops jararaca* venom. *Experientia*, **29**:1032–1035.

Das, M. and Soffer, R. L. (1975). Pulmonary angiotensin converting enzyme: Structural and catalytic properties. *J. Biol. Chem.*, **250**:6762–6768.

Deodhar, S. D. (1960). Immunologic production of angiotensin I and II. *J. Exp. Med.*, **111**:419–428, 429–439.

Depierre, D. and Roth, M. (1972). Activity of dipeptidylcarboxypeptidase (angiotensin converting enzyme) in lungs of different animal species. *Experientia*, **28**:154–155.

Dorer, F. E., Kahn, J. R., Lentz, K. E., Levine, M., and Skeggs, L. T. (1972). Purification and properties of angiotensin converting enzyme from dog lung. *Circ. Res.*, **31**:356–366.

Dorer, F. E., Kahn, J. R., Lentz, K. E., Levine, M., and Skeggs, L. T. (1974). Hydrolysis of bradykinin by angiotensin converting enzyme. *Circ. Res.*, **34**:824–827.

Dorer, F. E., Kahn, J. R., Lentz, K. E., Levine, M., and Skeggs, L. T. (1976). Kinetic properties of pulmonary angiotensin converting enzyme. Hydrolysis of hippurylglycylglycine. *Biochim. Biophys. Acta*, **429**:220–228.

Dorer, F. E., Skeggs, L. T., Kahn, J. R., Lentz, K. E., and Levine, M. (1970). Angiotensin converting enzyme: Method of assay and partial purification. *Anal. Biochem.*, **33**:102–113.

Elliott, D. G. and Peart, W. S. (1956). Aminoacid sequence in hypertension. *Nature*, **177**:527–528.

Erdös, E. G. (1975). Angiotensin I converting enzyme. *Circ. Res.*, **36**:247, 555.

Erdös, E. G. and Oshima, G. (1974). The angiotensin I converting enzyme of the lung and kidney. *Acta Physiol. Lat. Am.*, **24**:507–514.

Fanburg, B. L. and Glazier, J. B. (1973). Conversion of angiotensin I to angiotensin II in the isolated perfused dog lung. *J. Appl. Physiol.*, **35**:325–331.

Ferreira, S. H. (1965). A bradykinin potentiating factor (BPF) in the venom of *Bothrops jararaca*. *Br. J. Pharmacol. Chemother.*, **24**:163–169.

Ferreira, S. H., Greene, L. H., Alabaster, V. A., Bakhle, Y. S., and Vane, J. R. (1970). Activity of various fractions of bradykinin potentiating factor against angiotensin I converting enzyme. *Nature (Lond.)*, **225**:379–380.

Ferreira, S. H. and Vane, J. R. (1967). Disappearance of bradykinin and eledoisin in the circulation and vascular beds of the cat. *Br. J. Pharmacol. Chemother.*, **30**:417–424.

Fishman, A. P. and Pietra, G. G. (1974). Handling of bioactive materials by the lung (Parts I and II). *N. Engl. J. Med.*, **291**:884–890 and 953–959.

Fitz, A., Boyd, G. W., and Peart, W. S. (1971). Converting enzyme activity in human plasma. *Circ. Res.*, **28**:246–253.

Fitz, A., Overturf, M., and Wyatt, S. (1972). Human angiotensin I lung converting enzyme. *Circulation*, **46**:Suppl. 2:81.

Franklin, W. G., Peach, M. J., and Gilmore, J. P. (1970). Evidence for the renal conversion of angiotensin I in the dog. *Circ. Res.*, **27**:321–324.

Freer, R. J. and Stewart, J. M. (1972). In vivo metabolism of angiotensin I and 5-hydroxytryptamine in the rat. *Fed. Proc.,* **31**:512(abstr. 1686).

Freer, R. J. and Stewart, J. M. (1975). In vivo pulmonary metabolism of bradykinin, angiotensin I, and 5-hydroxytryptamine in the rat. *Arch. Int. Pharmacodyn. Ther.,* **217**:97–109.

Gillis, C. N. (1973). Metabolism of vasoactive hormones by lung. *Anesthesiology,* **39**:626–632.

Gilmore, N. J. and Vane, J. R. (1970). A sensitive and specific assay for vasopressin in the circulating blood. *Br. J. Pharmacol.,* **38**:633–652.

Goffinet, J. A. and Mulrow, P. J. (1965). Estimation of angiotensin clearance by an in vivo assay. *Clin. Res.,* **11**:408.

Green, E. L. J., Camargo, A. C. M., Krieger, E. M., Stewart, J. M., and Ferreira, S. H. (1972). Inhibition of the conversion of angiotensin I to II and potentiation of bradykinin by small peptides present in *Bothrops jararaca* venom. *Circ. Res.,* **30–31**:62–71.

Haber, E., Koerner, T., Page, L. B., Kliman, B., and Purnode, A. (1969). Application of a radioimmunoassay for angiotensin I to the physiologic measurement of plasma renin activity in normal human subjects. *J. Clin. Endocrinol. Metabol.,* **29**1349–1355.

Helmer, O. M. (1957). Differentiation between two forms of angiotensin by means of spirally cut strips of rabbit aorta. *Am. J. Physiol.,* **188**:571–577.

Hodge, R. L., Ng, K. K. F., and Vane, J. R. (1967). Disappearance of angiotensin from the circulation of the dog. *Nature (Lond.),* **215**:138–141.

Huggins, C. G., Corcoran, R. J., Gordon, J. S., Henry, H. W., and John, J. P. (1970). Kinetics of the plasma and lung angiotensin I converting enzyme. *Circ. Res.,* **27**:Suppl. 1:93–101.

Huggins, C. G. and Thampi, N. S. (1968). A simple method for the determination of angiotensin I converting enzyme. *Life Sci.,* **7**:633–639.

Igic, R., Yeh, H. S., Sorrells, K., and Erdös, E. G. (1972a). Cleavage of active peptides by A lung enzyme. *Experientia,* **28**:135–136.

Igic, R., Erdös, E. G., Yeh, H. S., Sorrells, K., and Nakajima, T. (1972b). Angiotensin I converting enzyme of the lung. *Circ. Res.,* **31**:Suppl. 2:51–61.

Jakschik, B. A., Marshall, G. R., Kourik, J. L., and Needleman, P. (1974). Profile of circulating vasoactive substances in hemorrhagic shock and their pharmacologic manipulation. *J. Clin. Invest.,* **54**:842–852.

Junod, A. F. and deHaller, R. (eds.) (1975). Lung metabolism: Proteolysis and antiproteolysis, biochemical pharmacology, handling of bioactive substances. *Academic Press, Inc.,* New York, London.

Khairallah, P. A. and Smeby, R. R. (1974). Bioassay of angiotensin. In I. H. Page and F. M. Bumpus (eds.): *Angiotensin, Handbook of Experimental Pharmacology.* Springer-Verlag, New York-Heidelberg-Berlin, pp. 227–239.

Khosla, M. C., Smeby, R. R., and Bumpus, F. M. (1974). Structure-activity relationship in angiotensin II analogs. In I. H. Page and F. M. Bumpus (eds.): *Angiotensin, Handbook of Experimental Pharmacology.* Springer-Verlag, New York-Heidelberg-Berlin, pp. 126–161.

Lanzillo, J. J. and Fanburg, B. L. (1974). Membrane-bound angiotensin converting enzyme from rat lung. *J. Biol. Chem.*, **249**:2312–2318.

Leary, W. P. and Ledingham, J. G. (1969). Removal of angiotensin by isolated perfused organs of the rat. *Nature (Lond.)*, **222**:959–960.

Ledingham, J. G. and Leary, W. P. (1974). Catabolism of angiotensin II. In I. H. Page and F. M. Bumpus (eds.): *Angiotensin, Handbook of Experimental Pharmacology*. Springer-Verlag, New York-Heidelberg-Berlin, pp. 111–125.

Lee, H. J., Larue, J. N., and Wilson, I. B. (1971). Angiotensin converting enzyme from guinea pig and hog lung. *Biochim. Biophys. Acta*, **250**:549–557.

Lentz, K. E., Skeggs, Jr., L. T., Woods, K., Kahn, J. R., and Shumway, N. P. (1956). Amino acid composition of hypertensin II and its biochemical relationship to hypertensin I. *J. Exp. Med.*, **104**:183–191.

Longenecker, G. L., Wiseman, M. T., and Huggins, C. G. (1976). In vitro inhibition of angiotensin converting enzyme by 1-Sar-8-Ala-angiotensin II. *Fed. Proc.*, **35**:646 (abstr. 24–28).

Lubran, M. M. (1973). Role of the lung in angiotensin metabolism. *Ann. Clin. Lab. Sci.*, **3**:235–241.

Luduena, F. P. (1940). Accion de los preparodos de hipertensina sobre los musculos lisas. *Rev. Soc. Argent. Biol.*, **16**:358–375.

Marshall, B. E. (1973). Non-respiratory functions of the lung. *Anesthesiology*, **39**:573–574.

Menard, J. and Catt, K. J. (1972). Measurement of renin activity concentration and substrate in rat plasma by radioimmunoassay of angiotensin I. *Endocrinology*, **90**:422–430.

Nakajima, T., Oshima, G., Yeh, H. S. J., Igic, R., and Erdös, E. G. (1973). Purification of the angiotensin I converting enzyme of the lung. *Biochim. Biophys. Acta*, **315**:430–438.

Needleman, P., Johnson, Jr., E. M., Vine, W., Flanigan, E., and Marshall, G. R. (1972). Pharmacology of antagonists of angiotensin I and II. *Circ. Res.*, **31**:862–867.

Ng, K. K. F. and Vane, J. R. (1967). Conversion of angiotensin I to angiotensin II. *Nature (Lond.)*, **216**:762–766.

Ng, K. K. F. and Vane, J. R. (1968). Fate of angiotensin I in the circulation. *Nature (Lond.)*, **218**:144–150.

Ng, K. K. F. and Vane, J. R. (1970). Some properties of the angiotensin converting enzyme in the lung in vivo. *Nature (Lond.)*, **225**:1142–1144.

Oates, H. F. and Stokes, G. S. (1974). Role of extrapulmonary conversion in mediating the systemic pressor activity of angiotensin I. *J. Exp. Med.*, **140**:79–86.

Ondetti, M. A., Williams, N. J., Sabo, E. F., Pluscec, J., Weaver, E. R., and Kocy, O. (1971). Angiotensin converting enzyme inhibitors from the venom of *Bothrops jararaca*. Isolation, elucidation of structure and synthesis. *Biochemistry*, **10**:4032–4039.

Oparil, S. and Haber, E. (1974). The renin-angiotensin system (Parts I and II). *N. Engl. J. Med.*, **291**:389–401 and 446–457.

Oparil, S., Sanders, C. A., and Haber, E. (1970). In vivo and in vitro conversion of angiotensin I to angiotensin II in dog blood. *Circ. Res.,* **26**:591–599.

Oparil, S., Tregar, G. W., Koerner, R., Barnes, B. A., and Haber, E. (1971). Mechanism of pulmonary conversion of angiotensin I to angiotensin II in the dog. *Circ. Res.,* **29**:682–690.

Osborn, E. C., Tildesley, G., and Pickens, P. T. (1972). Pressor response to angiotensin I and angiotensin II: the site of conversion of angiotensin I. *Clin. Sci.,* **43**:839–849.

Oshima, G. and Erdös, E. G. (1974). Inhibition of the angiotensin converting enzyme of the lung by a peptide fragment of bradykinin. *Experientia,* **30**: 733–734.

Oshima, G., Gecse, A., and Erdös, E. G. (1974). Angiotensin I converting enzyme of the kidney cortex. *Biochim. Biophys. Acta,* **350**:26–37.

Overturf, M., Wyatt, S., Boaz, D., and Fitz, A. (1975). Angiotensin I (Phe^8-His^9) hydrolase and bradykininase from human lung. *Life Sci.,* **16**:1669–81.

Page, I. H. and Bumpus, F. M. (eds.) (1974). *Angiotensin, Handbook of Experimental Pharmacology.* Springer-Verlag, New York-Heidelberg-Berlin, p. 37.

Page, I. H. and Helmer, O. M. (1940). A crystalline pressor substance (angiotonin) resulting from the reaction between renin and reninactivator. *Exp. Med.,* **7**:29–42.

Picarelli, Z. P., Kupper, R., Prado, E. S., Prado, J. L., and Valle, J. R. (1954). Assay of renin and hypertensin with isolated guinea pig ileum. *Circ. Res.,* **2**:354–358.

Piquilloud, Y., Reinharz, A., and Roth, M. (1970). Studies on the angiotensin converting enzyme with different substrates. *Biochim. Biophys. Acta,* **206**:136–142.

Regoli, D. and Vane, J. R. (1964). A sensitive method for the assay of angiotensin. *Br. J. Pharmacol.,* **23**:351–359.

Richardson, J. B. and Beaulines, A. (1971). The cellular site of action of angiotensin. *J. Cell. Biol.,* **51**:419–432.

Roth, M., Weitzman, A. F., and Piquilloud, Y. (1969). Converting enzyme content of different tissues of the rat. *Experientia,* **25**:1247.

Ryan, J. W., Roblero, J., and Stewart, J. M. (1968). Inactivation of bradykinin in the pulmonary circulation. *Biochem. J.,* **110**:795–797.

Ryan, J. W., Roblero, J., Stewart, J. M., and Leary, W. P. (1971). Metabolism of vasoactive polypeptides in the pulmonary circulation. *Chest,* **59**:8S–9S.

Ryan, J. W., Ryan, U. S., Schultz, D. R., Day, A. R., and Dorer, F. E. (1976). Further evidence on the subcellular sites of kininase II (angiotensin converting enzyme). *Adv. Exp. Med. Biol.,* **70**:235–243.

Ryan, J. W., Ryan, U. S., Schultz, D. T., Whitaker, C., and Chung, A. (1975). Subcellular localization of pulmonary angiotensin converting enzyme (kininase II). *Biochem. J.,* **146**:497–499.

Ryan, J. W., Smith, U., and Niemeyer, R. S. (1972). Angiotensin I: metabolism by plasma membrane of lung. *Science,* **176**:64–66.

Ryan, J. W., Stewart, J. M., Leary, W. P., and Ledingham, J. G. (1970). Metabolism of angiotensin I in the pulmonary circulation. *Biochem. J.,* **120**:221–223.

Said, S. I. (1970). Pulmonary responses to inhaled particles: role of vasoactive substances. *Arch. Intern. Med.,* **126**:475–476.

Sander, G. E. and Huggins, C. G. (1971). Subcellular localization of angiotensin I converting enzyme in rabbit lung. *Nature New Biol.,* **230**:27–29.

Sander, G. E. and Huggins, C. G. (1972). Vasoactive peptides. *Annu. Rev. Pharmacol.,* **12**:227–264.

Sander, G. E., West, D. W., and Huggins, C. G. (1971). Peptide inhibitors of pulmonary angiotensin I converting enzyme. *Biochim. Biophys. Acta,* **242**: 662–667.

Sander, G. E., West, D. W., and Huggins, C. G. (1972). Inhibitors of the pulmonary angiotensin I converting enzyme. *Biochim. Biophys. Acta,* **289**:392–400.

Scholz, H. W. and Biron, P. (1969). Non-identity between pulmonary bradykininase and converting enzyme activity. *Rev. Can. Biol.,* **28**:197–200.

Simmons, W. H., Burkholder, D. E., and Brecher, A. S. (1974). Effect of bovine lung thromboplastin on vasoactive peptides. *Fed. Proc.,* **33**:291.

Skeggs, L. T., Kahn, J. R., and Shumway, N. P. (1956). Preparation and function of the hypertensin converting enzyme. *J. Exp. Med.,* **103**:295–299.

Skeggs, Jr., L., Marsh, W. H., Kahn, J. R., and Shumway, N. P. (1954). Existence of two forms of hypertensin. *J. Exp. Med.,* **99**:275–282.

Smith, U. and Ryan, J. W. (1971). Pinocytotic vesicles of the pulmonary endothelial cell. *Chest,* **59**:Suppl.:12S–14S.

Soffer, R. L. (1976). Angiotensin converting enzyme and the regulation of vasoactive peptides. *Ann. Rev. Biochem.,* **45**:73–94.

Soffer, R., Reza, R., and Caldwell, P. R. B. (1974). Angiotensin converting enzyme from rabbit pulmonary particles. *Proc. Natl. Acad. Sci. U.S.A.,* **71**: 1720–1724.

Stevens, R. L., Micalizzi, E. R., Fessler, D. C., and Pals, D. T. (1972). Angiotensin I converting enzyme of calf lung. Method of assay and partial purification. *Biochemistry,* **11**:1999–3007.

Stewart, J. M. (1971). Role of the lungs in the metabolism of circulating hormones. *Chest,* **59**:7S–8S.

Tsai, B. S., Peach, M. J., Khosla, M. C., and Bumpus, F. M. (1975). Synthesis and evaluation of (des-Asp^1)angiotensin I as a precursor for (des-Asp^1)angiotensin II (angiotensin III). *J. Med. Chem.,* **18**:1180–1183.

Turker, R. K. (1973). Change of activity of angiotensins I and II in the isolated perfused guinea pig lung. *Arch. Intern. Physiol. Biochem.,* **81**:523–536.

Turker, R. K., Page, I. H., and Bumpus, F. M. (1974). Antagonists of angiotensin II. In I. H. Page and F. M. Bumpus (eds.): *Angiotensin, Handbook of Experimental Pharmacology.* Springer-Verlag, New York-Heidelberg-Berlin, pp. 162–169.

Turker, R. K., Yamamoto, M., Bumpus, F. M., and Khairallah, P. A. (1971). Lung perfusion with angiotensins I and II: evidence for release of myotropic and inhibitory substances. *Circ. Res.,* **28**:559–567.

Vane, J. R. (1968). The release and assay of hormones in the circulation. In *The Scientific Basis of Medicine Annual Reviews.* Athlone Press, London, pp. 336–358.

Vane, J. R. (1969). The release and fate of vasoactive hormones in the circulation. *Br. J. Pharmacol.,* **35**:209–242.

Worobec, R. B., Wallace, J. H., and Huggins, C. G. (1972). Angiotensin-antibody interaction. I. Induction of the antibody response. *Immunochemistry,* **9**: 229–238.

Yang, H. Y., Erdös, E. G., and Levin, Y. (1971). Characterization of a dipeptide hydrolase (kininase II: angiotensin I). *J. Pharmacol. Exp. Ther.,* **177**:291–300.

4

Prostaglandin Metabolism
in the Lung

RODERICK J. FLOWER

Wellcome Research Laboratories
Langley Court, Beckenham,
Kent, England

I. Introduction

Any contemporary account of the metabolic functions of the lung would be incomplete without a discussion of prostaglandin (PG) metabolism. The PGs possess a bewildering spectrum of biologic activity, including dramatic cardiovascular effects, in plasma concentrations often as low as 10^{-7} to 10^{-8} M, and it is therefore not surprising to discover that the lungs (whose ability to limit the access of vasoactive substances to the arterial circulation is discussed elsewhere in this book) possess extremely efficient enzymatic machinery for the rapid conversion of PGs to inactive metabolites; indeed, it is not unlikely that the pulmonary vascular bed constitutes the major inactivation mechanism for PGs liberated into the venous circulation.

Not only can the lung metabolize PGs but it can also synthesize them. Synthesis may be initiated by a variety of stimuli, both physiologic and pathogenic, and the PGs thus released can modify pulmonary function in a number of ways.

In this brief account of pulmonary PG metabolism, the author will outline the basic biochemistry of PG biosynthesis and catabolism, with special regard to work done with enzymes derived from lung tissue. A section at the end of this chapter is devoted to a consideration of some physiologic and pathologic processes in which these enzymes may play a part.

A.   Other Literature

A great deal of literature dealing with various aspects of PG biochemistry is currently available. Several reviews of PG metabolism have been published: Änggård and Samuelsson 1967, Samuelsson et al. 1967, Bergström et al. 1968, Samuelsson 1970, van Dorp 1971, Lands et al. 1971, Hinman 1972, Oesterling et al. 1972, Samuelsson 1972, Sih and Takeguchi 1973, Marazzi and Andersen 1974. The reader is referred to these reviews for a more complete account of PG biosynthesis and catabolism as well as for a comprehensive bibliography. A review dealing with the inhibition of PG synthesis and catabolism by inhibitors of all sorts was written by Flower (1974) and several other reviews by Vane and Ferreira (Vane 1973a,b, Ferreira and Vane 1973, 1974a,b) are available in which the thesis is developed that *aspirin-like drugs* exert their therapeutic action by inhibiting PG generation in vivo. Several reviews or papers dealing more specifically with the lung, also contain comments regarding the biosynthesis or metabolism of PGs (Vane 1969, Heinemann and Fishman 1969, Gillis 1973, Fanburg 1973, Said 1973, Tierney 1974, and Bakhle and Vane 1974).

B.   Prostaglandin Nomenclature

The PGs may be considered derivatives of prostanoic acid (Fig. 1) and the nomenclature is based on that carbon skeleton. There are several groups of PGs distinguished by the nature and geometry of the substituent groups in the ring (for example E, F, D) and the number of double bonds in the side chains (for example E_1, E_2, E_3, F_1, F_2, F_3, etc.). Figure 2 shows the structures of these primary PGs and Table 1 gives the systematic chemical nomenclature and the trivial abbreviations for the primary PGs and their major metabolites.

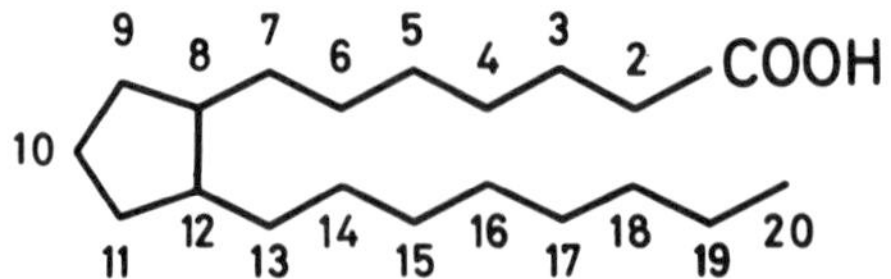

FIGURE 1   The skeleton structure of prostanoic acid.

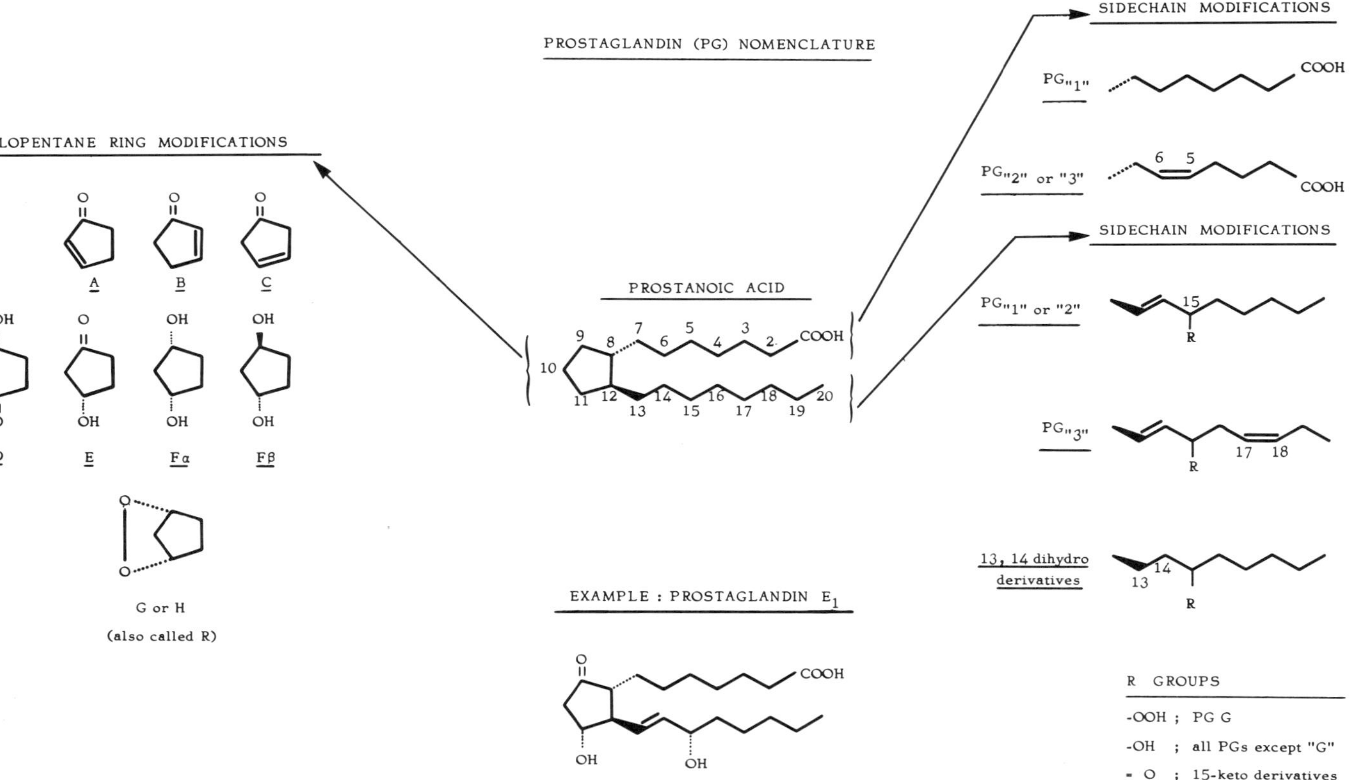

FIGURE 2 Structures of prostaglandins, prostaglandin intermediates, and major metabolites.

TABLE 1　Prostaglandin Nomenclature

Systematic name	Trivial name
11α-15-dihydroxy-9-ketoprost-13-enoic acid	PGE_1
11α-15-dihydroxy-9-ketoprosta-5,13-dienoic acid	PGE_2
9α,11α-15-trihydroxyprosta-13-enoic acid	$PGF_{1\alpha}$
9α,11α-15-trihydroxyprost-5,13-dienoic acid	$PGF_{2\alpha}$
15-hydroxy-9-ketoprosta-10,13-dienoic acid	PGA_1
15-hydroxy-9-ketoprosta-5,10,13-trienoic acid	PGA_2
15-hydroxy-9-ketoprosta-8(12),13-dienoic acid	PGB_1
15-hydroxy-9-ketoprosta-5,8(12),13-trienoic acid	PGB_2
9α,15-dihydroxy-11-ketoprosta-13-enoic acid	PGD_1
9α,15-dihydroxy-11-ketoprosta-5,13-dienoic acid	PGD_2
11α-hydroxy-9,15-diketoprost-13-enoic acid	15-keto PGE_1
11α-hydroxy-9,15-diketoprosta-5,13-dienoic acid	15-keto PGE_2
9α,11-dihydroxy-15-ketoprost-13-enoic acid	15-keto $PGF_{1\alpha}$
9α,11-dihydroxy-15-ketoprost-5,13-dienoic acid	15-keto $PGF_{2\alpha}$
9α-hydroxy-11,15-diketoprost-13-enoic acid	15-keto PGD_1
9α-hydroxy-11,15-diketoprost-5,13-dienoic acid	15-keto PGD_2
11α-15-dihydroxy-9-ketoprostanoic acid	dihydro PGE_1
11α-15-dihydroxy-9-ketoprosta-5-enoic acid	dihydro PGE_2
9α-11α-15-trihydroxyprostanoic acid	dihydro $PGF_{2\alpha}$
9α-11α-15-trihydroxyprosta-5-enoic acid	dihydro $PGF_{2\alpha}$
11α-hydroxy-9,15-diketoprostanoic acid	15-keto-dihydro PGE_1
11α-hydroxy-9,15-diketoprosta-5-enoic acid	15-keto-dihydro PGE_2
9α-11α-dihydroxy-15-ketoprostanoic acid	15-keto-dihydro $PGF_{2\alpha}$
9α-11α-dihydroxy-15-ketoprosta-5-enoic acid	15-keto-dihydro $PGF_{2\alpha}$

II.　Prostaglandin Biosynthesis

A.　Distribution of PG Synthetase

Prostaglandins are synthesized by a multienzyme complex referred to loosely as *PG synthetase.* This enzyme complex appears to be present in every mammalian tissue so far investigated (as well as in several nonmammalian tissues);

Horton (1969) and Ramwell and Shaw (1970) have published lists of tissue types from which PG release has been elicited after the application of suitable stimuli. Christ and van Dorp (1972, 1973) have conducted extensive investigations into the biosynthetic capacity of a wide range of tissues, including those from vertebrates, arthropods, molluscs, and coelenterates. These authors measured synthetase activity in a wide variety of mammalian tissues by measuring the conversion of labeled precursor acid to PGE_1 and classified tissues into three broad categories: (a) those, such as kidney medulla and lung, in which between 10% to 40% conversion occurred, (b) tissues, such as gut, in which only some 3% occurred, and (c) other tissues, such as spleen and aorta, in which the conversion was 1% or less. It is noteworthy that lungs are among the richest source of synthetic enzymes. These workers also found synthetase activity in the lung tissue or homologous structures of other vertebrates (i.e., frog lung and carp gills) and from members of other phyla. The gills are especially rich in synthetase. The presence of PGs in the lung, which may be taken as an indication of synthetic activity, has been confirmed by Bergstrom et al. (1963) and Samuelsson (1964) for sheep, cattle, and pig lung, and by Änggård (1965) for sheep, guinea pig, monkey, and man. The latter author found that $PGF_{2\alpha}$ was the main PG present, although some PGE_2 was found in sheep lung, and reported the following amounts (as $PGF_{2\alpha}/g$ of lung): sheep and guinea pig, 0.5 μg; human, 0.02 μg; monkey, 0.2 μg. Karim et al. (1967) reported the presence of PGE_2 and $PGF_{2\alpha}$ in human lung; more $PGF_{2\alpha}$ than PGE_2 was found (approximate ratio, 10 to 20:1). No PGE_1 or $PGF_{1\alpha}$ was detected.

The only tissues that seem to possess very high synthetic activity (75% conversion of substrate or more) are sheep and bovine seminal vesicles. For this reason, much of the experimental work on the biosynthetic mechanisms have been conducted using these tissues as a source of enzyme.

B.   Mechanism of Biosynthesis

The enzymatic conversion of certain essential fatty acids into prostaglandins was first demonstrated in 1964 by two groups of workers led by van Dorp in Holland and Bergstrom and Samuelsson in Sweden. Most of the subsequent work on the biochemistry of PG biosynthesis (and catabolism) has also been pioneered by these two groups. For the reasons stated earlier, much of the original experimental work on the reaction mechanism was conducted with a synthetase preparation derived from sheep or bovine seminal vesicles, but there is no reason to suspect that the reaction catalyzed by enzymes from other tissues proceeds by a radically different pathway.

Prostaglandin synthetase is located in the high-speed particulate fraction of cells, although it may be partially solubilized with detergents (Miyamoto et al. 1974). The actual number of component enzymes in the system is unknown, but the mechanism of the reaction is reasonably well elucidated. The initial step (Hamberg and Samuelsson 1967, Nugteren et al. 1966; Fig. 3) of this dioxygenase reaction is initiated by stereospecific (L) removal of the (ω-8) hydrogen and the conversion of the substrate to an (ω-10) hydroperoxide. This step is

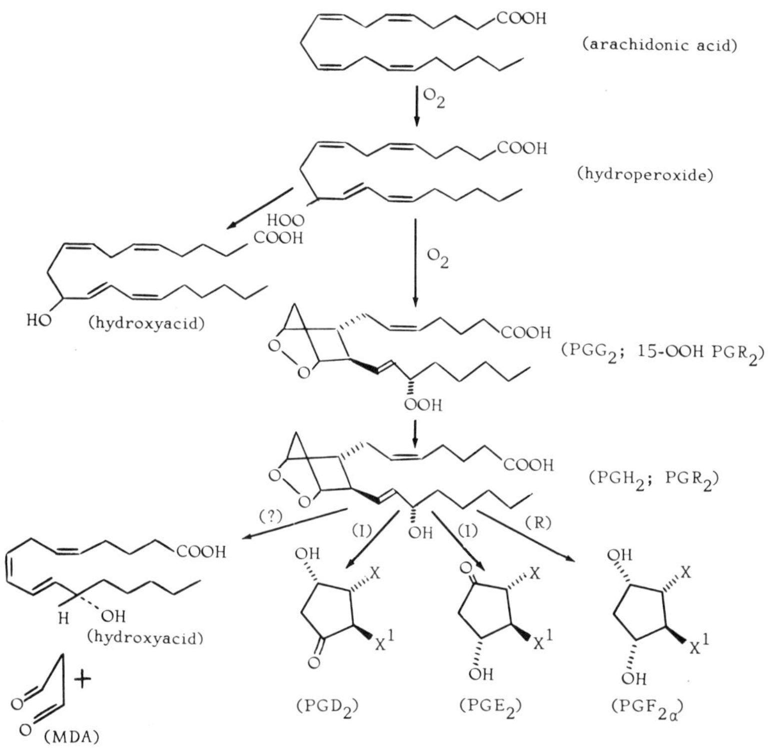

FIGURE 3 Proposed reactions for generation of cyclic endoperoxides and prostaglandins from arachidonic acid. This scheme is based largely on the work of Nugteren et al. (1966), Nugteren and Hazelhof (1973), and Samuelsson and Hamberg et al. (1974). Only the ring structures of the prostaglandins have been drawn; X and Y refer to appropriate hydrocarbon chains. I = isomerization; R = reduction; ? = enzymic or nonenzymic? MDA = malondialdehyde. Although this scheme shows the conversion of arachidonic acid into G_2, H_2, E_2, and so on, the conversion of the dihomo-γ-linoleic acid probably proceeds by an analogous pathway (data from Hamberg and Samuelsson 1974).

somewhat reminiscent of the reaction catalyzed by the plant enzyme soyabean lipoxidase, although in the latter case an ω-6 hydroperoxide is formed. The next stage is a concerted reaction; the addition of oxygen at C-15 is followed by an isomerization of the C-13 double bond, ring closure between C-8 and C-12, and an attack by an oxygen radical (of the C-11 hydroperoxide) at C-9, thus forming a *cyclic endoperoxide.* This intermediate is referred to as *PGG* by Samuelsson's group (see Hamberg and Samuelsson 1973, Hamberg et al. 1974) and as 15-hydroperoxy PG-R by Nugteren and Hazelhof (1973). The next stage involves the reduction of the hydroperoxy group at C-15 to a hydroxy group, giving rise to a compound known as PGH by Samuelsson's group and as PGR by Nugteren and Hazelhof. Both of these endoperoxide intermediates are rather unstable, spontaneously decomposing in aqueous solutions, although they can be isolated in organic solvents. They are stable in dry acetone at $-20°C$ for some weeks. The endoperoxide intermediates have distinct pharmacologic actions of their own, which are in some respects different from that of their endproducts, the prostaglandins. As Figure 3 shows, PGH_2 can be further modified in a number of ways, either by isomerization to PGE_2 or to PGD_2 or by reductive cleavage to $PGF_{2\alpha}$.

Under some conditions, the endoperoxide may break down into a 17-C hydroxy acid and malondialdehyde (MDA) (it is not known whether this is under enzymatic control) or even to other compounds, such as 15-keto PGE (Samuelsson and Hamberg 1974).

Two moles of oxygen are consumed per mole of product formed, and experiments in which the reaction mixture was incubated in an atmosphere of $^{18}O_2 - {}^{16}O_2$ have indicated that the oxygen substituents at C-9 and C-11 are both derived from the same molecule. Prostaglandin B and its isomer PGA (not shown in Fig. 3) are dehydration products of PGE and are easily formed by treating PGE with either base or acid, respectively. Prostaglandin C is an intermediate in the transformation of PGA to PGB by a plasma enzyme (Jones 1972). It is not unlikely that much of the PGA, which is often detected in tissues and enzyme incubations, arises nonenzymically during extractions and isolation procedures (Lee et al. 1967, Samuelsson 1970) that commonly involve acidification, although this PG does appear to occur naturally in seminal fluid. Despite numerous reports in the literature of the biologic activity of PGA (see Horton 1969, Hinman 1970, Weeks 1972) and its metabolic transformations (Horton et al. 1971, Jones 1972), the existence of an enzyme catalyzing the conversion of PGE to PGA (*PGE dehydratase*) has not been unequivocally demonstrated, although there have been some preliminary reports (Alam et al. 1973, Cammock 1973).

In light of the foregoing considerations, it is difficult to assign a definite role to either A or B type PGs at the moment. One may surmize, however, that unless some completely novel biosynthetic route is reported (perhaps from PGG or PGH?), PGE is most likely to be the precursor of PGA.

Although PG synthetase is located in the membranous fraction of cells, a heat-stable cofactor from the soluble fraction is required for appreciable activity (Samuelsson 1969, 1970). For in vitro studies, however, this cofactor is generally replaced by a source of reducing equivalents, often hydroquinone, adrenaline, or some other phenolic compound, and reduced glutathione (GSH) (Nugteren et al. 1966, van Dorp 1967). Two moles of reducing equivalents are required for the synthesis of PGF, but only one mole for PGE or PGD (Sih and Takeguchi 1973). The requirement for GSH seems to be rather specific (several other thiol compounds are inactive; van Dorp 1967, Sih and Takeguchi 1973), although the exact role played by this compound in the synthetic reaction is not yet clearly established. Possibly it may simply serve to keep the electron donor in a reduced state.

Only the nonesterified fatty acids are substrates for the enzyme (Lands and Samuelsson 1968), and since the cellular concentrations of free fatty acid precursors is generally rather low, it is likely that lipolytic enzymes, such as phospholipase A_2 are important in regulating the supply of substrate for biosynthesis.

C. Prostaglandin Biosynthesis in Lung

Although PG biosynthesis has received a great deal of attention, the amount of research work actually devoted to the enzyme from the lung has been disappointing. This is surprising considering that the lung contains a relative abundance of PG synthetase and that PGs are readily released from perfused lungs by such diverse stimuli as vasoactive peptides (Vargaftig and Dao Hai 1971), phospholipase A (Babilli and Vogt 1964), anaphylactic shock (Piper and Vane 1969, Liebig et al. 1974), histamine (Bakhle and Smith 1972, Liebig et al. 1974), 5-hydroxytryptamine and tryptamine (Alabaster and Bakhle 1970, 1976), and other mechanical or chemical stimulation (Piper and Vane 1971, Palmer et al. 1973).

Änggård and Samuelsson (1965) were the first workers to study the biosynthesis of PGs in the cell-free system of lung. They prepared a simple homogenate of guinea pig lungs, centrifuged it at low speed to remove coarse cellular debris, and mixed aliquots of the homogenate with tritiated arachidonic acid. After 30 min incubation at 37°C, the reaction was terminated and the reaction products extracted and separated by thin layer chromatography. Two compounds were formed, both more polar than arachidonic acid and representing approximately 10% conversion of the substrate. These products were later identified, on the basis of their chromatographic mobility, as being predominantly $PGF_{2\alpha}$, together with small quantities of PGE_2; some PGE_2 metabolites were also present (in these experiments homogenates were used which contained not only synthetic but also degrading enzymes). Parkes and Eling (1974) have further investigated characteristics of the PG synthetase system in guinea pig lungs. As in the case with other tissues, the enzyme system was principally concentrated in the microsomal ($100,000g$) fraction of cells, and by using such preparations the authors were able to study the synthesis of PGs in the absence of metabolizing enzymes present in the $100,000g$ supernatant. When studied under these conditions, the guinea pig lung synthetase produced predominantly $PGF_{2\alpha}$ together with an unidentified PG-like compound, which may have been PGD_2. Prostaglandin biosynthesis by this preparation was stimulated by the addition of hydroquinone, adrenaline, noradrenaline, and 5-hydroxytryptamine.

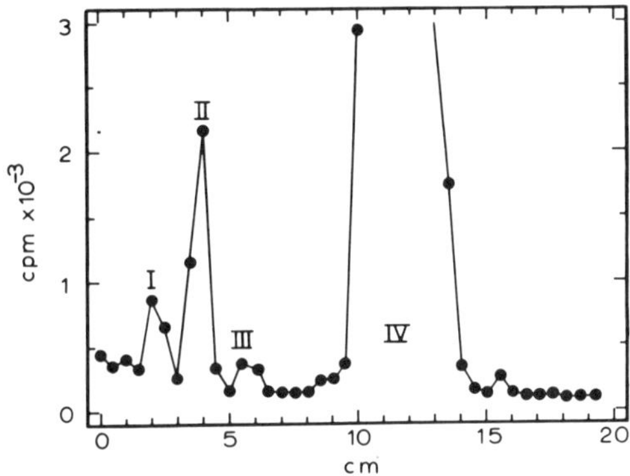

FIGURE 4 Biosynthesis of prostaglandins by lung homogenates. Guinea pig lungs were homogenized in ice cold phosphate buffer, pH 7.5, and centrifuged at $5,000g$ to remove coarse cellular debris. An aliquot of the supernatant was mixed with 0.1 μCi of $[1^{14}C]$ arachidonic acid and 20 μg of unlabeled PGE_1 to protect the newly formed radioactive prostaglandins from enzymatic degradation. The reaction mixture, which also included 1 mM adrenaline and 1 mM reduced glutathione was incubated at $37°C$ for 5 min in a shaking water bath, then acidified to pH 3 with 1 N HCl, and the prostaglandins and unreacted substrate extracted into ethyl acetate. The organic phase was then decanted, concentrated under reduced pressure, and the components separated by thin layer chromatography on silica gel. After development in the solvent system, iso-octane, acetic acid, ethyl acetate, water 5:2:11:10 (upper phase), the plate was divided into 0.5-cm sections and the radioactivity in each band estimated. Peaks I, II and III were cochromatographed with authentic prostaglandin $F_{2\alpha}$, E_2, and D_2, respectively. Peak IV represents unreacted substrate. In this experiment PGE_2 predominated (experiments performed in author's laboratory).

The biosynthesis of PGs by rat lung was studied by Nugteren and Hazelhof (1973). When ^{14}C-8,11,14-eicosatrienoic was incubated with rat lung homogenates, there was about 5% conversion to a PG-like material, most of which ($\sim$65%) was found to be PGD_1. The same authors also performed experiments in which radioactive endoperoxide intermediates (PGH_1 or H_2) were added to rat lung homogenates; again both H_1 and H_2 were metabolized chiefly to PGD_1 or D_2.

In summary, despite a certain amount of work, lung PG synthetase has not been completely characterized in the same way as the synthetase from (for example) bovine seminal vesicles (Flower et al. 1973), kidney (Blackwell et al. 1975) or heart (Limas and Cohn 1973). Such work as has been done, however, would suggest that it possess basically the same properties as other PG synthetase enzymes.

D.   Inhibition of PG Biosynthesis in the Lung

A wide variety of compounds are known to inhibit PG synthetase (Flower 1974), but perhaps the most significant of these are the so-called *aspirin-like* drugs. This group of agents, which comprises a chemically diverse group of compounds sharing to a greater or less degree the pharmacologic actions of aspirin, were simultaneously shown to inhibit PG release from human platelets by Smith and Willis (1971), PG release from the perfused dog spleen by Ferreira et al. (1971), and PG synthesis in cell-free homogenates of guinea pig lung by Vane (1971). In a typical experiment of the last type, an extract of guinea pig lungs was prepared, according to the method of Änggård and Samuelsson (1965), as mentioned earlier. After homogenization and centrifugation, the supernatant was decanted and mixed with arachidonic acid and various concentrations of aspirin, salicylic acid, or indomethacin. After a 30-min incubation, extraction, and, in some cases, separation by thin layer chromatography, the $PGF_{2\alpha}$ content was bioassayed, using the superfused rat colon preparation. Plotting the log dose-response curves, Vane calculated the following I_{50} concentrations: indomethacin 0.75 μM, aspirin 35 μM, and salicylate 750 μM.

Since this original discovery, inhibition by these and other aspirin-like agents have been demonstrated in over 30 different systems (Flower 1974), including tissue homogenates, subcellular fractions, and isolated tissues as well as whole animals. Thus all the evidence points to the effect being a general one, depending in vivo only on the drug reaching the enzyme.

In the first experiments PG synthetase was quantitated biologically, but subsequent workers have employed a variety of techniques, including radiometric, spectrophotometric, and polarographic assays as well as immunochemical techniques and gas-liquid chromatography-mass spectrometry. The basic findings are similar regardless of the assay method used (Flower 1974 and references therein).

Several fairly complete lists of I_{50} values for these drugs against the synthetase from different tissues have been published, allowing a direct comparison of activity (Flower 1974) and it is possible to deduce the following order of decreasing potency: meclofenamic acid, niflumic acid or indomethacin, mefenamic acid, flufenamic acid, naproxen, phenylbutazone, aspirin, or ibuprofen. This order of potency is, generally speaking, consistent with all data so far published, regardless of the source of synthetase, although some minor variations have been reported. Unfortunately, no complete lists of data are available for enzymes derived from lung tissue, although in light of what is already known about the inhibitory activity of these drugs, the order of potency may be assumed to be approximately the same as that given for other tissues (Table 2). Lee (1974) has confirmed the inhibitory activity of aspirin and indomethacin on guinea pig lung synthetase (I_{50}: aspirin 150 μM and indomethacin 3.6 μM), and also reported that psychotropic drugs inhibit this enzyme. Evidence exists that inhibition of PG formation is a peculiar and selective action of aspirin-like drugs (this has been discussed at some length by Flower 1974). In man there is now adequate evidence (Collier and Flower 1971, Smith and Willis 1971, Hamberg 1972, Horton et al. 1973) that aspirin-like drugs inhibit PG biosynthesis in clinical doses, and thus one might anticipate that the ability of lungs to synthesize PGs would be impaired during therapy with these agents.

A number of authors have reported that the release of PGs and rabbit aorta contracting substances (RCS) (a potent smooth muscle contracting factor), from isolated, perfused, or chopped lungs is abolished by aspirin-like drugs, whether

TABLE 2   Inhibition of Prostaglandin Biosynthesis by Aspirin-Like Drugs (I_{50} μM)

Drug	Spleen[a]	Kidney[b]	Seminal vesicle[c]	Lung[d]
Meclofenamic acid	0.1	1.4	15.0	NT
Indomethacin	0.17	3.7	34.0	0.75
Phenylbutazone	7.25	15.0	1,300.0	NT
Aspirin	37.0	2,800.0	10,000.0	35.0
Salicylic acid	~800.0	70,000.0	>5,000.0	750.0

[a] Flower et al. 1972
[b] Blackwell et al. 1975
[c] Flower et al. 1973
[d] Vane 1971

the stimulus is mechanical, chemical, or immunologic (Piper and Vane 1969, Palmer et al. 1973, Fjalland 1974). In cases such as this *release* may be equated with de novo synthesis, and it is evident that aspirin-like drugs are active inhibitors in lung tissue.

III.   Prostaglandin Inactivation

It is now clear that PGs can be synthesized by, and are released from, virtually all mammalian cells. Hamberg (1972) has estimated that the daily production rate of PGE_1 and PGE_2 in man is approximately 50 to 330 μg in males and 20 to 40 μg in females. Reliable estimates of PG levels in plasma, however, indicate concentrations of <50 pg/ml for E type PGs and <10 pg/ml for $PGF_{2\alpha}$ (Dray and Charbonnel 1974). Such observations would seem to indicate that rapid mechanisms exist for PG metabolism. This assumption is born out by the observation of Ferreira and Vane (1967), who found that more than 95% of infused PGE_2 was inactivated during one circulation through the lungs, and of Hamberg and Samuelsson (1971), who showed that only 3% of the original injected tritiated E_2 remained in the plasma after 90 sec. After 4½ min, there was no detectable PGE_2.

The lungs are a rich source of PG catabolizing enzymes, and it seems likely that the pulmonary circulation is a major site of metabolism of blood-borne PGs. The next section will be devoted to a brief general discussion of PG inactivation in the whole animal in order to gain some perspective of the problem.

A.   Mechanism of PG Catabolism

It is now clear (at least for PGs of the E and F series) that enzymatic mechanisms exist whereby the biologic activity of the PG molecule is rapidly destroyed, the metabolite being excreted in the urine after several successive modifications of the native structure. Broadly speaking, these reactions are of two types: an initial rapid step whereby PGs lose most of their biologic activity, which is catalyzed by PG-specific enzymes, and a second step in which metabolites formed are subsequently oxidized by enzymes probably identical to those involved in the β and ω oxidation of other fatty acids. This sequence of reactions has been investigated in man (Hamberg and Samuelsson 1971) and is summarized for PGE_2 in Figure 5.

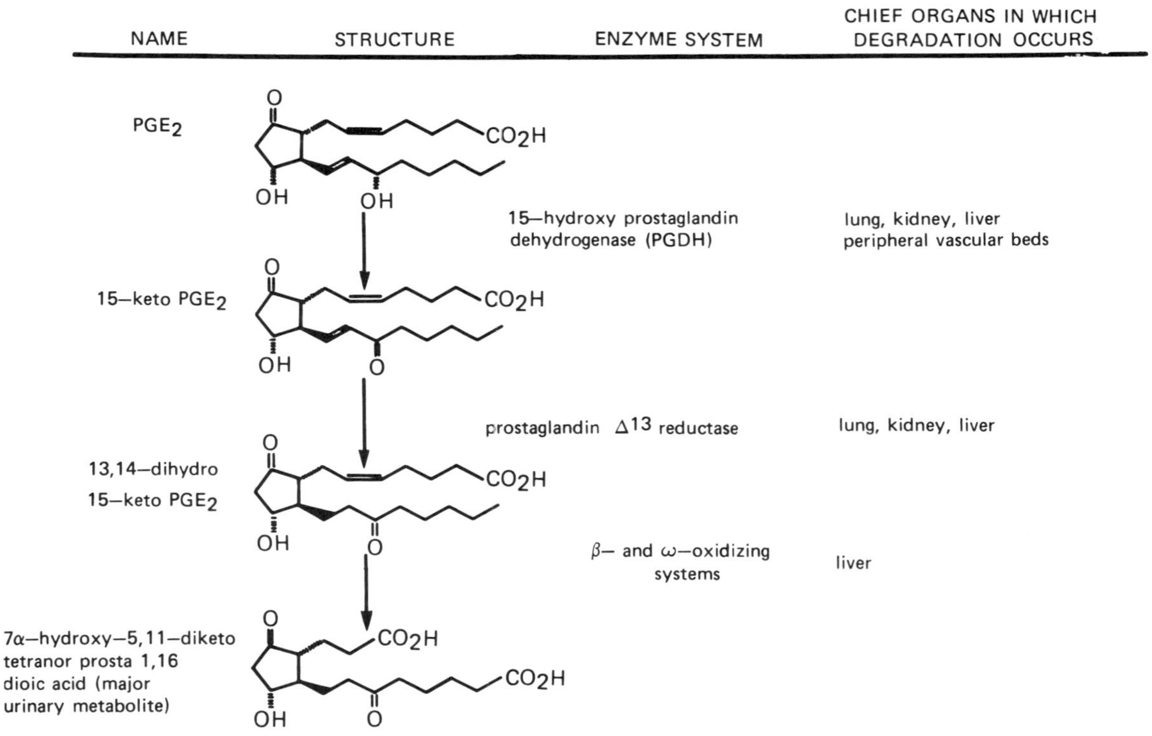

FIGURE 5 Metabolism of prostaglandin E₂ in man (data from Hamberg and Samuelsson 1974).

The initial step in the degradation of PGE_2 is the oxidation of the 15-hydroxyl group to the corresponding ketone under the influence of the enzyme 15-hydroxyprostaglandin dehydrogenase (PGDH). The 15-keto compound is then transformed into the 13,14-dihydro compound, a reaction catalyzed by the enzyme prostaglandin Δ^{13} reductase. While the foregoing steps are relatively rapid, the last steps in the metabolism are probably fairly slow. These consist of oxidation of the β- and ω-side chains of the PGs giving rise to a more polar product (a dicarboxylic acid) that is excreted in urine as the major metabolite of both PGE_1 and PGE_2. The kinetics of these reactions is of interest; in the experiments of Hamberg and Samuelsson (1971) only 3% of the original tritiated PGE_2 injected was present in blood after 90 sec, the bulk of the radioactivity in the plasma being present as the 13,14-dihydro-15-keto metabolite, although this metabolite itself had a half-life of only some 8 min in the circulation. Samuelsson et al. (1971) administered 9β-$[^3H]\,PGF_{2\alpha}$ to human subjects and measured the excretion rate of tritium (present mainly as the dioic acid metabolite) into urine. Approximately 40% was excreted during the first 30 min, almost 80% after 2 hr and maximal excretion (about 90%) occurred after 4 hr. Studies similar to these have been performed in animals, such as the rat (see for example Gréen and Samuelsson 1971, Sun 1974) and in guinea pig (Hamberg and Samuelsson 1972). In each case the initial transformations (i.e., oxidation of the C-15 hydroxyl group and saturation of the 13,14 double bond) appeared to be identical, although the final product of the ω- and β-oxidizing systems, while similar to that in man, was not identical. After the injection of tritiated PGE_1 (Hansson and Samuelsson 1965) and $F_{2\alpha}$ (Gréen et al. 1967) into mice, high concentrations were found in the kidney, liver, and connective tissue with smaller amounts in the lung.

B.   Distribution of Enzymes

Enzymes that catalyze PG degradation are widely distributed throughout different tissues of the body, such as the kidney (Änggård and Samuelsson 1966, Nissen and Andersen 1968, 1969, Nakano 1970, Nakano and Prancan 1971) and intestine of guinea pig (Änggård and Samuelsson 1966), isolated rat liver and testicle (Dawson et al. 1968, Nakano and Prancan 1971) as well as guinea pig lung (Ängård and Samuelsson 1964). Ängård et al. (1971) studied the distribution of PGDH and PG-Δ^{13}-reductase in swine tissue and found that both of the enzymes were located in the $100,000g$ supernatant of cell-free homogenates. Tissues with the highest dehydrogenase activity were the lung, spleen, and kidney, and those with the highest reductase activity were the spleen, kidney, liver, adrenals, and small intestine. The highest activity of PGDH per gram of tissue, however, was found in adipose tissue.

Enzymes responsible for β or ω oxidation are found in the liver (Samuelsson 1970, Samuelsson et al. 1971), in lung and kidney (Nakano and Morsey 1971), and in intestine (Parkinson and Schneider 1969). Probably, however, the liver is the major site of side-chain oxidation.

Various other metabolic transformations of PGE have been reported. In some tissues PGE may be transformed by a *9-keto reductase* to $PGF_{2\alpha}$. Leslie and Levine (1973) investigated the distribution of this enzyme in tissues of the rat; the heart was found to contain the highest specific activity followed by the kidney, brain, liver, and adrenal tissue. Uterus, blood, and lung tissue had approximately equivalent (small) amounts. None was found in striated muscle, spleen, or ileum. Although present in rat lung, no 9-keto reductase activity was detectable in guinea pig lung homogenates.

C.   Properties of PG Catabolizing Enzymes in the Lung

As pointed out earlier, the lungs are a rich source of both the PGDH and the Δ^{13} reductase enzymes. Not only were lungs the first tissue in which metabolism of PG was elucidated, but they have subsequently received most attention. Because of the reduction in biologic activity, which is a consequence of metabolism, and the unique position of the lungs, situated as they are between the venous and the arterial circulation, it would seem that the pulmonary circulation constitutes an important barrier through which PGs, having potent smooth muscle stimulating or cardiovascular actions, cannot pass and are thus prevented from reaching target organs via the arterial circulation.

In 1964 Änggård and Samuelsson first reported that enzymes in the particle-free supernatant of guinea pig lung homogenates converted labeled PGE_1 to the 13,14-dihydro and 15-keto-13,14-dihydro derivatives. Two years later the same authors reported that in swine lung only the 15-keto derivative was found, and it was therefore deduced that these transformations involved first an oxidation of the C-15 alcohol followed by a reduction of the C-13 double bond. Later work has demonstrated that the reduction at C-13 cannot occur without prior formation of the 15-keto group. However, 13,14-dihydro derivatives of PGs are found, and these appear to arise by a reduction of the 15-keto group after the 13,14 double bond has been saturated (Hamberg 1972, Hamberg and Samuelsson 1971, Samuelsson et al. 1971). Further studies by Änggård et al. (1965) and by Änggård and Samuelsson (1965), using guinea pig lung homogenates, suggested that PGE_2 and PGE_3 were metabolized in a similar fashion. Änggård and Samuelsson also investigated the metabolism of $PGF_{2\alpha}$ in the guinea pig lung system and found a slow conversion to one product, which was not identical to PGE_2 or its metabolites.

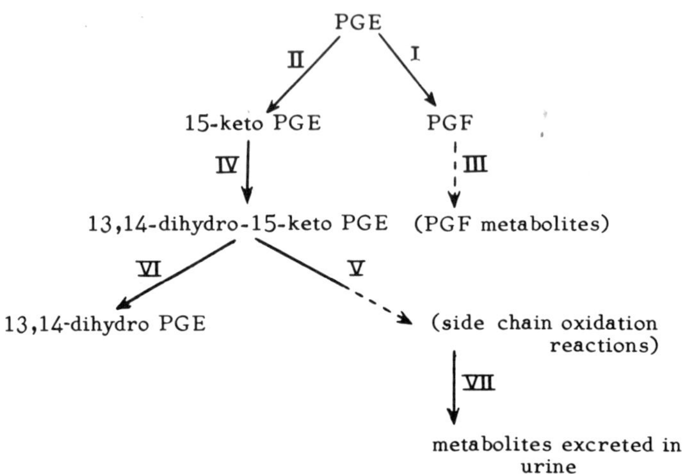

FIGURE 6   Possible routes of metabolism of prostaglandin E in the lung (see text for explanation and references).   Reaction I: transformation of PGE to PGF by 9-ketoreductase. This enzyme has been reported in rat but not guinea pig lungs. Reaction II: transformation of PGE to the 15-keto metabolite. This reaction is catalyzed by prostaglandin 15-hydroxydehydrogenase, an enzyme that exists in particularly high concentrations in the lung. Reaction III: PGF may be metabolized by pathways similar to those of PGE_2. Reaction IV: Saturation of the 13,14 double bond by prostaglandin $\Delta 13$ reductase. This enzyme is also present in high concentrations in lung tissue, except in the swine, and the principal metabolite in swine is therefore the 15-keto derivative. Reaction V: β- and ω-oxidation reactions. These occur in several tissues, including the lung, but probably occur chiefly in the liver. Reaction VI: A small amount of 13,14-dihydro-15-keto PGE can be reduced back to 13,14-dihydro-PGE by an enzyme known as 15-keto prostaglandin reductase. Reaction VII: The β- and ω-oxidized metabolites are eventually excreted in the urine.

Granström (1971) found that $PGF_{2\alpha}$ was metabolized in the guinea pig lung by pathways similar to those of the E series.

Änggård and Samuelsson (1966) were also the first workers to isolate and purify PGDH from swine lung. Using ammonium sulfate and column chromatography (TEAE-cellulose, Sephadex G100, hydroxyapatite, and DEAE Sephadex), they were able to isolate an enzyme that was shown to be NAD^+ dependent and specific for the C-15 hydroxyl group of PGs. Prostaglandin E_1 was the best substrate tested, the relative reaction rates of PGE_2 and PGE_3 being 0.97 and 0.6, respectively ($PGE_1 = 1$). The reaction rate of 13,14-dihydro PGE_1 was 0.2 compared to PGE_1. Among the F series, $PGF_{1\alpha}$ had a relative reaction rate of 0.75, $F_{2\alpha}$ and $F_{3\alpha}$, 0.62. Dehydration products of PGEs had the following relative reaction rates, PGA_1 0.45 and PGA_2 0.33; PGB_1 or B_2 were not substrates for the enzyme. Several other compounds, such as steroids, alcohols, hydroxy acids, and carbohydrates, were not oxidized at all, indicating good specificity. The reaction rate rose with increasing temperatures up to a maximum of 55°C after which denaturation occurred; little dependence on pH between 6 and 8 was noted. Vonkeman et al. (1969) have extended this work on the specificity of the enzyme to include several PGs that do not occur naturally and concluded that a fixed length of carboxyl and/or alkyl chain of PGs was unimportant for oxidation. Thus PGs, which are biologically active yet not known to occur naturally, are metabolized and lose biologic activity in the same way as do the native compounds. Shio et al. (1970) have published data on the specificity of the swine lung enzyme. They noted that the enzyme was stereospecific for the C-15 (S)-configuration, thus confirming the observations of Nakano et al. (1969). The latter authors also noted that while the constituents of the cyclopentane ring were relatively unimportant, the nature of the carboxyl side chain was.

Marrazzi and Matschinsky (1972) published a careful study of the PGDH from swine lung and elucidated its structural requirements for substrate bind-

TABLE 3   Some Properties of Lung PGDH

	Source			
Parameter	Swine lung[a]	Swine lung[b]	Beef lung[c]	Beef lung[d]
pH optimum	8.5–9.0	>8.0	~9.0	–
Approximate molecular weight (Daltons)	$60-70 \times 10^3$	20×10^3	20×10^3	40×10^3
Specific activity (nmol) NAD^+ reduced/min/mg protein)	$0.13-0.65 \times 10^{-3}$	4.2	1.0	1.4 mU/mg[e]
K_m PGE_1 (μm)	~10.0	1.14	4.0	3.4
K_m NAD^+ (μm)	200.0	60.0	–	110.0

[a] Änggård 1971
[b] Marazzi and Matschinsky 1972
[c] Shanahan et al. quoted in Marrazzi and Anderson 1974.
[d] Hansen 1974
[e] 1 unit here is identified as the amount of enzyme that oxidizes 1 μmol PGE_1/min at saturating PGE_1 and NAD^+ concentrations.

ing as well as for inhibition by substrate and cofactor analogs. Unlike that of
Änggård and Samuelsson their enzyme preparation was very sensitive to
changes of pH between 6 and 8. Marrazzi et al. (1972) found that swine lung
PGDH was reversible and could catalyze the reduction of 15-keto PGE_1. During the reaction, however, an inhibitor accumulated, which rendered the reaction quasi-irreversible.

A serious drawback to experimental work with this enzyme, as well as
to its use as an assay tool (Marrazzi and Andersen 1974), has been its lack of
stability on storage.

Purified PGDH has been isolated from beef lungs by Saeed and Roy
(1972) who reported an increased specific activity over the swine lung enzyme.
Shannahan et al. (1974) have also reported purification of a beef lung enzyme.
Table 3 gives a brief resume of the biochemical properties of some lung PGDH
enzymes.

Metabolism of PGE_1 occurs in homogenates of human lung (Nakano and
Greenfield 1970).

Little is known about the properties of the Δ^{13} reductase.

D.   Prostaglandin Inactivation by Intact Lung

In Vivo

The significance of the lungs as sites of PG inactivation in vivo was first demonstrated by Ferreira and Vane (1967). Although stable in blood, greater
than 95% of infused PGE_1 or PGE_2 (0.5 to 1 μg/min) was removed during

---

FIGURE 7   Conversion of radioactive prostaglandins to less polar metabolites
during passage through isolated, perfused guinea pig lungs. PGE_2, $F_{2\alpha}$, or A_2,
0.1 μCi, was injected into the pulmonary artery of isolated lungs from guinea
pigs, perfused with Krebs solution at 37°C. The effluent was collected, acidified to pH 3, extracted into ethyl acetate, and the products separated on a
silica gel thin-layer chromatogram in the solvent system water, acetic acid, isooctane, ethyl acetate 10:2:5:11. The chromatogram was cut into 0.5-cm sections and the radioactivity in each band estimated. The percent total activity
in each 0.5-cm strip was plotted as shown. Small aliquots of PGE_2, $F_{2\alpha}$, and
A_2 were also extracted from Krebs solution and chromatographed alongside.
Dotted lines show the position of authentic tritiated PGE_2, $F_{2\alpha}$, and A_2,
while the black circles and continuous line represent the pattern obtained of
the passage through guinea pig lungs. Transformation to a less polar metabolite is observed in each instance, the conversion being approximately 82% of
injected PGE_2, 50% of injected $F_{2\alpha}$, and 38% A_2 (experiments performed in
author's laboratory).

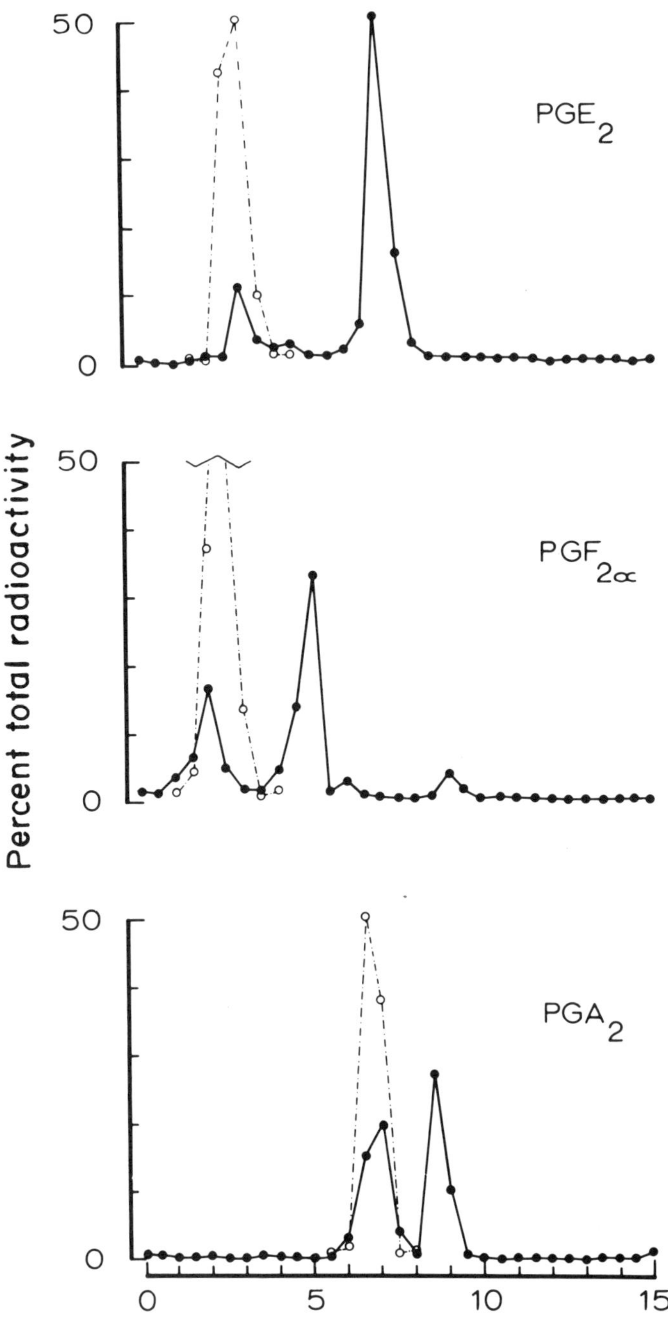

50
0
50
0
50
0
PGE$_2$
PGF$_{2\alpha}$
PGA$_2$
Percent total radioactivity
0
5
10
15
cm

one passage through cat lungs, as determined by bioassay. Using similar infusion rates, the same effects were demonstrated in dogs and rabbits. Other
vascular beds, such as those of liver and hind quarters, also inactivated prostaglandins, although not to the same degree. Two years later McGiff et al.
(1967), using changes in dog renal blood flow as an index of PG concentration in arterial blood, confirmed that PGE_1 and PGE_2 were rapidly inactivated
by the lung, whereas PGA_1 and A_2 were not. This finding was in qualitative,
if not quantitative, agreement with kinetic data obtained in vitro. On the
basis of these results the authors suggested that PGs of the A series are the
only PGs likely to be circulating hormones. Horton and Jones (1969) have
confirmed that a single passage through the pulmonary circulation of the cat or
dog causes substantial losses of the vasodilator activity of PGE_1 but not of PGA_1.

In Isolated Lungs

In 1970 Piper et al., speculating that *inactivation* in vivo could be due to
either uptake of prostaglandins into the cells of the lung or blood, binding to
plasma or other proteins, or metabolism per se, investigated the mechanisms
by which isolated, perfused guinea pig lungs inactivated PGs. Substantial
(>90%) inactivation of PGE_1, E_2, and $F_{2\alpha}$ occurred in one passage through
guinea pig lungs, but PGA_2 was only inactivated to the extent of about 30%.
These authors ruled out the possibility that PGs were taken up by, and stored
within, the lung and demonstrated instead that the inactivation was a temperature-dependent (and therefore probably enzymic) process and that PGA_2 was
metabolized at a slower rate than PGE_1, E_2, or $F_{2\alpha}$. Thin layer chromatography revealed that the PGs were converted to less polar derivatives, and the
authors concluded that PGDH was probably the enzyme responsible for inactivation. Parallel with, and complementary to these observations are the
findings of Horton et al. (1965) and Carlsson and Oro (1966) that the hypotensive action of PGs in the ewe and in the dog are greater when PGs are
given intraarterially than when given intravenously.

Pace-Asciak and Miller (1973), measuring metabolic activity in tissue
homogenates, found that the 15-PGDH and the Δ^{13} reductase activity in rat
lung varied with age. High reductase activity was found in fetal and early
newborn animals (compared with adults) but decreased thereafter. Dehydrogenase activity was found to be maximal at about 19 days after birth. The
ratio of 15-keto-13,14-dihydro to 15-keto metabolites in fetal and neonatal
rats was five to six times adult levels. The authors conclude that high reductase activity in lung is essential for the efficient metabolism of 15-keto and
naturally occurring PGs. Enzyme levels measured by in vitro and in vivo
techniques were also found to alter during pregnancy in the rabbit (Sun and
Armour 1974, Bedwani and Marley 1974).

E. Biologic Activity of PG Metabolites

Prostaglandins possess extremely potent pharmacologic activity and an important question is at which stage of the metabolic degradation this loss occurs.

Änggård and Samuelsson (1967) synthesized the 13,14-dihydro PGE_1, and 15-keto-13,14-dihydro PGE_1 and compared the biologic activity (smooth muscle contractile and vasodepressor effects in the guinea pig and rabbit) with that of the parent molecule. Figure 8 shows the loss of biologic activity, which occurs on successive modifications of the PGE_1 molecule in the guinea pig. It

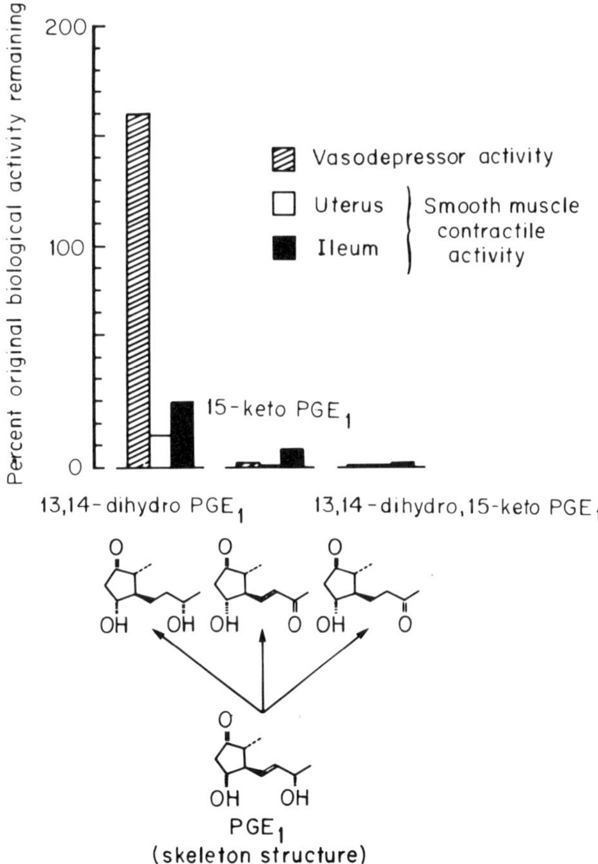

FIGURE 8   Loss of vasodepressor and smooth muscle contracting activity (guinea pig) after metabolic transformation (data from Änggård and Samuelsson (1971).

is evident that after saturation of the 13,14 double bond, the molecule still retains a significant proportion of its biologic activity and indeed, the depressor effect is somewhat augmented. Biologic activity is greatly attenuated when the 15-hydroxyl group is oxidized and virtually disappears when both modifications are introduced. Qualitatively similar results were seen when the metabolite was tested for contractile activity on rabbit duodenum and for vasodepressor actions on rabbit blood pressure. Nakano (1971) reported that the vasodilator actions of 13,14-dihydro E_1, 15-keto E_1, and 15-keto-13,14-dihydro PGE_1 were approximately 1/4, 1/80, and 1/100 of PGE_1 in dog hind-limb preparations. Similarly Kloeze (1969) found that the 13,14-dihydro derivative of PGE_1 had an activity of 0.64, relative to the parent molecule, as an inhibitor of platelet aggregation and that the 15-keto compound was inactive. The 15-keto derivative of PGE_2 was likewise inactive as an inducer of platelet aggregation. 15-keto-13,14-dihydro $PGF_{2\alpha}$ has been shown by Pike et al (1967) to have little spasmogenic activity on many smooth muscle preparations, 15-keto $F_{2\alpha}$ however, has up to ten times the contractile activity of the parent molecule on smooth muscle preparations, including human bronchial muscle and guinea pig trachea (Dawson et al. 1974) and is also a more potent pressor agent (Jones 1975). Jones (1975) has analyzed the cardiovascular responses to PGs and postulated the existence of two systems on which PGs can act: one pressor and the other depressor. He concluded that (a) oxidation of the 15-hydroxyl group to a ketone results in a loss of depressor activity of PGs and (b) saturation of the 13,14 (trans) or 5,6 (cis) double bond results in a loss of pressor activity but has little effect on depressor activity.

No data are at present available for the ω- or β-oxidized metabolites.

It is evident from the foregoing discussion that the lung enzymes are capable of transforming biologically active PGs into inactive metabolites and that moreover this can occur within the transit time through the pulmonary circulation.

F. Inhibition of PG Inactivation
   by the Lung

If the lungs are an important site of metabolism, which prevent the access of biologically active PGs to the arterial circulation, then inhibitors of the dehydrogenase could have far-reaching effects on the physiology (especially the cardiovascular physiology) of animals. This is a fairly new concept, and not much relevant data have been published.

Obvious candidates for inhibitors of all enzymes are substrate analogs. Nakano et al. (1969) found that swine lung PGDH was noncompetitively inhibited by a synthetic epimer of PGE_1, 15-R-PGE_1 and that the B-type PGs (though not substrates) were also noncompetitive inhibitors; dihydro PGE_1 and 8-iso PGE_1 were inactive. Fried et al. (1973) found that several PG analogs were active against the dehydrogenase from human placenta. Marrazzi and Matschinsky (1972), using swine lung, found that a derivative of $PGF_{1\alpha}$, 7-oxa $PGF_{1\alpha}$ (oxygen substituted at C-7), had the same V_{max} as the original substrate (but much lower affinity), and various stereoisomers of this derivative (15-epimer, the optical antipode, and an analog with both of these modifica-

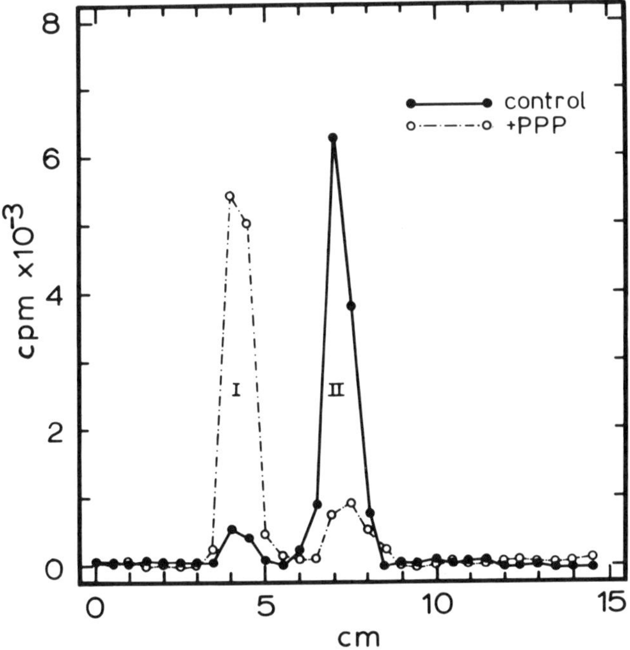

FIGURE 9 Blockade of prostaglandin destruction by polyphloretin phosphate. Tritiated PGE_2, 0.1 μCi, was injected into the pulmonary artery of lungs isolated from guinea pigs and perfused with Krebs solution at $37°C$. The effluent was collected, acidified to pH 3, extracted into ethyl acetate, the organic phase evaporated, and the components separated by thin layer chromatography on silca gel, using the solvent system ethyl acetate, water, iso-octane, acetic acid 10:11:5:2. The thin layer chromatogram was cut into 0.5-cm sections and the radioactivity in each estimated by liquid scintilation counting. The unbroken line and the black circles show that PGE_2 is transformed almost completely to a single metabolite (II) during a single passage through the lungs. The broken line and open circles (I) represent the pattern obtained when 10 μg/ml polyphloretin phosphate was infused simultaneously with the injection of tritiated E_2 (Bakhle and Flower 1973, unpublished observations).

tions) all showed mixed inhibition of PGDH, as did several fatty acids (arachidonic, linolenic, and oleic, and their respective coenzyme A derivatives). Polyphloretin phosphate (PPP), a high molecular weight polymer of phloretin (which antagonizes some of the actions of PGs on smooth muscle, Bennett 1975) was also a competitive inhibitor of the enzyme but SC19222, another antagonist, (Bennett 1975) was not.

The foregoing compounds were inhibitors at the substrate site of the enzyme. With regard to the cofactor site, Marazzi and Matschinsky found that certain NAD^+ analogs or derivatives were inhibitory and a range of substituted pyridines were noncompetitive inhibitors. Several nucleosides and nucleotides, in concentrations of 3 to 10 mM, were also active, as were the methylxanthines, caffeine, and theophylline as well as aminophylline. Among compounds inactive against the preparation were the barbiturates.

The aspirin-like drugs are inhibitors of PG synthesis (see above), and it has been subsequently found that indomethacin inhibits the NAD^+-dependent destruction of PGE_1 or E_2 by the high-speed supernatant of dog spleen (Flower 1974). Cheung and Cushman (unpublished observations 1972) found that some other aspirin-like drugs inhibited the rabbit lung dehydrogenase. Indomethacin, in concentrations of 1 mM, gave a 93% inhibition of PGE_2 metabolism, niflumic acid in a concentration of 0.5 mM inhibited 38% and meclofenamic acid in the same concentration inhibited 14%. Aspirin, naproxen, ibuprofen, phenylbutazone, and benzydamine were inactive. Hansen (1974) reported inhibition of a purified bovine lung PGDH by indomethacin ($K_i = 1.4 \times 10^{-4}$ M) and aspirin. Indomethacin inhibition was noncompetitive.

One study supports the concept that aspirin-like drugs can inhibit lung dehydrogenase in vivo. Jackson and associates (1973) studied the pulmonary inactivation of $PGF_{2\alpha}$ during one passage through the pulmonary circulation of dogs. In these experiments the mean inactivation of $PGF_{2\alpha}$ on passage through the lungs (6 dogs) was 91.9%. After treatment with aspirin, 50 mg/ kg repeated hourly, there was a small but statistically highly significant decrease (almost 10%) in the inactivation. When the same experiment was performed in sheep, however, aspirin was inactive, indicating perhaps a species difference. Against these results one must balance the results of Hamberg and Samuelsson (1972) who found that administration of indomethacin (50 mg/ day) to guinea pigs did not change the in vivo metabolism of tritiated PGE_2.

It is not known how aspirin-like drugs inhibit PGDH. However, the salicylates are known to inhibit several dehydrogenases (Smith and Dawkins 1971), probably by competing for the cofactor site, so possibly a similar action could account for the inhibition of PGDH. It seems, from what limited data are available, that the concentrations required to inhibit the synthetase are considerably less than those that produce a corresponding inhibition of the dehydrogenase.

Crutchley and Piper (1974) performed parallel investigations on the inhibition of pulmonary removal of prostaglandins by isolated guinea pig lungs and the inhibition of prostaglandin metabolism by a crude enzyme preparation from guinea pig lung homogenates. Polyphloretin phosphate as well as diphloretin phosphate (DPP), in doses of 0.1 to 5 μg/ml of the perfusing fluid, inhibited the inactivation of PGE_2, $F_{2\alpha}$, and $F_2\beta$ and therefore increased the amount of PGs surviving passage through the lungs. Both agents also inhibited the crude enzyme preparation. Polyphloretin phosphate had no effect on the pulmonary inactivation of bradykinin or 5-hydroxytryptamine by isolated guinea pig lungs. A number of metabolic inhibitors and sulphydryl binding reagents were also tested: 2,4 dinitrophenol was inactive at doses of 0.5 mM, whereas iodoacetate was inactive at 0.25 mM but showed weak activity (about 10%) at 0.5 mM. In doses of 3 mM 2:3-dimercaptopropanol was inactive; disulfiram showed no significant inhibition at 6 μM. Two sulphydryl binding agents sodium *p*-chloromercuriphenylsulphonate and *N*-ethylmaleimide were, however, active, having an ID_{50} of 0.6 mM and 70 μM, respectively. Both these agents were also active against the crude enzyme preparation. The same authors also tried some antiinflammatory agents: phenylbutazone (50 μg/ml) and indomethacin (20 μg/ml) showed slight activity (a reduction of 40% and 10%, respectively) but aspirin, paracetamol, ibuprofen, and meclofenamic acid were inactive.

In a later paper the same authors (Crutchley and Piper 1975) investigated the actions of one of these agents (DPP) in the rabbit in vivo. By infusing PGE_2 and $PGF_{2\alpha}$ into the superior vena cava and comparing the response with that of an infusion into the aorta, a measure of pulmonary inactivation was obtained. Diphloretin phosphate potentiated, 25 to 100 times, the depressor effects of the PGs and also the effects on gastrointestinal motility, as measured by a balloon in the jejunum.

G. Problems Associated with PG Inactivation

The exact mechanics of PG metabolism by the lung are not entirely clear. It seems very likely that the hydrolytic enzymes responsible for the metabolism of AMP, angiotensin I, bradykinin, and ATP (Ryan et al. 1972, see also Ryan and Ryan, this volume) are located close to the luminal surface of the pulmonary vascular endothelium. Sander and Huggins (1971) have suggested that the angiotensin I converting enzymes are located on the external surface of the plasma membrane. As mentioned before, PGDH resists sedimentation at 100,000 X *g* and is therefore presumably a soluble cytoplasmic enzyme. This being the case, it would seem that at least three steps are involved in the metabolism of PGs by the lung: (a) entry of PGs into the cell cytoplasm, (b) metabolism per se, and (c) release of metabolites from the cell. Because of the complexity of this process, one might anticipate a delay in the clearance of PGs and their metabolites from the lung when compared, for example, to the passage of a high molecular weight compound unlikely to leave the vascular space. Ryan et al. (1972) have shown that such delay does indeed occur in the washout of labeled PG metabolites from rat lungs. Exactly how PGs enter the cells and PG metabolites leave is not clear. Transport mechanisms for PGs are thought to exist in some tissues (Bito 1972), but while metabolism is a temperature-dependent process (Piper et al. 1970), it is not sensitive to metabolic poisons (Crutchley and Piper 1974) so presumably the transport process (if there is one) is not directly energy linked.

IV. Prostaglandin Metabolizing Enzymes in the Placenta

For most of the gestation period, the placenta serves as the *fetal lung* and as such is germane to our discussion. That this surrogate function of the placenta does not extend only to the gas exchange mechanism has been suggested by the finding that metabolic machinery for the uptake and removal of several vasoactive substances is present in the placenta and is analogous to mechanisms present in the lung. It is not surprising to find, therefore, that the placenta is a rich source of PGDH even in the early stages of gestation, although there appear to be kinetic differences between the placental and lung enzymes (Jarabak 1972, Schlegel et al. 1974). Schlegel and his coworkers have partially purified the placental enzyme by column chromatography and ammonium sulfate fractionation. Polyacrylamide gel electrophoresis of the final product suggested that isoenzymic forms of PGDH might exist. The maternal steroids, estrogen and progesterone, exerted some inhibitory effect on the enzyme.

Alam and associates (1973) have reported the existence of a *dehydratase* enzyme in human placenta, catalyzing the conversion of PGE to PGA. Comparisons of placentas from normal or toxemic patients revealed that the metabolism of PGE_2 by the crude enzyme preparation (15,000g supernatant) derived from toxemic patients was much less than that of corresponding control placentas. The ability to metabolize PGs appeared to be inversely proportional to the severity of the toxemia, suggesting that the biochemical lesion in toxemia may involve the PG system.

V. Significance of PG Synthesis and Catabolism in Lung

At the time of writing (November 1974) it is extremely difficult to delineate the role played by PGs in the normal physiology of animals or man, although there seems to be no doubt of their pathologic significance. The fact that PG synthetase is found in the respiratory exchange organs and gills of lower animals (see Section IV) tempts speculation that PGs are involved in oxygen or ion transport mechanisms. There is, however, no evidence for the former, and the latter suggestion would not seem to be applicable to mammalian lungs.

The mere presence of endogenous substances possessing high pharmacologic activity within a tissue is certainly no guarantee of their having a physiologic function; PGs do, however, have dramatic effects on pulmonary hemodynamics (Hauge et al. 1967, Hyman 1968, 1969, Said 1968) as well as respiratory smooth muscle both in vivo and in vitro (see Cuthbert 1971 for a review). Since the effects of PGs on pulmonary smooth muscle are not blocked by adrenergic or cholinergic blockers (Strong and Bohr 1967), ganglion blocking agents, or botulinum toxin (Carlsson and Oro 1966, Myazaki et al. 1967), it has been speculated that they may act on the lung cyclic AMP system (Cuthbert 1973). Edmonds et al. (1969) have demonstrated the release of PGs from perfused guinea pig lungs in response to inflation, and since certain PGs dilate the pulmonary vasculature, several authors (Edmonds et al. 1969, Cuthbert 1973) have suggested that PGs might be responsible for maintaining the correct ventilation/perfusion ratio in pulmonary tissue.

There is a great deal of experimental evidence that PGs are released from lungs by a variety of traumatic stimuli (see above, and Piper and Said, this volume), and it has been suggested that PGs may be important in the development of the clinical picture associated with immunologic reactions or embolism and even with migraine (Sandler 1972). The suggestion that PGs play a part in bronchial asthma has been widely canvassed (for a review see Parker and Snider 1973, Cuthbert 1973); $PGF_{2\alpha}$ is a bronchoconstrictor (Sweatman and Collier 1968), furthermore, Dawson et al. (1974) have observed that 15-keto $F_{2\alpha}$ (i.e., the product of PGDH) has two to three times the biologic activity of $PGF_{2\alpha}$ on the guinea pig trachea and one to two times the activity on human bronchial muscle, suggesting that the metabolites may be important mediators in asthma. The same authors also observed that PGD_2 was a potent bronchoconstrictor, having approximately the same order of potency as $PGF_{2\alpha}$. The idea that $PGF_{2\alpha}$ or a metabolite may be an important mediator in asthma and that this disease may therefore be a consequence of aberrant PG production is certainly very attractive but has at least two serious flaws: (a) PGs of the E series, which would presumably be synthesized alongside the

F-type, have opposite activity and have in fact been used as bronchodilators for asthmatics (Cuthbert 1971), and (b) if $PGF_{2\alpha}$ is a mediator in asthma, then aspirin-like drugs that inhibit PG biosynthesis could be of some therapeutic value; however, the majority of asthmatics do not respond to aspirin-like drugs. A possible counter argument to these objections is that if E- and F-type PGs are released simultaneously, then their effects on the bronchial tree would tend to cancel out, and in the small proportion of asthmatics who do respond to aspirin-like drugs the predominant PG released is $F_{2\alpha}$, which maintains a constrictor tone. Thus, by removing this, aspirin has a beneficial effect. The reverse may also obtain if the predominant PG released is PGE_2 (bronchodilator); then one would expect such asthmatics to be extremely sensitive to aspirin. Indeed, there appears to be a small population of asthmatics who are hypersensitive to aspirin and other PG synthetase inhibitors (Smith 1971). Another possible explanation is that the lung tissue of asthmatics is more sensitive to the bronchoconstrictor actions of $PGF_{2\alpha}$. This idea has been supported by the work of Mathe et al. (1973) who found that asthmatics were substantially (8,000 times) more sensitive to $F_{2\alpha}$ than normal controls and that bronchoconstriction induced by $F_{2\alpha}$ was of a long duration.

Further evidence against the involvement of prostaglandins in asthma comes from the work of Dawson and Tomlinson (1974) who found that disodium cromoglycate, which is therapeutically active in asthma, prevented the release of SRS-A but not of PGs from sensitized guinea pig lungs; indomethacin prevented the release of PG but not of SRS-A.

Whatever the function (or lack of function) of PG synthetase in the lung, there seems to be no doubt of the role of PGDH, which must now be regarded as belonging to that class of enzymes (which include inter alia phosphodiesterase, cholinesterase, and monoamine oxidase) that inactivate compounds of high biologic activity and thus limit their tissue distribution (Marrazzi and Matschinsky 1972). If, for some reason, inactivation of PGs by the lung is diminished, then PGs might accumulate in the circulation in sufficient quantities to cause panpharmacologic effects. The concept that a specific disease state may be a reflection of altered PG metabolizing enzymes in the lung is relatively new, although analogous ideas have been postulated for 5-HT as well as for other vasoactive peptides also removed or inactivated by the lung (Vane 1969). The possibility that PGs are involved in endotoxin shock and that this is secondary to an impaired degradation mechanism has been investigated by Nakano and Prancan (1973); plasma levels of PGs are elevated in endotoxin shock (Scarnes and Harper 1972, Anderson et al. 1973, Kessler et al. 1973) and there is evidence that these increased levels of PGs could account for some of the circulatory and other changes that are a feature of this condition (Parrott and Sturgess 1974). Nakano and Prancan (1973) investigated the hypothesis that this could be due to impaired metabolism of PGs by the lung (and kidney). Eight hours after endotoxin shock was induced in rats, the lungs and kidneys were removed and the metabolism of PGE_2 measured. The capacity of the lungs (and to a lesser extent the kidneys) of these animals to metabolize PGs was greatly impaired.

VI. Summary

In the preceding pages evidence has been presented that PGs are not only synthesized but also rapidly catabolized by the lungs in vivo and in vitro. The biologic activity of PG metabolites in the lung effluent represents only a fraction of that of the native molecule, and since many of the PGs have potent pharmacologic actions in the arterial circulation, the lung may serve as a continuous attenuator of arterial blood levels. Should this mechanism become imbalanced, pathologic conditions could arise.

Note: Since this chapter was written, two novel pathways of arachidonic acid metabolism have been reported in the lung (Hamberg and Samuelsson (1974). *Biochem. Biophys. Res. Commun.,* **61**:942–949. One of these products, a hydroperoxide of arachidonic acid, is formed by an enzyme in the cell cytoplasm. The other pathway transforms the endoperoxide PGG_2 (see Section IVB) to "PHD," a hemiacetal derivative of 8-(1-hydroxy-3-oxopropyl)-9,12-dihydroxy-5,10-heptadecadienoic acid. It appears that this new pathway may constitute the major route of PGG_2 metabolism in the lung, the other metabolites (already described) accounting (in toto) for about half as much PGG_2 as does PHD. The metabolism and biologic activity of this new product is not yet clearly understood, and it will be some while before its significance (if any) in pulmonary physiology is understood.

References

Alabaster, V. A. and Bakhle, Y. S. (1970). The release of biologically active substances from isolated lungs by 5-hydroxytryptamine and tryptamine. *Br. J. Pharmacol.,* **40**:582–583P.

Alabaster, V. A. and Bakhle, Y. S. (1976). Release of smooth muscle contracting substances from isolated perfused lungs. *Eur. J. Pharmacol.,* **35**:349–360.

Alam, N. A., Clary, P., and Russell, P. T. (1973). Depressed placental prostaglandin E_1 metabolism in toxemia of pregnancy. *Prostaglandins,* **4**:363–370.

Anderson, F. L., Jubiz, W., Kralios, A. C., and Tsagaris, T. G. (1973). Plasma prostaglandin E levels during endotoxin shock in dogs. *Clin. Res.,* **21**:194.

Änggård, E. (1965). The isolation and determination of prostaglandins in lungs of sheep, guinea pig, monkey and man. *Biochem. Pharmacol.,* **14**:1507–1516.

Änggård, E. (1966). The biological activities of three metabolites of prostaglandin E_1. *Acta Physiol. Scand.*, **66**:509–510.

Änggård, E. (1971). Studies on the analysis and metabolism of the prostaglandins. *Ann. N. Y. Acad. Sci.*, **180**:200–217.

Änggård, E., Gréen, K., and Samuelsson, B. (1965). Synthesis of tritium-labeled
prostaglandin E_2 and studies on its metabolism in guinea pig lung. *J. Biol.
Chem.*, **240**:1932–1940.

Änggård, E., Larsson, C., and Samuelsson, B. (1971). The distribution of 15-
hydroxyprostaglandin dehydrogenase and prostaglandin Δ^{13} reductase in
tissues of the swine. *Acta Physiol. Scand.*, **81**:396–404.

Änggård, E. and Samuelsson, B. (1964). Prostaglandins and related factors. 28.
Metabolism of prostaglandin E_1 in guinea pig lung: the structures of two
metabolites. *J. Biol. Chem.*, **239**:4087–4102.

Änggård, E. and Samuelsson, B. (1965). Biosynthesis of prostaglandins from
arachidonic acid in guinea pig lung. *J. Biol. Chem.*, **240**:3518–3521.

Änggård, E. and Samuelsson, B. (1965). Prostaglandins and related factors.
XLII. Metabolism of prostaglandin E_3 in guinea pig lung. *Biochemistry*,
4:1864–1871.

Änggård, E. and Samuelsson, B. (1966). Purification and properties of a 15-
hydroxy prostaglandin dehydrogenase from swine lung. Prostaglandins
and related factors 55. *Arkiv. Chemi.*, **25**:293–300.

Änggård, E. and Samuelsson, B. (1967). The metabolism of prostaglandins in
lung tissue. In S. Bergstrom and B. Samuelsson (eds.): Nobel Symposium,
vol. 2, Prostaglandins. Interscience, New York, pp. 97–105.

Babilli, S. and Vogt, W. (1965). Nature of the fatty acids acting as 'slow reacting
substance' (SRC-C). *J. Physiol. (Lond.)*, **177**:31–32.

Bakhle, Y. S. and Smith, T. W. (1972). Release of spasmogenic substances induced by vasoactive amines from isolated lungs. *Br. J. Pharmacol.*, **46**:
543–544P.

Bakhle, Y. S. and Vane, J. R. (1974). Pharmacokinetic function of the pulmonary circulation. *Physiol. Rev.*, **54**:1007–1045.

Bedwani, J. R. and Marley, P. B. (1974). Increased inactivation of prostaglandin
E_2 by the rabbit lung during pregnancy. *Br. J. Pharmacol.*, **50**:459P.

Bennett, A. (1975). Prostaglandin antagonists. In A. B. Simmonds (ed.): Advances in Drug Research. Academic Press, London, pp. 83–118.

Bergström, S., Carlsson, L. A., and Weeks, J. R. (1968). The prostaglandins: a
family of biologically active lipids. *Pharmacol. Rev.*, **20**:1–48.

Bergström, S., Danielsson, H., and Samuelsson, B. (1964). The enzymatic formation of prostaglandin E_2 from arachidonic acid. Prostaglandins and related
factors. *Biochim. Biophys. Acta*, **90**:207–210.

Bergström, S., Dressler, F., Krabisch, L., Ryhage, R., and Sjövall, J. (1962). The
isolation and structure of a smooth muscle stimulating factor in normal
sheep and pig lungs, Prostaglandins and related factors 9. *Arkiv. Kemi.*, **20**:
53–66.

Bito, L. Z. (1972). Accumulation and apparent active transport of prostaglandins
by some rabbit tissues in vitro. *J. Physiol.*, **221**:371–387.

Blackwell, G. J., Flower, R. J., and Vane, J. R. (1975). Studies on the prostaglandin synthesizing system in rabbit kidney microsomes. *Biochim. Biophys. Acta,* **398**:178–190.

Cammock, S. (1973). Conversion of PGE_1 to a PGA_1 like compound by rat kidney homogenates. In S. Bergström and S. Bernhard (eds.): Supplement to Advances in the Biosciences, vol. 9. International Conference on Prostaglandins, Vienna, Pergamon Press, Viewig, Braunschweig, p. 10.

Carlsson, L. A. and Oro, L. (1966). Effect of PGE_1 on blood pressure and heart rate in the dog. *Acta Physiol. Scand.,* **67**:89–99.

Cheung, H. S. and Cushman, D. W. (1972). Unpublished observations.

Christ, E. J. and van Dorp, D. A. (1972). Comparative aspects of prostaglandin biosynthesis in animal tissues. *Biochim. Biophys. Acta,* **270**:537–545.

Christ, E. J. and van Dorp, D. A. (1973). Comparative aspects of prostaglandin biosynthesis in animal tissue. In S. Bergström and S. Bernhard (eds.): Supplement to Advances in the Biosciences, vol. 9. International Conference on Prostaglandins, Vienna, Pergamon Press, Viewig, Braunschweig, pp. 35–38.

Collier, J. G. and Flower, R. J. (1971). Effect of aspirin on human seminal prostaglandins. *Lancet* **2**:852–853.

Crutchley, D. J. and Piper, P. J. (1973). Inhibition of the inactivation of prostaglandins in guinea pig lungs. *Naunyn Schmiedebergs Arch. Pharmakol.,* **279**:R20.

Crutchley, D. J. and Piper, P. J. (1974). Prostaglandin inactivation in guinea pig lung and its inhibition. *Br. J. Pharmacol.,* **52**:197–203.

Crutchley, D. J. and Piper, P. J. (1975). Inhibition of the pulmonary inactivation of prostaglandins in rabbit in vivo. *Br. J. Pharmacol.,* **53**:467P.

Cuthbert, M. F. (1971). Bronchodilator activity of aerosols of prostaglandins E_1 and E_2 in asthmatic subjects. *Proc. R. Soc. Med.,* **64**:15–16.

Cuthbert, M. F. (1973). Prostaglandins and respiratory smooth muscle. In M. F. Cuthbert (ed.): The Prostaglandins: Pharmacological and Therapeutic Advances. London, Heinemann, pp. 253–285.

Dawson, W., Lewis, R. L., MacMahon, R. E., and Sweatman, W. J. F. (1974). Potent bronchoconstrictor activity of 15-keto prostaglandin $F_{2\alpha}$. *Nature,* **250**:331–332.

Dawson, W., Ramwell, P. W. and Shaw, J. (1968). Metabolism of prostaglandins by rat isolated liver. *Br. J. Pharmacol.,* **34**:668–669.

Dawson, W. and Tomlinson, R. (1974). Effect of cromoglycate and eicosatetraynoic acid on the release of prostaglandins and SRS-A from immunologically challenged guinea pig lungs. *Br. J. Pharmacol.,* **52**:107–108.

Van Dorp, D. A. (1967). Aspects of the biosynthesis of prostaglandins. *Prog. Biochem. Pharmacol.,* **3**:71–82.

Van Dorp, D. A. (1971). Recent developments in the biosynthesis and analyses of prostaglandins. *Ann. N. Y. Acad. Sci.,* **180**:181–199.

Dray, F. and Charbonnel, B. (1974). Letter to the Editor. Radioimmunoassay of PGF_α in human plasma: Very low levels. *Prostaglandins,* **5**:173–174.

Edmonds, J. F., Berry, E., and Wyllie, J. H. (1969). Release of prostaglandins caused by distension of the lungs. *Br. J. Surg.,* **56**:622–623.

Fanburg, B. L. (1973). Prostaglandins and the lung. *Am. Rev. Resp. Dis.,* **108**: 482–489.

Ferreira, S. H. and Vane, J. R. (1967). Prostaglandins; their disappearance from and release into the circulation. *Nature,* **216**:868–873.

Ferreira, S. H. and Vane, J. R. (1973). Inhibition of Prostaglandin biosynthesis: an explanation of the therapeutic effects of nonsteroid anti-inflammatory agents. In *Seminar Inserm Prostaglandins.* Editions Inserm, Paris, pp. 345–357.

Ferreira, S. H. and Vane, J. R. (1974a). Aspirin and prostaglandins. In P. W. Ramwell (ed.): *The Prostaglandins,* vol. 2. Plenum Press, New York, pp. 1–47.

Ferreira, S. H. and Vane, J. R. (1974b). New aspects of the mode of action of non-steroid anti-inflammatory drugs. *Ann. Rev. Pharmacol.,* **14**:57–73.

Ferreira, S. H., Moncada, S., and Vane, J. R. (1971). Indomethacin and aspirin abolish prostaglandin release from the spleen. *Nature New Biol.,* **231**:237–239.

Fjalland, B. (1974). Inhibition by non-steroidal anti-inflammatory agents of the release of rabbit aorta contracting substance and prostaglandins from chopped guinea pig lungs. *J. Pharm. Pharmacol.,* **26**:448–451.

Flower, R. J. (1974). Drugs which inhibit prostaglandin biosynthesis. *Pharmacol. Rev.,* **26**:33–67.

Flower, R. J., Cheung, H. S., and Cushman, D. W. (1973). Quantitative determination of prostaglandins and malondialdehyde formed by the arachidonate oxygenase system of bovine seminal vesicle. *Prostaglandins,* **4**:325–341.

Flower, R. J., Gryglewski, R., Herbaczynska-Cedro, K., and Vane, J. R. (1972). The effects of anti-inflammatory drugs on prostaglandin biosynthesis. *Nature New Biol.,* **238**:104–106.

Flower, R. J. and Vane, J. R. (1972). Inhibition of prostaglandin synthetase in brain explains the anti-pyretic activity of paracetamol (4-acetamidophenol). *Nature (Lond.),* **240**:410–411.

Fried, J., Mehrer, M. M., and Gaede, B. J. (1973). Novel selective inhibitors of human placental PG-15-dehydrogenase. In S. Bergström and S. Bernhard (eds.): Supplement to Advances in the Biosciences, vol. 9. International Conference on Prostaglandins, Vienna, Pergamon Press, Viewig, Braunschweig, p. 18.

Gillis, C. N. (1973). Metabolism of vasoactive hormones by the lung. *Anesthesiology,* **39**:626–632.

Granström, E. (1971). Metabolism of prostaglandin $F_{2\alpha}$ in guinea pig lung. *Eur. J. Biochem.,* **20**:451–458.

Gréen, K., Hansson, E., and Samuelsson, B. (1967). *Prog. Biochem. Pharmacol.,* **3**:85–88.

Gréen, K. and Samuelsson, B. (1971). Quantitative studies on the synthesis in vivo of prostaglandins in the rat. Cold stress induced stimulation of synthesis. *Eur. J. Biochem.,* **22**:391–395.

Hamberg, M. (1972). Inhibition of prostaglandin synthesis in man. *Biochem. Biophys. Res. Commun.,* **49**:720–726.

Hamberg, M., Israelsson, U., and Samuelsson, B. (1971). Metabolism of prostaglandin E_2 in guinea pig liver. *Ann. N. Y. Acad. Sci.*, **180**:164–180.

Hamberg, M. and Samuelsson, B. (1967). On the mechanism of the biosynthesis of prostaglandins E_1 and $F_{1\alpha}$. *J. Biol. Chem.*, **242**:5336–5343.

Hamberg, M. and Samuelsson, B. (1971). On the metabolism of prostaglandins E_1 and E_2 in man. *J. Biol. Chem.*, **246**:6713–6721.

Hamberg, M. and Samuelsson, B. (1972). On the metabolism of prostaglandins E_1 and E_2 in the guinea pig. *J. Biol. Chem.*, **247**:3495–3502.

Hamberg, M. and Samuelsson, B. (1971). Metabolism of prostaglandin E_2 in guinea pig liver. 2. Pathways in the formation of the major metabolites. *J. Biol. Chem.*, **246**:1073–1077.

Hamberg, M. and Samuelsson, B. (1973). Detection and isolation of an endoperoxide intermediate in prostaglandin biosynthesis. *Proc. Natl. Acad. Sci. USA*, **70**:899–903.

Hamberg, M., Svensson, J., Wakabayashi, T., and Samuelsson, B. (1974). Isolation and structure of two prostaglandin endoperoxides that cause platelet aggregation. *Proc. Natl. Acad. Sci. USA*, **71**:345–349.

Hansen, H. S. (1974). Inhibition by indomethacin and aspirin of 15-hydroxy prostaglandin dehydrogenase in vitro. *Prostaglandins*, **8**:95–105.

Hansson, E. and Samuelsson, B. (1965). Autoradiographic distribution studies of ^{3}H-labeled prostaglandin E in mice: Prostaglandins and related factors 31. *Biochim. Biophys. Acta*, **106**:379–385.

Hauge, A., Lunde, P. K. M., and Waaler, B. A. (1967). Effects of prostaglandin E_1 and adrenaline on the pulmonary vascular resistance (PVR) in isolated rabbit lungs. *Life Sci.*, **6**:673–680.

Heinemann, H. O. and Fishman, A. P. (1969). Non-respiratory functions of mammalian lung. *Physiol. Rev.*, **49**:1–47.

Hinman, J. W. (1970). Prostaglandins: a report on early clinical studies. *Postgrad. Med. J.*, **46**:562–575.

Hinman, J. W. (1972). Prostaglandins. *Ann. Rev. Biochem.*, **41**:161–178.

Horton, E. W. (1969). Hypothesis on physiological roles of prostaglandins. *Physiol. Rev.*, **49**:122–161.

Horton, E. W. and Jones, R. L. (1969). Prostaglandins A_1, A_2 and 19-hydroxy A_1; their actions on smooth muscle and their inactivation on passage through the pulmonary and hepatic portal vascular beds. *Br. J. Pharmacol.*, **37**:705–722.

Horton, E. W., Jones, R. L., and Marr, G. G. (1973). Effects of aspirin on prostaglandin and fructose levels in human semen. *J. Reprod. Fert.*, **33**:385–392.

Horton, E. W., Jones, R., Thompson, C., and Poyser, N. (1971). Release of prostaglandins. *Ann. N. Y. Acad. Sci.*, **180**:351–362.

Horton, E. W., Maine, I. H. M., and Thompson, C. J. (1965). Effects of prostaglandins on the oviduct, studied in rabbits and ewes. *J. Physiol.*, **180**:514–528.

Hyman, A. L. (1968). Active responses in pulmonary veins. *Clin. Res.*, **16**:71.

Hyman, A. L. (1969). The active responses of pulmonary veins in intact dogs to prostaglandins $F_{2\alpha}$ and E_1. *J. Pharmacol. Exp. Ther.*, **165**:267–273.

Jackson, H. R., Hall, R. D., Hodge, R. L., Gibson, E. L., Katik, F. P., and
Stevens, M. (1973). The effect of aspirin on the pulmonary extraction of
$PGF_{2\alpha}$ and the cardiovascular response to $PGF_{2\alpha}$. *Aust. J. Exp. Biol. Med.
Sci.,* **51**:837–846.

Jarabak, J. (1972). Human placental 15-hydroxyprostaglandin dehydrogenase.
Proc. Natl. Acad. Sci. USA, **69**:533–534.

Jones, R. L. (1972). 15-hydroxy-9-oxoprosta-11, 13-dienoic acid as the product
of a prostaglandin isomerase. *J. Lipid. Res.,* **13**:511–518.

Jones, R. L. (1975). Actions of prostaglandins on the arterial system of the
sheep: some structure-activity relationships. *Br. J. Pharmacol.,* **53**:464P.

Karim, S. M. M., Sandler, M., and Williams, E. D. (1967). Distribution of prostaglandins in human tissues. *Br. J. Pharmacol.,* **31**:340–344.

Kessler, E., Hughes, R. C., Bennett, E. N., and Nadella, E. (1973). Evidence for the
presence of prostaglandin-like material in the plasma of dogs with endotoxin shock. *J. Lab. Clin. Med.,* **81**:85–94.

Kloeze, J. (1969). Relationship between chemical structures and platelet-aggre-
gation activity of prostaglandins. *Biochem. Biophys. Acta,* **187**:285–292.

Lands, W., Lee, R., and Smith, W. (1971). Factors regulating the biosynthesis of
various prostaglandins. *Ann. N. Y. Acad. Sci.,* **180**:107–122.

Lands, W. E. M. and Samuelsson, B. (1968). Phospholipid precursors of prostaglandins. *Biochim. Biophys. Acta,* **164**:426–429.

Lee, J. B., Crowshaw, K., Takman, B. H., and Attrep, K. A. (1967). The identification of prostaglandins E_2, $F_{2\alpha}$, and A_2 from rabbit kidney medulla.
Biochem. J., **105**:1251–1260.

Lee, R. E. (1974). The influence of psychotropic drugs on prostaglandin biosynthesis. *Prostaglandin,* **5**:63–68.

Liebig, R., Bernhauer, W., and Peskar, B. A. (1974). Release of prostaglandins, a
prostaglandin metabolite, slow-reacting substance and histamine from anaphylactic lungs, and its modification by catecholamines. *Naunyn Schmiedebergs Arch. Pharmacol.,* **284**:279–293.

Limas, C. J. and Cohn, N. H. (1973). Isolation and properties of myocardial
prostaglandin synthetase. *Cardiovasc. Res.,* **7**:623–628.

Leslie, C. A. and Levine, L. (1973). Evidence for the presence of a prostaglandin
E_2 – 9-keto reductase in rat organs. *Biochem. Biophys. Res. Commun.,*
52:717–724.

Marrazzi, M. A. and Andersen, N. H. (1974). Prostaglandin dehydrogenase. In
P. Ramwell (ed.): The Prostaglandins, vol. 2. Plenum Press, New York,
pp. 99–155.

Marrazzi, M. A. and Matschinsky, F. M. (1972). Properties of 15-hydroxyprosta-
glandin dehydrogenase: structural requirements for substrate binding.
Prostaglandins, **1**:373–388.

Marrazzi, M. A., Shaw, J. E., Tao, F. T., and Matschinsky, F. M. (1972). Reversibility of 15-hydroxy prostaglandin dehydrogenase from swine lung. *Prostaglandins,* **1**:389–395.

Mathé, A. A., Hedquist, P., and Holmgren, A. (1973). Bronchial hyperreactivity
to prostaglandin $F_{2\alpha}$ and histamine in patients with asthma. *Br. Med. J.,*
1:193–196.

McGiff, J. C., Terragno, N. A., Strand, J. C., Lee, J. B., Lonigro, A. J., and Ng, K. K. F. (1967). Selective passage of prostaglandins across the lung. *Nature*, 223:742–745.

Miyamoto, T., Yamamoto, S., and Hayaishi, O. (1974). Prostaglandin synthetase system-resolution into oxygenase and isomerase components. *Proc. Natl. Acad. Sci. USA*, 71:3645–3648.

Myazaki, E., Ishizawa, M., Simano, S., Syato, B., and Sakazami, T. (1967). Stimulatory action of prostaglandins on the rabbit duodenal muscle. In S. Bergstrom and B. Samuelsson (eds.): Prostaglandins, Proceedings of the second Nobel symposium, Stockholm, June 1967. Almqvist and Wicksell, Stockholm, Interscience, Publishers, Inc., New York, pp. 277.

Nakano, J. (1970a). Metabolism of Prostaglandin E_1 (PGE_1) in kidney and lung. *Fed. Proc.*, 29:746 (abstr. 2828).

Nakano, J. (1970b). Metabolism of prostaglandin E_1 in dog kidneys. *Br. J. Pharmacol.*, 40:317–325.

Nakano, J. (1971). Effects of the metabolites of prostaglandin E_1 of the systemic and peripheral circulation in dogs. *Proc. Soc. Exp. Biol. Med.*, 136:1265–1268.

Nakano, J., Änggård, E., and Samuelsson, B. (1969). 15-hydroxy-prostanoate dehydrogenase. Prostaglandins as substrates and inhibitors. *Eur. J. Biochem.*, 2:386–389.

Nakano, J. and Greenfield, L. J. (1970). Metabolic degradation of prostaglandin E_1 in human lungs and plasma. *J. Lab. Clin. Med.*, 76:1018.

Nakano, J. and Kessinger, J. M. (1970). Cardiovascular effects of the metabolites of prostaglandin E_1 (PGE_1) in dogs. *Clin. Res.*, 18:595.

Nakano, J. and Morsey, N. H. (1971). Beta-oxidation of prostaglandins E_1 and E_2 in rat lung and kidney homogenates. *Clin. Res.*, 19:142.

Nakano, J., Montague, B., and Darrow, B. (1971). Metabolism of prostaglandin E_1 in human plasma, uterus and placenta in swine ovary and in rat testicle. *Biochem. Pharmacol.*, 20:2512–2514.

Nakano, J. and Prancan, A. V. (1971). Metabolic degradation of prostaglandin E_1 in the rat plasma and in the rat brain, heart, lung, kidney and testicle homogenates. *J. Pharm. Pharmacol.*, 23:231–232.

Nakano, J. and Prancan, A. V. (1973). Metabolic degradation of prostaglandin E_1 in the lung and kidney of rats in endotoxin shock. *Proc. Soc. Exp. Biol. Med.*, 144:506–508.

Nissen, H. M. and Andersen, H. (1968). On the localization of a prostaglandin-dehydrogenase activity in the kidney. *Histo Chemie.*, 14:189–200.

Nissen, H. M. and Andersen, H. (1969). On the activity of prostaglandin dehydrogenase system in the kidney. A histochemical study during hydration-dehydration and salt-repletion salt-depletion. *Histo Chemie.*, 17:241–247.

Nugteren, D. H., Beerthuis, R. K., and Van Dorp, D. A. (1966). The enzymic conversion of all-*cis* 8, 14 eicosatrienoic acid into prostaglandin E_1. *Rec. Trav. Chim. Pays-Bas*, 85:405–419.

Nugteren, D. H. and Hazelhof, E. (1973). Isolation and properties of intermediates in prostaglandin biosynthesis. *Biochem. Biophys. Acta*, 326:448–461.

Oesterling, T. O., Morozowich, W., and Roseman, T. J. (1972). Prostaglandins. *J. Pharm. Sci.,* **61**:1861–1895.

Pace-Asciak, C. and Miller, D. (1973). Prostaglandins during development. I. age dependent activity profiles of prostaglandin 15 hydroxydehydrogenase and 13,14-reductase in lung tissue from late pre-natal, early post-natal and adult rats. *Prostaglandins,* **4**:351–362.

Palmer, M., Piper, P., and Vane, J. R. (1973). Release of rabbit aorta contracting substance (RCS) and prostaglandins induced by chemical or mechanical stimulation of guinea pig lungs. *Br. J. Pharmacol.,* **49**:226–242.

Parker, C. W. and Snider, D. E. (1973). Prostaglandins and asthma. *Ann. Intern. Med.,* **78**:963–965.

Parkinson, T. M. and Schneider, J. C. (1969). Absorption and metabolism of prostaglandin E_1 by perfused rat jejunum in vitro. *Biochem. Biophys. Acta,* **176**:78.

Parkes, D. G. and Eling, T. E. (1974). Characterization of prostaglandin synthetase in guinea pig lung. Isolation of a new prostaglandin derivative from arachidonic acid. *Biochemistry,* **13**:2598–2604.

Parrott, J. R. and Sturgess, R. M. (1974). Evidence that prostaglandin release mediates pulmonary vascular constriction induced by endotoxin. *J. Physiol.,* 84p.

Pike, J. E., Kupiecki, F. P., and Weeks, J. R. (1967). In S. Bergstrom and B. Samuelsson (eds.): *Prostaglandins, Nobel Symposium 2.* Interscience, New York, p. 21.

Piper, P. J. (1972). Distribution and metabolism. In M. F. Cuthbert (ed.): *The Prostaglandins, Pharmacological and Therapeutic Advances.* Heinemann Medical Books, London, pp. 125–150.

Piper, P. J. and Vane, J. R. (1969). Release of additional factors in anaphylaxis and its antagonism by anti-inflammatory drugs. *Nature,* **233**:29–35.

Piper, P. J., Vane, J. R., and Wyllie, J. H. (1970). Inactivation of prostaglandins by the lungs. *Nature,* **225**:600–604.

Piper, P. J. and Vane, J. R. (1971). The release of prostaglandins from lung and other tissues. *Ann. N. Y. Acad. Sci.,* **180**:363–385.

Piper, P. J. and Walker, J. L. (1973). The release of spasmogenic substances from human chopped lung tissue and its inhibition. *Br. J. Pharmacol.,* **47**:291–304.

Ramwell, P. W. and Shaw, J. E. (1970). Biological significance of the prostaglandins. *Rec. Prog. Hormone Res.,* **26**:139–187.

Ryan, J. W., Niemeyer, R. S., and Goodwin, D. W. (1972). Metabolic rates of bradykinin, angiotensin I, adenine nucleotides and prostaglandins E_1 and $F_{1\alpha}$ in the pulmonary circulation. *Adv. Exp. Med. Biol.,* **21**:259–265.

Saeed, S. A. and Roy, A. C. (1972). Purification of 15-hydroxy prostaglandin dehydrogenase from bovine lung. *Biochem. Biophys. Res. Commun.,* **47**:96–102.

Said, S. I. (1968). Some respiratory effects of prostaglandins E_2 and $F_{2\alpha}$. In P. W. Ramwell and J. R. Shaw (eds.): Prostaglandin Symposium of the Worcester Foundation for Experimental Biology. Interscience, New York, pp. 267–289.

Said, S. I. (1973). The lung in relation to hormones. *Resp. Care,* **18**:722–730.

Samuelsson, B. (1964). Indentification of prostaglandin $F_{3\alpha}$ in bovine lung: prostaglandins and related factors 26. *Biochim. Biophys. Acta,* **84**:707–713.

Samuelsson, B. (1969). Biosynthesis of prostaglandins. *Prog. Biochem. Pharmacol.,* **5**:109–128.

Samuelsson, B. (1970). Structures, biosynthesis and metabolism of prostaglandins. In S. Wakil (ed.): *Lipid Metabolism.* Academic Press, New York, London, pp. 107–153.

Samuelsson, B. (1972). Biosynthesis of prostaglandins. *Fed. Proc.,* **31**:1442–1450.

Samuelsson, B., Granström, E., and Hamberg, M. (1967). On the mechanism of biosynthesis of prostaglandins. In S. Bergström and B. Samuelsson (eds.): *Prostaglandins, Nobel Symposium 2.* Interscience, New York, p. 21.

Samuelsson, B., Granström, E., Gréen, K., and Hamberg, M. (1971). Metabolism of prostaglandins. *Ann. N. Y. Acad. Sci.,* **180**:138–163.

Samuelsson, B. and Hamberg, M. (1974). Role of endoperoxides in the biosynthesis and action of prostaglandins. In H. J. Robinson and J. R. Vane (eds.): *Prostaglandin Synthetase Inhibitors.* Raven Press, New York, pp. 107–119.

Sander, G. E. and Huggins, C. G. (1971). Subcellular localization of angiotensin I converting enzyme in rabbit lung. *Nature, New Biol.,* **230**:27–29.

Sandler, M. (1972). Migraine, a pulmonary disease? *The Lancet,* 618–619.

Scarnes, R. C. and Harper, M. J. K. (1972). Relationship between endotoxin induced abortion and synthesis of prostaglandin F. *Prostaglandins,* **1**:191–203.

Schlegel, W., Demers, L. M., Hildebrandt-Stark, H. E., Behrmann, H. R., and Greep, R. O. (1974). Partial purification of human placental 15-hydroxyprostaglandin dehydrogenase. Kinetic properties. *Prostaglandins,* **5**:417–433.

Schoenemann, D., Ellermann, J., and Matschinsky, F. M. (1974). An improved procedure for the enzymatic analysis of prostaglandins in the nanogram range, quoted in: Marrazzi and Andersen 1974.

Shio, H., Ramwell, P. W., Andersen, N. A., and Corey, E. J. (1970). Stereospecificity of the prostaglandin 15-dehydrogenase from swine lung. *Experientia,* **26**:335–357.

Sih, C. J., and Takeguchi, C. A. (1973). In P. W. Ramwell (ed.): *Biosynthesis in the Prostaglandins,* chap. 3. Plenum Press, New York, London, pp. 83–100.

Smith, A. P. (1971). Response of aspirin-allergic patients to challenge by some analgesics in common use. *Br. Med. J.,* **2**:494–496.

Smith, M. J. H. and Dawkins, P. D. (1971). Salicylate and enzymes. *J. Pharm. Pharmacol.,* **23**:729–744.

Smith, J. B. and Willis, A. L. (1971). Aspirin selectively inhibits prostaglandin production in human platelets. *Nature, New Biol.,* **231**:235–237.

Strong, C. J. and Bohr, D. F. (1967). Effects of prostaglandin E_1, E_2, A_1 and F_1 on isolated vascular smooth muscle. *Am. J. Physiol.,* **213**:725–733.

Sun, D. D. (1974). Metabolism of prostaglandin $F_{2\alpha}$ in the rat. *Biochem. Biophys. Acta,* **348**:249–262.

Sun, F. F. and Armour, S. B. (1974). Prostaglandin 15-hydroxy dehydrogenase and 13 reductase levels in the lungs of maternal fetal, and neonatal rabbits. *Prostaglandins*, 7:327–338.

Sweatman, W. J. F. and Collier, H. O. J. (1968). Effects of prostaglandins on human bronchial muscle. *Nature*, 217:69.

Tierney, D. F. (1974). Lung metabolism and biochemistry. *Ann. Rev. Physiol.*, 36:209–231.

Vane, J. R. (1970). The alteration or removal of vasoactive substances by the pulmonary circulation. In T. H. Tedeschi and R. E. Tedeschi (eds.): Importance of Fundamental Principles in Drug Evaluation. Raven Press, New York, pp. 217–235.

Vane, J. R. (1969). The release and fate of vasoactive hormones in the circulation. *Br. J. Pharmacol.*, 35:209–242.

Vane, J. R. (1971). Inhibition of prostaglandin synthesis as mechanism of action for aspirin-like drugs. *Nature, New Biol.*, 231:232–235.

Vargaftig, B. B. and Dao Hai, N. (1971). Selective inhibition by mepacrine of the release of "rabbit aorta contracting substance" evoked by the administration of bradykinin. *J. Pharm. Pharmacol.*, 24:159–161.

Vonkeman, H., Nugteren, D. H., and Van Dorp, D. A. (1969). The action of prostaglandin 15-hydroxy dehydrogenase on various prostaglandins. *Biochim. Biophys. Acta*, 187:581–583.

Weeks, J. R. (1972). Prostaglandins. *Annu. Rev. Pharmacol.*, 12:317–336.

5

Uptake, Accumulation, and Metabolism of Chemicals by the Lung

RICHARD M. PHILPOT, MARSHALL W. ANDERSON,
and THOMAS E. ELING

National Institute of Environmental Health Sciences
Research Triangle Park, North Carolina

I. Introduction

Investigations of the pharmacokinetics of drugs and chemicals, i.e., the absorption, distribution, metabolism, and excretion of chemicals in animals, have often overlooked the lung as an organ of importance. In recent years, the lung's ability to metabolize chemicals has been investigated and this is discussed in detail later in this chapter. However, the lung's ability to concentrate and store chemicals has received little attention. Our purpose is not to review all literature on this subject (see recent review, Brown 1974) but to bring together information on the mechanisms responsible for the accumulation of chemicals in the lung and to discuss the toxicologic implications of such accumulations.

II. Accumulation of Chemicals by Lung

An examination of the chemicals and drugs that preferentially accumulate in the lung, resulting in high tissue-to-blood concentration ratios, reveals a wide diversity of chemical structures and pharmacologic or biologic activities (Table 1). Chemicals with biologic activity, which accumulate in the lung, include antihistamines, CNS-active drugs, such as narcotics and antidepressants, and herbicides, such as paraquat, which induce lung damage (Clark et al. 1966, Robertson et al. 1971). A careful examination of the chemical structures of such compounds indicates that, except for the herbicide paraquat, all chemicals listed in Table 1 are amines with pK_as greater than 8. These chemicals will be referred to as *basic amines,* to differentiate them from amines with pK_as less than 8. Furthermore, some of these basic amines also contain large hydrophobic moities.

Cyclizine, chlorcyclizine, diphenhydramine, tripelennamine, fluphenazine, chlorpromazine, promazine, imipramine, desipramine, methadone, propranolol, and chlorphentermine can be considered amphiphilic compounds, compounds that contain both a large hydrophobic region and a group ionized at physiologic pH. Amphetamine and its derivatives, listed in Table 1, are lipophilic basic amines but should not be considered amphiphilic chemicals. The herbicide paraquat is a dipyridyl derivative and should not be considered a basic amine. Differences in the chemical structures of the basic amines may provide a clue to mechanisms responsible for the localization of these compounds in the lung. The time course for the uptake and release of basic amines by the lung is different for each compound. For example, 1 hr after injection, the concentration ratio (tissue-to-blood) of chlorphentermine in the lung (Table 1) was 53 compared to a concentration ratio of 40 for phentermine. However, 24 hr after injection, the concentration ratio of chlorphentermine had decreased to 30, while the concentration ratio of phentermine had decreased to 3. This illustrates that investigation of the localization of basic amines in the lung must be considered from two standpoints, accumulation and persistence. The mechanisms responsible for the accumulation and persistence of basic amines in the lung may be different and may be important in relating localization of basic amines to chemically induced toxicities.

A. Mechanisms of Uptake, Accumulation, and Persistence

Many basic amines accumulate and persist in lung tissue. Mechanisms responsible for this have been studied primarily in isolated, perfused lung (IPL) preparations. The IPL is perhaps the best system available for examining these mechanisms, since organ interactions inherent in in vivo studies are eliminated, while the physiologic functions and biochemical integrity of the lung are either maintained or can be simulated. The results we have obtained, using the IPL for the study of the mechanisms by which basic amines accumulate and persist in the lung, are presented in the following section.

TABLE 1 Accumulation of Chemicals by the Lung

Chemical	Lung/blood concentration ratio	Species	References
Antihistamines			
Cyclizine	112(4)[a]	Rat	Kuntzman et al. 1965
Chlorcyclizine	107(3)	Rat	Kuntzman et al. 1965
Diphenhydramine	100(1)	Guinea pig	Glazko et al. 1949
Tripelennamine	17(1)	Rat	Way et al. 1950
Antipsychotics			
Fluphemazine	100(19)	Dog	Dreyfuss et al. 1971
Tricyclic antidepressants			
Imipramine	150(10),10(24)	Rabbit	Wilson et al. (unpublished observation)
Desimpramine	400(10),20(24)	Rabbit	Wilson et al. (unpublished observation)
Desimpramine	400(2),150(12)	Rat	Bickel and Weder 1968
Anorectic drugs			
Chlorphentermine	53(1),30(24)	Rat	Lullmann et al. 1973b
Phentermine	40(1), 3(24)	Rat	Lullmann et al. 1973b
Amphetamines			
Amphetamine	33(1)	Rat	Fuller et al. 1973b
β-monofluoramphetamine	20(1)	Rat	Fuller et al. 1973b
β,β-difluoramphetamine	4(1)	Rat	Fuller et al. 1973b
Chloramphetamine	30(1)	Rat	Fuller et al. 1973a
Analgesics			
Methadone	100(3)	Rat	Richards et al. 1950
β-Adrenergic blocking agents			
Propranolol	25(1/2)	Monkey	Hayes and Cooper, 1971
Propranolol	125(1)	Rabbit	Black et al. 1965
KO 592	44(2)	Rat	Stock and Westerman 1965
Herbicide			
Paraquat	4(1),14(32)	Rat	Sharp et al. 1972

[a]Numbers in parentheses are hours after injection.

Uptake

Carrier-mediated, sodium-dependent transport systems in the lung remove 5-hydroxytryptamine (5-HT) and noradrenaline from the pulmonary circulation (Bakhle and Vane 1974). It is possible that some exogenous basic amines are also removed from the circulation by these transport systems and accumulated in the lung in concentrations in excess of those found in blood. Rates of removal of basic amines from the circulation into the lung were measured in the IPL for imipramine, methadone, and amphetamine over wide perfusate concentration ranges. For methadone and imipramine, the unidirectional flux of the chemical into the lung was equal to the rate at which the chemical was supplied to the lung (perfusate conc. × flow rate, Fig. 1; Wilson et al. 1976). These results suggest that imipramine and methadone are not removed from the

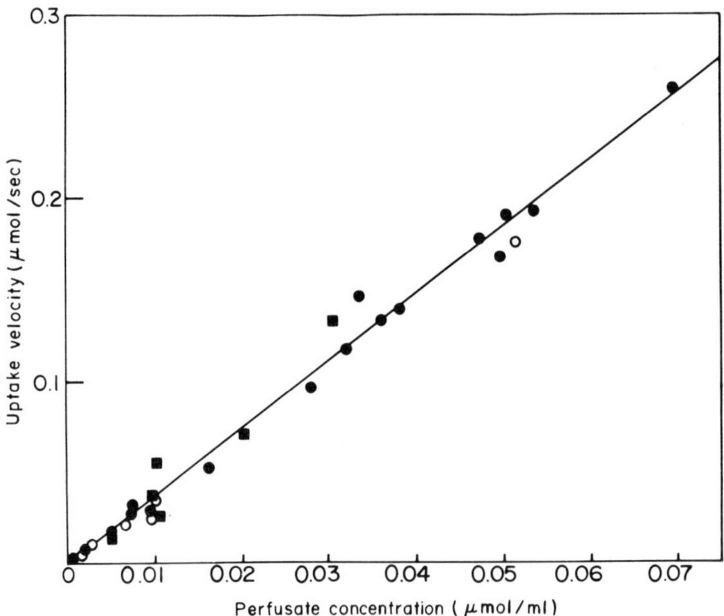

FIGURE 1   The concentration dependence of the velocity of [^{14}C] methadone accumulation in isolated perfused lungs. The vertical axis is the velocity of [^{14}C] methadone uptake (μmol/sec); the horizontal axis is the perfusate concentration (μmol/ml). Racemic methadone (●) (n = 18); D-methadone (■) (n = 8); and L-methadone (○) (n = 6). The line was obtained by least squares regression analysis of all points. Slope = 3.7; correlation coefficient = 0.99. For clarity some data points have been omitted (Reprinted by permission from Wilson et al. (1976). *J. Pharmacol. Exp. Thera.,* **199**:360–367.

circulation by a carrier-mediated transport system. It appears that imipramine and methadone diffuse into the lung and accumulate there as a result of binding. In contrast to imipramine and methadone, one component of the removal of amphetamine by lung tissue was saturable with respect to perfusate concentration, suggesting the presence of a carrier-mediated transport process in the lung (Eling and Anderson, unpublished observation). This type of relationship between the rate of removal and the perfusate concentration was also observed in the IPL with 5-HT (Pickett et al. 1975). The existence of a transport system in lung tissue for 5-HT has been confirmed by several independent investigations (Bakhle and Vane 1974). Because of structural similarities, amphetamine may be accumulated in lung tissue by the noradrenaline transport system.

The herbicide paraquat is known to accumulate in lung tissue and to cause pulmonary edema. From studies with rat lung slices, Rose et al. (1974) proposed that paraquat is accumulated by means of a carrier-mediated transport system. The rate of removal of paraquat by the lung is very slow in comparison to chemicals such as imipramine or 5-HT. Whereas greater than 50% of these chemicals are removed in a single pass through the pulmonary circulation, less than 0.5% of paraquat is removed at the same pulmonary arterial perfusate concentration (Pickett et al. 1975, Eling et al. 1975, Orton et al. 1973, Wilson et al., unpublished observation). Using IPLs of rats and rabbits, we are currently investigating the mechanism(s) responsible for the removal of paraquat and the related herbicide diquat by lung. These mechanisms could help explain the differences between the toxicities of these compounds, paraquat being toxic while diquat is not, and the species differences in the toxicity of paraquat.

Accumulation

Steady-state accumulations of various basic and nonbasic amines were measured in the IPL. Table 2 shows that the steady-state concentrations of the basic amines are much greater than those of the nonbasic amines. The steady-state accumulation of the nonbasic amines imidazole, promazine, and aniline was linearly related to the perfusate concentration, with tissue-to-blood ratios of approximately 1. In contrast, the accumulation of the basic amines, imipramine, methadone, amphetamine, and chlorcyclizine was curvilinearly related to the perfusate concentration, with tissue-to-blood ratios exceeding 200 at the lower perfusate concentrations (Anderson et al. 1974). This clearly suggests that specific mechanisms exist for the accumulation of basic, but not nonbasic, amines in the lung.

TABLE 2   Steady-state Accumulation of Various Compounds in the Isolated Perfused Rabbit Lung

Drug	Accumulation[a]		
	μmol/g	μmol/organ	Percentage of dose
Imipramine	0.27 ± 0.02 [6]	2.80 ± 0.14 [6]	93.3 ± 2.6 [6]
Amphetamine	0.24 ± 0.01 [6]	2.23 ± 0.11 [6]	74.4 ± 3.5 [6]
Methadone	0.27 ± 0.04 [3]	2.43 ± 0.11 [3]	81.0 ± 2.0 [3]
Chlorcyclizine	0.28 ± 0.27 [3]	2.74 ± 0.04 [3]	91.4 ± 1.2 [3]
Imidazole	0.05 ± 0.01 [3]	0.48 ± 0.09 [3]	16.1 ± 2.1 [3]
Aniline		0.30–0.65[b]	<20[b] [3]
Prometone		0.25–0.50[b]	<15[b] [2]
Propazine		0.25–0.50[b]	<15[b] [2]

[a] After a 10-min equilibration period, 3 μmol of drug were added to the reservoir of the perfused lung preparation. The accumulation at steady state, usually after 60 min perfusion, was determined from time-dependent uptake curves. Results are expressed as mean ± SD. Numbers in brackets refer to the number of experiments.
[b] Tubing uptake prevented more quantitative determination. The values are an approximation obtained by subtracting tubing uptake from apparent lung uptake. (Reproduced with permission from Orton et al. (1973), *J. Pharmacol. Exp. Ther.*, **186**:482–497.

The steady-state accumulation of basic amines in the lung consisted of a saturable and a nonsaturable component (Fig. 2, Anderson et al. 1974). The magnitude of the nonsaturable (linear) component was too large to be accounted for solely by diffusion into the extracellular space. These components were further examined by determining the rates of efflux of accumulated chemicals into chemical-free perfusate. Figure 3 shows the variation with time of the rate of [^{14}C]imipramine efflux from the lung into the perfusate. This decay curve was resolved into the sum of three exponential functions (Fig. 3, Eling et al. 1975). This suggests that at least three distinct pools of accumulated imipramine exist in lung tissue. By integrating these rate expressions, it can be shown that the linear component of *accumulation* (Fig. 2) corresponds to the two components of efflux that have short half-lives, 18 and 58 sec. It is suggested that this component of accumulation represents partitioning of imipramine into cellular membranes bathed by extracellular fluids. The component of efflux that has the longest half-life, ~8 min, is included in the saturable component of accumulation in Figure 2. It can be further demonstrated that this component of efflux consists of two distinct types of binding and we argue that this binding is intracellular (Eling et al. 1975). Similar conclusions can be drawn concerning the nature of methadone accumulation in lung tissue (Wilson et al. 1976).

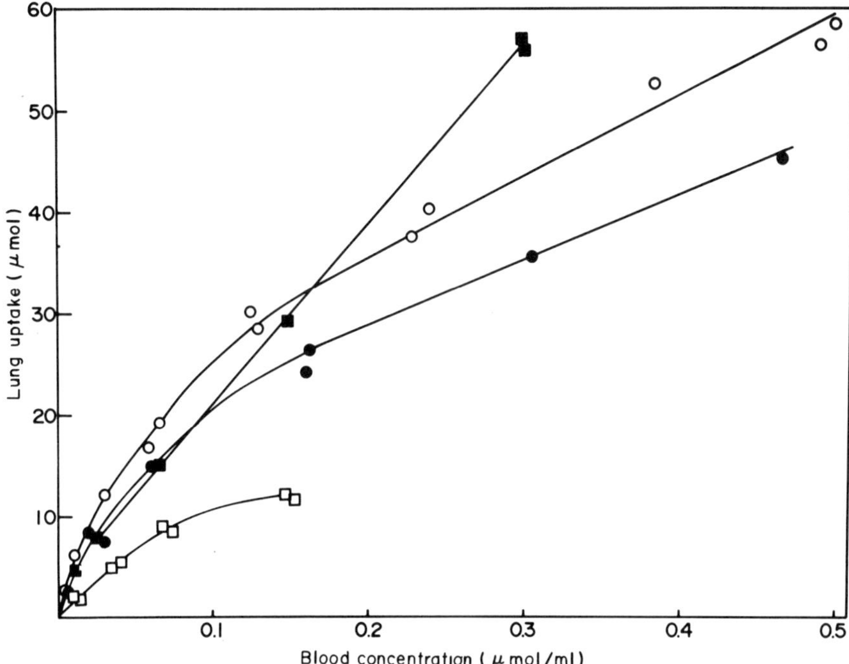

FIGURE 2 The relationship at steady state between lung accumulation (UL) and blood concentration (CB). On the ordinate is accumulation (μmol); on the abscissa is blood concentration (μmol/ml). Each curve was constructed from the results of at least 16 animals. Curves were obtained by a nonlinear regression analysis, with the formula UL = mC_B + (UL'$_{max}$ · C_B)/(K + C_B). For clarity, some points have been omitted from the figure. $\square$ = amphetamine; ● methadone; ■ = chlorcyclizines; ○ = imipramine. (Reprinted by permission from Anderson, M. W. et al. (1974). *J. Pharmacol. Exp. Ther.*, **189**:456–466.)

Persistence

For imipramine and methadone, the amount of chemical remaining in the lung during an efflux study appears to approach a constant value (Fig. 4, Law et al. 1976, Eling et al. 1975). Thus, a portion of the chemical accumulated in the IPL appears to be in a noneffluxable or persistent pool. This persistent pool is not observed with amphetamine. We have also shown that the persistent pool is formed in vivo after a single intravenous dose of imipramine in the rabbit and that it decays biphasically with half-lives of approximately 1 and 10 hr.

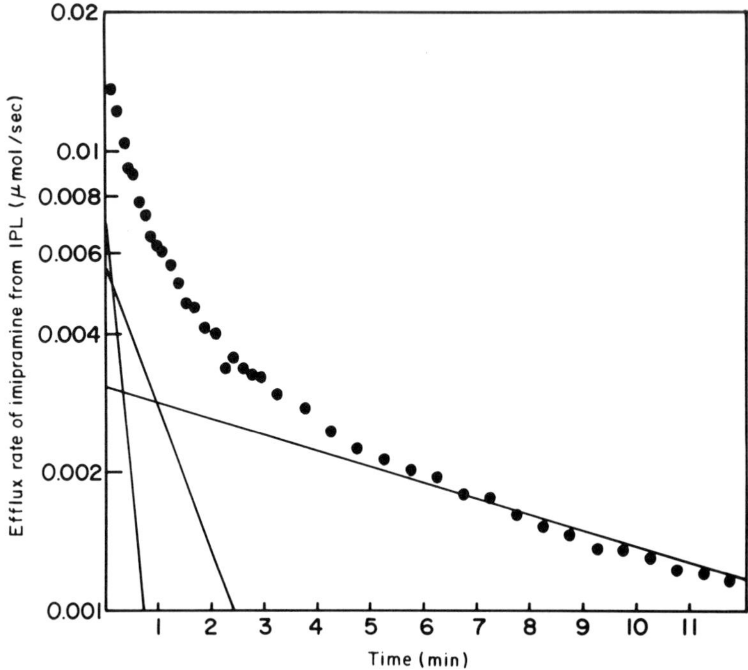

FIGURE 3   Variation with time of efflux rate of [^{14}C]imipramine from isolated perfused rabbit lung.   The vertical axis is the efflux rate (on logarithmic
scale) (μmol/sec) after infusion of [^{14}C]imipramine into pulmonary artery at
a concentration of 0.0048 μmol/ml.   Solid lines represent exponential components obtained by nonlinear regression analysis.   (Reprinted by permission
from Eling, T. E. et al. (1975). *Drug Metab. Disposition,* **3**:389–400.)

Irreversible binding of imipramine (or methadone) to tissue is not responsible for the persistent pool.   We have speculated that the persistent pool
could result from the formation of an imipramine-surfactant complex.   The
lipophilic character and existence of a positively charged nitrogen atom on
imipramine at physiologic pH suggest that an interaction between the amphiphilic phospholipid and imipramine is likely.   This would explain why the
molecules with amphiphilic character, imipramine and methadone, form a persistent pool, whereas amphetamine does not.

To summarize, basic amines are accumulated in lung tissue by a multicomponent accumulation system.   The high tissue-to-blood concentration
ratios result from several types of binding.   Partitioning (linear relationship between steady-state tissue concentration and blood concentration) and a more
specific type of binding with a limited capacity are both exhibited (Fig. 2).

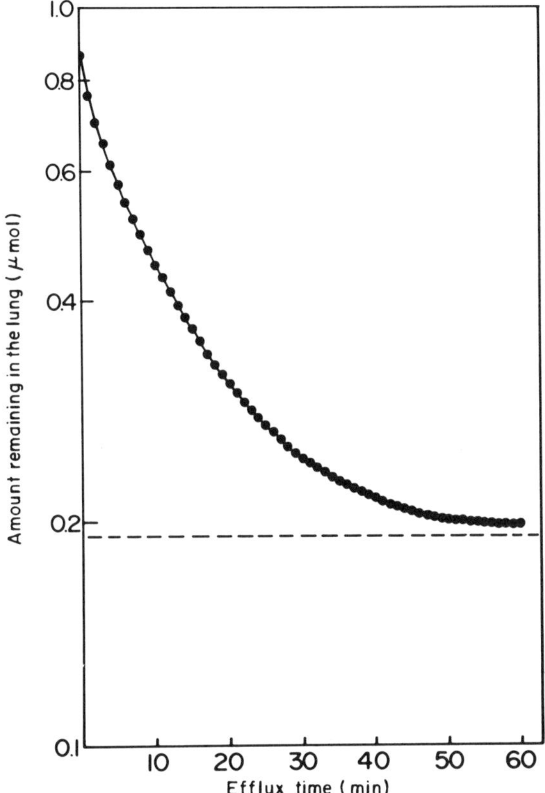

FIGURE 4   Time dependence of imipramine efflux from isolated perfused rabbit lung. Lungs were infused with imipramine at a concentration of 0.0048 μmol/ml for 8 min, and the efflux of accumulated imipramine examined after infusion ceased. On the vertical axis is the amount of [^{14}C] imipramine in the lung. On the horizontal axis is the time of efflux. (Reprinted by permission from Eling, T. E. et al. (1975). *Drug Metab. Disposition,* **3**:389–400.)

Basic amines with amphiphilic character tend to have higher tissue-to-blood concentration ratios than do other basic amines. In contrast to the endogenous amines, a carrier-mediated transport system is not involved in the removal and accumulation of the basic amines studied except for amphetamine.

The noneffluxable pool observed in the IPL could be responsible for the persistence of basic amines in lung tissue (Fig. 4, Wilson et al. 1976, Eling et al. 1975). This pool is formed in vivo. It appears that only those basic amines with amphiphilic character form this pool. Table 3 summarizes the mechanisms of accumulation for some of the basic amines studied.

TABLE 3 Summary of Mechanisms of Accumulation in Lung Tissue
(Measured in Isolated Perfused Lungs)

Chemical	Mechanisms of accumulation	Persistence	Metabolism
Methadone	Diffusion and binding	$t_{1/2}$ = 0.4, 1.65, and 8.9 min and 'noneffluxable' pool (approx 30% of total accumulated).	Metabolism by MFO
Imipramine	Diffusion and binding	$t_{1/2}$ = 0.3, 1.0, and 8.25 min and 'noneffluxable' pool (approx 30% of total accumulated).	None detectable
5-HT	Carrier-mediated sodium dependent transport	$t_{1/2}$ = 0.3 and 5.4 min	Extensively degraded by MAO
Amphetamine	Carrier-mediated transport and binding	$t_{1/2}$ = 0.1, 0.4, and 3.0 min	Possibly a small amount

The fact that neither the highly lipophilic nonionized amines nor the hydrophilic nonionized amines accumulate in lung tissue indicates that the charge on the nitrogen is a prerequisite for accumulation (Table 2). For a series of fluorinated amphetamine derivatives, accumulation in the lung was more dependent upon the degree of protonation than upon lipophilic properties (Anderson et al. 1974). Distribution studies with phenothiazines, by Huang et al. (1970), demonstrated that tertiary amines accumulate in lung tissue, whereas their quaternary ammonium derivatives do not. These observations suggest that the uptake of basic amines depends not only on the charge but also on the protonation of the nitrogen atom.

B. Toxicity from Accumulation and Persistence of Chemicals in Lung

Chemically-Induced Pulmonary Phospholipidosis

Chronic injection into or feeding animals a number of amphiphilic drugs produces a condition, particularly in the lung, termed *drug-induced phospholipidosis* (Lüllmann-Rauch et al. 1973a). This condition is characterized by an increase in lung phospholipids (Schmien et al. 1974) and the appearance of *foamy cells* in the lung (Lüllmann-Rauch et al. 1973a). Table 4 is a partial list of chemicals that induce phospholipidosis in lung tissue. The most studied

TABLE 4   Chemicals That Induce Lung Phospholipidosis

Chemical	Animal	Reference
Chlorphentermine	Guinea pig, mouse, rabbit, rat	Lüllmann-Rauch et al. 1973a Lüllmann-Rauch & Reil 1974
Triparanol	Rat	Lüllmann et al. 1973a
AY-9944	Rat	Kikkawa and Suzuki 1972
Chlorcyclizine	Rat	Hruban et al. 1973
4,4'-diethyl amino-ethoxyhexstrol	Rat, man	Shikata et al. 1972
Iprindole	Rat	Vijeyaratnam and Corrin 1972
l-chloroamitryptyline	Rat	Theiss et al. 1973
Imipramine	Rat	Lüllmann-Rauch et al. 1973a
Chloripramine	Rat	Lüllmann-Rauch et al. 1973a
Chloroquine	Rat	Hruban et al. 1973

inducer of phospholipidosis in the lung is the drug chlorphentermine. The persistence of chlorphentermine in lung and the induction of phospholipidosis appear to be related. Chlorphentermine persists in lung and increases lung phospholipids, while the structurally similar phentermine does not persist and does not produce phospholipidosis (Lüllmann et al. 1973b). Chlorphentermine interacts with phospholipid, while phentermine does not as shown by NMR spectroscopy (Seydel and Wassermann 1973), using synthetic lecithin.

After treatment with chlorphentermine, the total phospholipid of rat lung increased threefold (Schmien et al. 1974). The phospholipid in lung appears as lamellated inclusion bodies in alveolar epithelial cells, vascular endothelial cells, smooth muscle cells, bronchiolar epithelium, and in alveolar macrophages. Type II alveolar epithelial cells did not show significant increases in lamellated bodies (Lüllmann-Rauch and Reil 1974). The phospholipid content of alveolar macrophages isolated from chlorphentermine-treated rats was increased by 70% (Schmien et al. 1974). In addition, the concentrations of phosphatidyl ethanolamine and phosphatidyl serine were markedly elevated, while the relative content of phosphatidyl choline was unchanged (Schmien et al. 1974).

Mechanism(s) that account for the observed accumulation of phospholipids in lung remain obscure. We think there is a relationship between phospholipidosis and the formation of the noneffluxable pool found for imipramine and methadone in IPL. Our interpretation is as follows: (a) these amphiphilic chemicals interact with phospholipid in the lung to form micelles with specific chemical to lipid ratios. Of particular importance is the association of chemical with phospholipid secreted by the type II cell into the alveolar space (Buckingham et al. 1966). (b) These chemical-phospholipid micelles are not degraded by enzymes responsible for the degradation of surfactant and thus lipids are engulfed by lung macrophages. It is also possible that macrophages are the normal means of removing phospholipid from the alveolus and thus nondigestable phospholipids accumulate in macrophages.

Lecithin and imipramine have been shown to form micelles with a specific chemical-to-lecithin ratio in vitro (Bickel and Minder 1970). In addition, the ratio of chlorphentermine to phospholipid in the lung appears to be constant during continuous feeding with chlorphentermine (Lüllmann-Rauch, personal communication).

Further experimental evidence is needed to fully understand and evaluate the relationship of persistence of basic amines in the lung to phospholipidosis.

Inhibition of Pulmonary Detoxication
of Vasoactive Substances

The accumulation of basic amines in lung could alter ability to metabolize (both activate and detoxify) vasoactive substances (see review by Bakhle and Vane 1974). Alteration of these metabolic systems could change concentrations of vasoactive substances in venous blood. Increased concentrations of 5-HT or noradrenaline in venous blood would result in direct effects on the cardiovascular system. Imipramine (Roth and Gillis 1974) and iprindole (Roth and Gillis 1975) are inhibitors of lung MAO, and thus can prevent the metabolic degradation of 5-HT and NE by the lung.

Cardiovascular toxicities have been reported for various tricyclic antidepressants (Thorstrand 1974) and frequent cardiovascular complications have been seen in poisoning by antidepressants. Pulmonary hypertension observed with the use of the anorexic drug Amorex can be related to inhibition of the detoxication of vasoactive substances by the lung (Fishman 1974). The effect that accumulated amines have on other nonrespiratory functions has received little attention but deserves more study in view of the serious toxicity (both acute and chronic) that may result.

Pulmonary Toxicity of Paraquat

Toxicity produced by paraquat is characterized by lung fibrosis and death (Clark et al. 1966, Robertson et al. 1971). This toxicity appears to be related to both accumulation of paraquat in the lung and the generation of lipid peroxidation. Several investigators (Sharp et al. 1972, Murray and Gibson 1972) have reported that high concentrations of paraquat are found in the lung and that paraquat is accumulated in the lung by a carrier-mediated system (Rose et al. 1974). The mechanism by which the accumulated paraquat exerts its toxic effect is unclear, but lipid peroxidation may be involved (Bus et al. 1974). It has been proposed that paraquat is converted into a free radical that initiates the process of lipid peroxidation (Bus et al. 1974). Other dipyridyls, diquat and morfamquat, also produce free radicals (Baldwin et al. 1975) and damage to the lens of the eye (diquat) and kidney tubules (morfamquat) rather than to the lung. However, neither diquat nor morfamquat appears to accumulate in lung tissue (Smith and Rose, unpublished observation) and thus the selectivity of these toxicants may be related to selective accumulation. The role of accumulation in the mechanism of pulmonary damage by paraquat requires further study.

III. Metabolism of Chemicals by Lung Tissue

A. Cytochrome P-450-Dependent Mixed Function Oxidase System

The oxidative metabolism of a multitude of xenobiotics is now recognized as a requisite step in the biologic process responsible for the conversion of hydrophobic compounds into excretable products. This process has received a great deal of attention during the past 20 years, the majority of which has been directed towards the study of the oxidative metabolism of drugs by the liver (Estabrook et al. 1972, Fouts 1971, Gillette 1963, 1966, 1971, Gillette et al. 1957, 1969, 1972, La Du et al. 1971, Parke 1968, Williams 1959). It has been clearly established that the liver has the ability to metabolize oxidatively an astounding variety of compounds; a determination that has been instrumental in the understanding of drug interactions and disposition. Because it was also determined that the oxidative metabolites of most foreign compounds are relatively inactive, the oxidative process was generally characterized as a detoxication system.

It was soon realized, however, that the oxidative metabolism of certain compounds could have deleterious consequences, not due to a malfunction or alteration of the system but rather to the production of metabolites more active than the parent compounds. It is now hypothesized that oxidative metabolism is responsible for the activation of many carcinogenic, mutagenic, and necrosis-causing compounds. At present, the toxication aspect of the metabolism of xenobiotics, an unavoidable result of the nonspecificity of the oxidative process, is receiving as much, if not more, attention than detoxication.

Increased interest in the oxidative metabolism of xenobiotics in tissues other than the liver, particularly tissues that serve as targets for the action of activated metabolites, has resulted from the realization that drug metabolism is not wholly an innocuous process. In addition, the identification of numerous compounds in the environment which are candidates for metabolic activation, has led to an expanded effort directed toward the study of tissues associated with *portals of entry*. It is not surprising, therefore, that study of the oxidative metabolism of foreign compounds in the lung, a target and portal of entry tissue, has become the primary concern of a number of investigators.

Characteristics and Components

In the past few years it has become evident that a pulmonary mixed-function oxidase (MFO) system with the ability to metabolize oxidatively a variety of compounds exists in a number of species (see Table 5 for details) and that the

TABLE 5   The Metabolism of Various Compounds by Pulmonary Mixed-function Oxidase Systems from Various Species and a Comparison of Activities with those Obtained Using Hepatic Mixed-function Oxidase Systems

Substrate	Reaction	Species	Tissue fractions utilized	Ratio of activities (liver/lung)	References
Acetophenetidin	Hydroxylation	Rat	Homogenate	8.1 (per gm tissue)	Welch et al. 1972
Aminopyrene	N-Demethylation	Rabbit	Microsomes	2.5, 3.3 (per mg protein)	Bend et al. 1972; Hook et al. 1972[b]
		Rat	Microsomes	25 (per mg protein)	Oppelt et. al. 1970
		Rat	9000g S	10 (per mg protein)	Klinger, 1973
		Guinea pig	Microsomes	10 (per mg protein)	Oppelt et al. 1970
Aniline	Hydroxylation	Rabbit	Microsomes	1.7−2.5 (per mg protein)	Bend et al. 1972; Hook et al. 1972[b] Oppelt et al. 1970; Matsubara and Tochino 1971
		Rat	Microsomes	10 (per mg protein)	Oppelt et al. 1970
		Guinea pig	Microsomes	10 (per mg protein)	
Benzanthracene	Epoxidation	Human	Microsomes	−	Grover et al. 1973
Benzphetamine	N-Demethylation	Rabbit	Microsomes	0.8−1.0 (per mg protein)	Bend et al. 1972; Hook et al. 1972[b] Fouts and Devereux 1972; Hook et al. 1975; Philpot and Bend, unpublished data
		Rabbit	9000g S	0.9	Fouts and Devereux 1972
		Rabbit	Homogenate	1.4 (per g tissue) 1.0 (per mg protein)	
		Rabbit	Reconstituted[a]	−	Philpot et al. 1975
		Rat	Microsomes	10.7 (per mg protein)	Grasso et al. 1971
		Rat	Microsomes	6.4 (per mg protein)	Chhabra and Fouts 1974
		Rat (female)	Microsomes	2.8 (per mg protein)	Matsubara et al. 1974

TABLE 5 (continued)

Substrate	Reaction	Species	Tissue fractions utilized	Ratio of activities (liver/lung)	References
Benzene	Hydroxylation	Rabbit	Microsomes	0.5 (per mg protein)	Harper et al. 1975
		Rat	Microsomes	2.0 (per mg protein)	
Benzpyrene (see Table 3)					
Biphenyl	4-Hydroxylation	Rabbit	Microsomes	0.7−1.0 (per mg protein)	Bend et al, 1972; Hook et al. 1972[b] Hook et al. 1975
		Rat	Microsomes	5.7, 1.7 (per mg protein)	Hook et al. 1975; Matsubara et al. 1974
	2-Hydroxylation	Guinea pig	Microsomes	16 (per mg protein)	Hook et al. 1975
		Rabbit	Microsomes	2.5 (per mg protein)	
		Rat	Microsomes	2.0 (per mg protein)	
		Guinea pig	Microsomes	4.7 (per mg protein)	
o-Chloroaniline	p-Hydroxylation	Rabbit	Microsomes	3.0 (per mg protein)	Ichikawa et al. 1969
Decane	Hydroxylation	Rabbit	Microsomes	0.6 (per mg protein)	Ichikawa et al. 1969
		Rat	Microsomes	10 (per mg protein)	
		Mouse	Microsomes	1.0 (per mg protein)	
		Bovine	Microsomes	1.1 (per mg protein)	
Dimethylaminoazobenzene	N-Demethylation	Rat	Microsomes	−	Gilman and Conney 1963
Dimethylaniline	N-Demethylation	Rabbit	Microsomes	1.1−1.6 (per mg protein)	Devereux and Fouts 1974; Devereux and Fouts 1975
Dimethylaniline N-oxide	N-Demethylation	Rat	Microsomes	12.5 (per mg protein)	Machinist et al. 1968
		Pig	Microsomes	50 (per mg protein)	
7-Ethoxycoumarin	o-Deethylation	Rabbit	Microsomes	−	Philpot et al. 1975
			Reconstituted[a]	−	

Chemical	Reaction	Species	Preparation	Activity	Reference
Ethylmorphine	N-Demethylation	Rabbit	Microsomes	1.7 (per mg protein)	Machinist et al. 1968
		Rat	Microsomes	—	Stripp et al. 1973
17-Hydroxyprogesterone	21-Hydroxylation	Rabbit	Microsomes	1 (per mg protein)	Ichikawa et al. 1969
Imipramine	N-Demethylation	Rabbit	Microsomes	—	Law et al. 1974
		Rat	9000g S	50 (per g tissue)	Minder et al. 1971
N-Methylaniline	N-Demethylation	Rabbit	IPL[b]	2 (per organ)	Uehleke 1968
		Cat		—	Kiese and Uehleke 1961
		Rabbit	Homogenate	1 (per mg protein)	
		Rabbit	Microsomes	7.5 (per mg protein)	
	p-C-Hydroxylation	Rabbit	IPL	2.5 (per organ)	
		Rabbit	Homogenate	1 (per mg protein)	
		Rabbit	Microsomes	5.9 (per mg protein)	
N-Methyl-p-chloroaniline	N-Demethylation	Rabbit	Microsomes	0.7 (per mg protein)	Bend et al. 1972
p-Nitroanisole	Demethylation	Rabbit	Microsomes	4 (per mg protein)	Ichikawa et al. 1969
Parathion	(to Paraoxon)	Rabbit	Microsomes	4 (per mg protein)	Neal 1972; Poore and Neal 1972
	(to Diethyl phosphorothioic acid)	Rabbit	Microsomes	4 (per mg protein)	
p-Xylene	Hydroxylation	Rabbit	Microsomes	0.25 (per mg protein)	Harper et al. unpublished data
		Rat	Microsomes	2.0 (per mg protein)	

[a] Activity reconstituted by combining solubilized pulmonary cytochrome P-450, NADPH cytochrome c reductase and lipid fractions.
[b] Isolated perfused lung

pulmonary MFO system is similar in many ways to the system found in liver. This similarity was initially suggested by a number of factors that were the same for the pulmonary and hepatic systems: (a) a requirement for NADPH for maximum activity, (b) similar reactions (e.g., *N*-demethylation and ring hydroxylation), (c) the production of the same metabolites, and (d) the presence of cytochrome P-450 in both tissues. Cytochrome P-450 is known to be the terminal oxidase of the hepatic MFO system and it has been identified in lung tissue preparations from a number of species (see Table 6 for details). Detailed studies of the rabbit pulmonary MFO system in our laboratory have confirmed the similarity between pulmonary and hepatic MFO systems (Bend et al. 1972, 1973, Hook et al. 1972b, Philpot et al. 1975).

Like the hepatic system, the pulmonary MFO system is localized in the microsomal fraction (100,000g pellet) obtained from homogenized tissue by centrifugation. Cytochrome P-450 and NADPH-cytochrome c reductase, known to be the enzyme components of the hepatic system, are also localized in the pulmonary microsomal fractions from rabbits (Bend et al. 1972, Matsubara and Tochino 1971) and rats (Matsubara et al. 1974). Electron micrographs of rabbit pulmonary microsomal preparations differ from those obtained from hepatic preparations in that the vesicles formed from the lung endoplasmic reticulum are not evenly spaced but appear in *clumps*. Also, particles resembling ribosomes in lung preparations are associated with a fibrillar matrix, which is not evident in micrographs of hepatic preparations (Hook et al. 1972b). Pulmonary MFO activity can be further localized by fractionation of the 100,000g pellet on a discontinuous sucrose gradient. Fractions obtained in this manner are morphologically similar to the hepatic microsomal fraction (G. E. R. Hook, personal communication). Thus, it is safe to conclude that the pulmonary MFO system, like that of the liver, is associated with endoplasmic reticulum.

Localization of the pulmonary MFO system within specific cells is a different matter. Forty-two cell types have been identified in lung (Sorokin 1970) and only one, the alveolar macrophage, has been investigated specifically for MFO activity. Although NADPH-cytochrome c reductase activity was found to be present in microsomes prepared from rabbit alveolar macrophages, little MFO activity was demonstrable (Hook et al. 1972a). Cytochrome b$_5$ and NADPH-cytochrome c reductase, enzymes that may play a role in the metabolism of xenobiotics, were also found to be present in alveolar macrophages but cytochrome P-450 was not (Hook et al. 1972a). Benzpyrene hydroxylase activity has been reported in homogenates of alveolar macrophages from humans (Cantrell et al. 1973). Histochemical evidence suggests that hydroxylation of aniline takes place in the bronchiolar epithelium (Grasso et al. 1971) and that the oxidative metabolism of benzpyrene occurs in the alveolar walls (Wattenberg and Leong 1962).

TABLE 6 Pulmonary Microsomal Cytochrome P-450 Concentrations in Untreated and Treated Animals

Species[a]	Cytochrome P-450 Concentration (nmol/mg protein)				Reference
	Untreated	Treated[b]			
		PB	3-MC or BP	Other	
Cock	0.03				Ichikawa et al. 1969
Guinea pig	0.065				Oppelt et al. 1970
	0.16				Ichikawa et al. 1969
Mouse (C57BL)	0.034		0.054	0.058 (TCDD)	Poland et al. 1974
(DBA)	0.038		0.044	0.060 (TCDD)	
Oxen	0.21				Ichikawa et al. 1969
Pig	0.04				Machinist et al. 1968
	0.04				Ichikawa et al. 1969
Rabbit	0.49		0.51		Philpot and Bend, unpublished
	0.26	0.33			Uehleke 1968
	0.35				Matsubara and Tochino 1971
	0.27	0.38	0.38	0.51 (CP)	Oppelt et al. 1970
	0.17	0.18			Ichikawa et al. 1969
Rabbit (female)	0.25				Devereux and Fouts 1975
(pregnant)[c]	0.44				

TABLE 6 (continued)

| Species[a] | Cytochrome P-450 Concentration (nmol/mg protein) | | | | Reference |
| | Untreated | Treated | | | |
		PB	3-MC or BP	Other	
Rat	0.05				Hrycay and O'Brien 1974
	0.035				Oppelt et al. 1970
	0.06				Ichikawa et al. 1969
	nd[d]				Machinist et al. 1968
	0.045				Stripp et al. 1973
	0.033	0.028	0.132		Matsubara et al. 1974
Rat (female)	0.053				Stripp et al. 1973

[a] All animals examined were male unless otherwise noted.
[b] Abbreviations used are: PB = phenobarbital; 3-MC = 3-methylcholanthrene; BP = benzpyrene; TCDD = 2,3,7,8-tetrachlorodibenzo-p-dioxin; CP = chlorpromazine.
[c] Rabbits at day 28 of pregnancy used.
[d] Not detectable.

In addition to similar subcellular localizations, the rabbit pulmonary and hepatic MFO systems have been shown to have similar cofactor requirements, pH optima, responses to inhibitors, and substrate-elicited spectral interactions (Bend et al. 1972). Inhibition of pulmonary mixed-function oxidations by carbon monoxide and cytochrome c indicated that cytochrome P-450 and NADPH-cytochrome c reductase, respectively, were required components of the system (Bend et al. 1972). Requirements for these two enzymes have also been suggested for the rat pulmonary MFO system (Matsubara et al. 1974).

Recently, Philpot and associates (1975) have solubilized and separated the membrane-bound components of the rabbit pulmonary MFO system. Definitive evidence for the participation of cytochrome P-450 and NADPH-cytochrome c reductase in the rabbit system was obtained when both of these enzymes were found to be required for reconstitution of MFO activity (Philpot et al. 1975). In agreement with studies on the reconstitution of hepatic MFO systems (Lu and Levin 1974), the presence of a lipid-containing fraction was also required for maximum activity in the reconstituted pulmonary system.

Thus it appears that both the pulmonary and hepatic MFO systems obtain electrons from NADPH, which initially reduce the flavoprotein, NADPH-cytochrome c reductase. The reductase, in turn, reduces a cytochrome P-450-substrate complex, which then combines with O_2 and a second electron to produce an hydroxylated product or intermediate and H_2O.

Substrate Specificity

Notwithstanding the many similarities between the pulmonary and hepatic MFO systems, some significant differences between substrate specificities of the lung and liver have been noted. If the two systems were identical in a given species, it might be expected that the rates of oxidative metabolism of various substrates in lung and liver preparations would be proportional to the cytochrome P-450 concentrations. Four to five times more cytochrome P-450 (per milligram microsomal protein) is found in rabbit liver as compared to rabbit lung. The liver-to-lung ratio for the rates of metabolism of a number of substrates reflects this difference in cytochrome P-450 concentrations (Table 5). Aniline, aminopyrine, biphenyl (2-hydroxylation), parathion, *p*-nitroanisole, *o*-chloroaniline, and *N*-methylaniline are all metabolized two to seven times faster in rabbit liver preparations than in similar preparations from rabbit lung (Table 5). However, benzphetamine, benzene, biphenyl (4-hydroxylation), decane, and *N*-methyl-*p*-chloroaniline are metabolized by rabbit pulmonary microsomes at rates equal to or greater than those obtained with hepatic microsomes. *p*-Xylene, in fact, is hydroxylated four times faster in rabbit pulmonary microsomes as compared to rabbit hepatic microsomes per milligram protein and 16 to 20 times faster per nanomole of cytochro.ne P-450 (Harper et al., unpublished). On the other hand, perazine can be converted to hydroxyperazine in rat hepatic microsomal preparations but not in pulmonary microsomal preparations from rab, rabbit, or pig (Breyer 1971).

The question of what is responsible for the observed differences in substrate specificity between hepatic and pulmonary MFO systems has not been answered. Substrate specificity in hepatic MFO systems appears to be determined by the cytochrome P-450 component (Lu and Levin 1974), and differences between hepatic and pulmonary cytochrome P-450s could account for the substrate specificities associated with these tissues. Spectra of rabbit pulmonary cytochrome P-450, purified free from contaminating pigments, do not reveal any differences when compared to the spectra of purified rabbit hepatic cytochrome P-450 (Arinc and Philpot, unpublished). Attempts to compare the catalytic properties of pulmonary and hepatic cytochrome P-450s directly have been hampered by a lack of success in obtaining a single NADPH-cytochrome c reductase preparation that will interact with both cytochromes. Reductase solubilized from pulmonary microsomes by the method generally used to obtain the hepatic reductase (digestion of microsomes with deoxycholate) will support hydroxylase activity when combined with hepatic cytochrome P-450 but is inactive when combined with pulmonary P-450. Conversely, reductase prepared by digestion of rabbit pulmonary microsomes with sodium cholate will support hydroxylase activity when combined with the pulmonary cytochrome but is inactive in combination with the hepatic cytochrome (Philpot et al. 1975, Arinc and Philpot, unpublished data). These results suggest that a difference between rabbit pulmonary and hepatic cytochrome P-450s does indeed exist but give little hint as to the nature of the difference. Rat pulmonary cytochrome P-450 has also been solubilized, but, as yet, the rat pulmonary MFO system has not been reconstituted due to difficulties in obtaining NADPH-cytochrome c reductase from rat lung that will support hydroxylase activity (Jernstrom et al. 1975). Clearly, a great deal of additional effort will be required before the factors responsible for the substrate specificity differences between hepatic and pulmonary MFO systems are fully elucidated.

Induction, Inhibition, and Development

A number of factors are known to influence the capability of MFO systems to metabolize both exogenous and endogenous compounds. Age, sex, species, strain, tissue, and nutrition are but a few of the parameters that exert control over mixed-function oxidations. The inductive effects of many xenobiotics on MFO systems are perhaps the most thoroughly studied and among the most important of these factors. The number of components known to increase

MFO activity following in vivo administration is impressive and continually growing (Sher 1971). As is the case with most aspects of MFO reactions, the vast majority of information on induction pertains to hepatic systems. Inducers of hepatic MFO activities are generally classified into two groups. One group, exemplified by phenobarbital (PB), gives rise to increases in a wide range of activities and causes a proliferation of the endoplasmic reticulum of hepatic parenchymal cells. The second group, exemplified by 3-methylcholanthrene (3-MC) and benzpyrene (BP) and comprised mainly of polycyclic aromatic hydrocarbons, induces a narrow range of activities, including the metabolism of benzpyrene and other carcinogens, and leads to the formation of a form of cytochrome P-450 known as P-448 (Alvares et al. 1967).

With the exception of inductive effects on benzpyrene hydroxylase activity (aryl hydrocarbon hydroxylase, AHH, the pulmonary MFO systems of various species do not appear to be as responsive to inducers as are the hepatic systems. (The induction of AHH is covered in the following section.)

Little or no increase in the concentration of pulmonary cytochrome P-450 is observed following the treatment of animals with PB (see Table 6 for data on the induction of pulmonary cytochrome P-450 by various compounds). Slight increases in pulmonary aniline hydroxylase (60%) and aminopyrine N-demethylase (90%) have been observed following the treatment of rabbits with PB (Oppelt et al. 1970). Similar increases were noted in rabbits treated with chlorpromazine, although this compound appeared to be a better inducer of pulmonary cytochrome P-450 than was PB (Oppelt et al. 1970, Table 6). Phenobarbital has also been reported to increase slightly the metabolism of parathion to paraoxon and diethylphosphorothioic acid in rabbit pulmonary microsomes (Poore and Neal 1972); however, similar treatment of rabbits did not elicit significant changes in the rates of pulmonary N-demethylation of p-C-hydroxylation of N-methyl-aniline or in the concentration of pulmonary cytochrome P-450 (Uehleke 1968). Treatment of rats with PB did not stimulate pulmonary N-demethylation of 3-methyl-4-monomethylaminoazobenzene, while this reaction was markedly enhanced by treatment with 3-MC (Gilman and Conney 1963). On the other hand, 3-MC treatment of rabbits had no effect on the pulmonary metabolism of parathion (Poore and Neal 1972), benzphetamine, or benzpyrene (Philpot and Bend, unpublished data) or on the cytochrome P-450 concentration (Philpot and Bend, unpublished data).

Devereux and Fouts (1975) have observed increased rates of N-demethylation of dimethylaniline in pulmonary microsomes from 20- to 28-day pregnant rabbits as compared to nonpregnant rabbits. This *inductive* effect of pregnancy may be due to increased levels of certain steroids, since administration of dexamethasone, hydrocortisone, or deoxycorticosterone to nonpregnant rabbits mimicked the effect of pregnancy. It is interesting that the hepatic N-

demethylation of dimethylaniline did not increase during pregnancy even though dexamethasone and hydrocortisone induced the hepatic activity in non-pregnant rabbits (Devereux and Fouts 1975).

Few studies on the inhibition of pulmonary MFO activities have been reported. Those that have been reported have dealt with inhibition in vitro. The effects of in vivo administration of known inhibitors of hepatic mixed-function oxidations, such as methylenedioxyphenyl compounds (Hodgson and Philpot 1974), have not been investigated. The two most widely used in vitro inhibitors of hepatic MFO reactions, carbon monoxide and cytochrome c, also inhibit MFO activities in lung preparations. It is reasonable to conclude that the mechanisms of inhibition for these compounds (the binding of CO to the P-450 heme and the competition of cytochrome c with cytochrome P-450 for electrons from NADPH-cytochrome c reductase) are the same in both tissues. SKF-525A, another commonly used inhibitor, also has the same effect in liver and lung preparations (Bend et al. 1972, Machinist et al. 1968) as does Hg^{2+} (Devereux and Fouts 1975). In contrast, 1 to 10 mM Mg^{2+} slightly stimulates the N-demethylation of dimethylaniline in rabbit hepatic microsomes but inhibits this reaction in rabbit pulmonary microsomes (Devereux and Fouts 1974), and substrate inhibition of pulmonary but not hepatic aminopyrine N-demethylation has been described (Klinger 1973).

Developmental studies have suggested a major difference between pulmonary and hepatic MFO systems, at least in the rabbit. Rabbit pulmonary cytochrome P-450, cytochrome b_5, NADPH-cytochrome c reductase, benzpyrene hydroxylase, and benzphetamine and dimethylaniline N-demethylases increase linearly (per milligram microsomal protein) from 3 days of age to adult levels at 4 to 6 weeks of age. In rabbit liver gradual increases in cytochrome b_5 and NADPH-cytochrome c reductase to adult levels at 30 days are observed, while cytochrome P-450, benzpyrene hydroxylase and benzphetamine and dimethylaniline N-demethylases increase slowly during the first 15 days of life and then sharply rise to adult levels by day 30 (Fouts and Devereux 1972, Devereux and Fouts 1975).

Another interesting difference between hepatic and pulmonary MFO systems has been reported by Chhabra and Fouts (1974) who showed that the differences between the activities of the hepatic systems of male compared with female rats are not evident when the pulmonary activities are compared.

Oxidation of Polycyclic Hydrocarbons;
Aryl Hydrocarbon Hydroxylase

Higginson (1972) has estimated that 80% to 90% of all human cancers are the result of exposure to environmental compounds. Among the classes of carcinogenic chemicals that have been identified, the polycyclic hydrocarbons may be the most important in the etiology of lung cancer (Wynder and Hoffman 1968). Pulmonary carcinomas, morphologically similar to human lung cancers, have been experimentally produced in laboratory animals by exposing them to the polycyclic hydrocarbons, 3-methylcholanthrene, and benzpyrene (Kuschner et al. 1957, Saffiotti et al. 1968). Benzpyrene appears to be nearly ubiquitous in nature and its occurrence in tobacco smoke may be particularly important.

The molecular mechanisms involved in chemical carcinogenesis are not understood. However, certain aspects of the behavior of polycyclic hydrocarbons in biologic systems that may be responsible for their carcinogenic activity have been elucidated. Polycyclic hydrocarbons are metabolically activated to compounds that can covalently bind to DNA and other macromolecules (Grover and Sims 1968, Gelboin 1969). Several lines of evidence suggest that the active metabolites of polycyclic hydrocarbons are K-region epoxides. Boyland (1950) has postulated that epoxide intermediates could give rise to the metabolic products (phenols, trans-dihydrodiols, and glutathione conjugates) produced from polycyclic hydrocarbons. K-region epoxides of phenanthrene and dibenzanthracene covalently bind to DNA and proteins in cell culture (Grover et al. 1971) and in the test tube (Grover and Sims 1970). And K-region epoxides of dibenzanthracene (Selkirk et al. 1971), benzanthracene, pyrene, and benzpyrene (Grover et al. 1972) have been detected in hepatic microsomal incubations supplemented with NADPH.

The metabolism of polycyclic hydrocarbons in the lung appears to follow the same pathways as in the liver. 7-Methylbenzanthracene-5,6-oxide, benzpyrene 4,5-oxide, and benzanthracene 5,6-oxide have been identified in rat pulmonary microsomal incubations (Grover 1974) and the ability of human lung to form benzanthracene-5,6-oxide and the corresponding dihydrodiol and glutathione conjugate from benzanthracene has been demonstrated (Grover et al. 1973).

The initial step (activation) in the metabolism of polycyclic hydrocarbons is affected by the cytochrome P-450-dependent mixed-function oxidase system. Usually, this activity is determined using benzpyrene as the substrate. The rate of reaction is ascertained from changes in fluorescence and quantified by comparison with the fluorescence of known amounts of 3-hydroxybenzpyrene, one of the products of the reaction. This activity is generally referred to as aryl hydrocarbon hydroxylase (AHH) and has been extensively investigated in lung preparations.

Aryl hydrocarbon hydroxylase activity in the lung is highly species-dependent, as shown in Table 7. Microsomal rates as high as 330 pmol/min/ mg protein have been reported for rabbit, while for the rat the reported rates

TABLE 7 Benzpyrene Hydroxylase (AHH) Activity in Lung Tissue Preparations from Various Species

Species	Tissue fraction utilized	Benzpyrene hydroxylase (pmol product/min)	Ratio of activities (Liver/lung)	Reference
Guinea pig	Microsomes	70/mg protein	7.5	Hook et al. 1975
Hamster	Homogenate	+	—	Okamoto et al. 1972
Human	Homogenate (fetal)	+		Juchau et al. 1972
	Homogenate (PAMs of nonsmokers)[a]	$0-0.02/10^6$ cells	—	Cantrell et al. 1973
	Homogenate (PAMs of smokers)[a]	$0.03-0.25/10^6$ cells	—	Cantrell et al. 1973
Mouse (see Table 5)				
Rabbit	Microsomes	+	8 (per mg protein)	Fouts and Devereux 1972
	Microsomes	330/mg protein	2	Hook et al. 1975
	Microsomes	330/mg protein	1.5	Philpot and Bend, unpublished data

Rat (male)	Microsomes	8.7/mg protein	15.1	Wiebel et al. 1971
	Microsomes	1/mg protein	370	Matsubara et al. 1974
	Microsomes	$<$10/mg protein	$>$58	Hook et al. 1975
	Microsomes	—	165 (per mg protein)	Chhabra and Fouts 1974
(female)	Microsomes	—	9.4 (per g tissue)	Wang et al. 1971
	Microsomes		22 (per mg protein)	Chhabra and Fouts 1974
(male)	Homogenate	35/g tissue	—	Welch et al. 1971, 1972
	Homogenate	15/g tissue	~10	Gelboin and Blackburn 1964
	Homogenate	1–4/mg protein	10–15	Marcotte and Witschi 1972
(female)	Homogenate	215/g tissue	24	Wattenberg et al. 1968a
	Homogenate	325/g tissue	15	Wattenberg et al. 1968b
	Homogenate	300/g tissue	19	Wattenberg and Leong 1965
	Homogenate	3/mg protein	—	Wattenberg et al. 1968c
(pregnant)		36/g tissue	70	Welch et al. 1971, 1972
	Cell culture	2.9/mg protein	—	Wattenberg et al. 1968c

[a]PAM = pulmonary alveolar macrophage.

range from 1 to 16. Pulmonary AHH activity is highly inducible in the rat, hamster, and some strains of mice but not in the rabbit or guinea pig (Tables 8 and 9). Compounds capable of inducing pulmonary AHH activity in the rat include polycyclic hydrocarbons, flavones, and phenylbenzothiazoles while phenobarbital and steroids appear to be ineffective (Table 8). The importance of inducer compounds in the control of rat pulmonary AHH activity may be absolute; this activity essentially disappears in starved rats (Wattenberg 1972) or rats fed on purified diets (Wattenberg 1971). In fact, Wattenberg (1971) has shown that rat pulmonary AHH activity can vary significantly in animals fed different commercial laboratory chows. With the exception of tobacco smoke (Welch et al. 1971, 1972, Marcotte and Witschi 1972) and a few derivatives of 2-phenylbenzothiazole (Wattenberg et al. 1968c), particularly 2-(4'-cyanophenyl)-benzothiazole, the diet appears to contain the only factors that have a more significant effect on pulmonary than hepatic AHH activity (Wattenberg 1971). Some question remains about the relative effects of polycyclic hydrocarbons on AHH activity in the lung and liver. Compared with hepatic AHH activity, 3-methylcholanthrene has been reported to be both a more (Matsubara et al. 1974, Wiebel et al. 1971) and less (Gelboin and Blackburn 1964) potent inducer of pulmonary activity, while β-naphthoflavone (Wattenberg et al. 1968b) and benzpyrene (Wang et al. 1971) appear to have a greater effect in the liver. The induction of AHH activity by polycyclic hydrocarbons in various mouse tissues is under genetic control and is apparently inherited as a simple autosomal dominant trait (Gielen et al. 1972). This strain-dependent response is clearly shown in Table 9 for the induction of hepatic AHH activity. Benzanthracene and 3-methylcholanthrene both induce hepatic AHH activity in C57BL mice but not in DBA, NZB, or NZW mice. Pulmonary AHH activity responds in the same manner to 3-methylcholanthrene, but benzanthracene significantly induces pulmonary AHH activity in all strains examined. In addition to being both strain- and tissue-dependent, the response of mice to inducers of AHH activity is also dependent on the inducer compound used. Tetrachlorodibenzo-*p*-dioxin (TCDD) treatment of mice leads to induction of both pulmonary and hepatic AHH activity in all strains tested (Table 9).

The ultimate problem associated with pulmonary AHH activity is to determine the relationship between the metabolism of polycyclic hydrocarbons and lung cancer. Certainly, if K-region epoxides, as highly reactive electrophiles, are the actual carcinogens, then metabolic activation of polycyclic hydrocarbons is a prerequisite to carcinogenesis. If this is true, then it should be expected that increases in AHH activity would result in increases in the formation of activated metabolites from polycyclic hydrocarbons. This appears to be the case. The formation of 7-methylbenzanthracene 5,6-oxide and benzpyrene 4,5-oxide consistently occurs in vitro in pulmonary microsomal preparations from 3-methylcholanthrene-treated rats but these epoxides cannot always be identified in incubations carried out with preparations from untreated rats (Grover 1974). Aryl hydrocarbon hydroxylase activity and covalent binding of benzpyrene metabolites in vitro are both increased in microsomal preparations from rats treated with benzpyrene (Wang et al. 1971). Studies of bromobenzene-induced hepatic and pulmonary necrosis suggest that similar results also occur in vivo. The necrosis resulting from bromobenzene administration is thought to be caused by the covalent binding of an MFO-activated metabolite, probably an epoxide, to cellular proteins (Brodie et al. 1970, Reid et al. 1973, Reid and Krishna 1973). Hepatic necrosis and in vivo covalent binding are increased in phenobarbital-treated animals. Consistent with this, the metabolism of bromobenzene and the covalent binding of bromobenzene metabolites occur at much greater rates in hepatic microsomes prepared from phenobarbital-treated mice as compared to preparations from untreated mice. Reid and associates (1973) have hypothesized that the increase in covalent binding of bromobenzene in the lung following treatment with phenobarbital is the result of metabolites of bromobenzene produced in the liver. This hypothesis is supported by their observation that covalent binding of bromobenzene metabolites in phenobarbital-treated mice also occurs in heart and spleen, organs that do not contain any demonstrable MFO activity (Reid et al. 1973).

Next, it must be determined whether or not increases in pulmonary AHH activity can be associated with increased susceptibility to lung cancer. Little doubt remains that cigarette smokers have a higher incidence of lung cancer than do nonsmokers. Do they have induced levels of pulmonary AHH activity? Experiments with laboratory animals have clearly demonstrated that cigarette smoke contains potent inducers of pulmonary AHH activity (Welch et al. 1971, 1972, Marcotte and Witschi 1972). And studies with humans have shown that AHH activity in alveolar macrophages of smokers is significantly higher than in alveolar macrophages of nonsmokers (Cantrell et al. 1973).

Speculation at this point is tempting: the pulmonary MFO system produces carcinogenic metabolites from polycyclic hydrocarbons, induction increases the production of the activated metabolites, cigarette smoke contains both inducers and carcinogens, therefore, cigarette smokers are more susceptible to lung cancer than are nonsmokers. Aside from being overly simplistic, such a hypothesis is easily challenged by existing evidence. In fact, at least two studies suggest that induction of AHH activity is a protective mechanism with respect to the formation of chemically-induced pulmonary adenomas. The formation of these cancers in A/HeJ mice resulting from the oral administration of benzpyrene (Wattenberg and Leong 1970) or 7,12-dimethylbenzanthracene (Wattenberg and Leong 1968) is significantly inhibited in animals treated with β-naphthoflavone, an inducer of AHH activity in various tissues, including the lung. The hypothesis of Dixon et al. (1970) that asbestos-mediated susceptibility to lung cancer is due to the inhibition of pulmonary

TABLE 8 Induction of Pulmonary Benzpyrene Hydroxylase (AHH) Activity in Species other than the Mouse

Species	Tissue fraction utilized	Inducer compound	Induced activity (times control) Lung	Liver	Reference
Rat	Microsomes	Benzpyrene	2.4	17.9	Wang et al. 1971
Rat (female)	Homogenate		5.2		Wattenberg et al. 1968c
Rat (female)	Cell culture		2.2		
Hamster	Homogenate		13.5		Okamoto et al. 1972
Rat	Homogenate	Cannabis sativa			
		Smoke	2–3	~1.5	Marcotte and Witschi 1972
		Smoke after extraction of cannabinoids	2–3	~1.5	
Hamster		Smoke condensate	4.9		Okamoto et al. 1972
Rat (female)	Homogenate	Chlorpromazine HCl	5.4		Wattenberg et al. 1968c
	Cell culture		3.1		
	Homogenate	Chlorpromazine Sulfoxide	6.6		
	Cell culture		3.1		
Rat (female)	Homogenate	Dietary Factors (control = purified diet)			
		Commercial laboratory chows	6–16	1.8–1.1	Wattenberg 1971
		Brussle sprouts	3–30		
		Cauliflower	5		
		Broccoli, cabbage, celery, dill, turnips, spinach	2–3		
Rat (female)	Homogenate	2,5-Diphenyltriazole	8.5		Wattenberg et al. 1968c
	Cell culture		2.5		

Rat (female)	Homogenate	Flavones and related compounds			Wattenberg et al. 1968a
		Flavone	2.8	4.0	
		4'-Fluoroflavone	3.7	5.4	
		4'-Bromoflavone	7.0	12.0	
		Hydroxyflavones	$<$1.0	$<$1.0	
		Methoxyflavones	$\geqslant$2.5	$\geqslant$3.2	
		Beta-Naphthoflavone	7.3	15.1	
			4.1		Wattenberg et al. 1968c
	Cell culture		3.7		
	Homogenate	Flavanone	1.5	0.7	Wattenberg et al. 1968a
		4'-Bromoflavanone	3.1	3.7	
		Hydroxyflavanones	$\leqslant$1.2	$\leqslant$0.9	
		Chalcone	1.2	2.2	
		2'-Hydroxy-4-bromochalcone	1.0	1.2	
		2'-Methoxychalcone	1.8	3.2	
Rat	Microsomes	3-Methylcholanthrene	15	3.1	Matsubara et al. 1974
			12−25	5−16	Wiebel et al. 1971
	Homogenate		4	9	Gelboin and Blackburn 1964
Rat (female)			7.9		Wattenberg et al. 1968c
	Cell culture		2.6		
Rabbit	Microsomes		NS[b]	NS	Philpot et al. unpublished data
Rat (female)	Homogenate	2-Phenylbenzothiazoles and Related Compounds			Wattenberg et al. 1968b
		2-Phenylbenzothiazole (2-PBT)	3.9	3.5	
		Halogenated 2-PBT			
		Bromo: 3' $<$ 2-PBT $<$ 2' $<$ 4' =	7.3		
		3' = 2-PBT $<$ 2' $<$ 4' =		8.0	
		Chloro: 3' $<$ 2-PBT $<$ 2' $<$ 4' =	6.4		
		3' $<$ 2' $<$ 2-PBT $<$ 4' =		7.8	
		4' Halogens: Br $>$ Cl $>$ I $>$ 2-PBT $>$ F	2.7	2.5	

TABLE 8 (continued)

Species	Tissue fraction utilized	Inducer compound	Induced activity (times control)		Reference
			Lung	Liver	
Rat (female) (continued)		4' Substitutions (non-halogens) Formyl $<$ Carboxy $<$ Hydroxy $<$ Methyl $<$ Methoxy $<$ 2-PBT $<$ Amino $<$ Cyano =	4.6		
		Formyl = Carboxy $<$ Hydroxy = Methyl $<$ Methoxy = Cyano $<$ 2-PBT $<$ Amino		4.2	
		Benzothiazole and Derivatives			
		Benzothiazole	1.5	2.0	
		2,2'-Thiobisbenzothiazole	1.0	2.4	
		2-Benzothiobenzothiazole	1.9	2.6	
		2-Benzyloxybenzothiazole	2.4	2.5	
		2-Benzamidobenzothiazole	2.7	2.4	
		2-(4'-Pyridyl)benzothiazole	2.4	2.5	
		(other benzothiazole derivatives were less active than the parent compound)			
Rat	Microsomes	Phenobarbital	NS NS	1.6 2.8	Matsubara et al. 1974 Wiebel et al. 1971
Rat	Homogenate	Phenothiazine	4.4	20.7	Wattenberg and Leong 1965
Rat (female)	Cell culture		8.3 3.8		Wattenberg et al. 1968c
Rat (female)	Homogenate Cell culture	10-Acetylphenothiazine	6.6 3.6		Wattenberg et al. 1968c

Rat	Microsomes	Steroids			Stripp et al. 1973
		Methyltestosterone	NS	NS	
Rat (female)			NS	1.6	
Rat		Spironolactone	0.7	0.5	
Rat (female)			NS	3.3	
Rat		PCN[c]	0.7	NS	
Rat (female)			NS	5.3	
Rat	Microsomes	TCDD[d]	4.0	2.7	Hook et al. 1975
Rabbit			NS	NS	
Guinea pig			NS	0.6	
Rat	Homogenate	Tobacco smoke			
		2 hr	1.3		Welch et al. 1972
		4 hr	2.9		
		6 hr	3.6	NS	Marcotte and Witschi 1972
		3 hr, 24 hr wait	27		Welch et al. 1972
Rat (pregnant)		5 hr × 3 days	13	2.2	
Hamster		condensate	3.9		Okamoto et al. 1972

[a] Animals used were males unless designated female.
[b] NS = not significant.
[c] PCN = pregnenolone-carbonitrile.
[d] TCDD = 2,3,7,8-tetrachlorodibenzo-*p*-dioxin.

TABLE 9   Induction of Benzpyrene Hydroxylase Activity (AHH) in Mice

| Strain | Tissue fraction utilized | Ratio of activities (Liver/lung) | Induction | | | Reference |
| | | | Times control activity | | | |
			Inducer[a]	Lung	Liver	
C57BL	Homogenate	16	3-MC	4.6	6.4	Gielen et al. 1972
		7.5	BA	2.6	3.7	Wiebel et al. 1973
		—	PB	NS[b]	—	Gielen et al. 1972
	10000g S	—	3-MC	—	5.2	Poland et al. 1974
		—	TCDD	—	9.3	Poland et al. 1974
	Microsomes	—	PB	—	1.8	Gielen et al. 1972
DBA	Homogenate	27	3-MC	NS	NS	Gielen et al. 1972
		16.4	BA	6.3	NS	Wiebel et al. 1973
		—	PB	NS	NS	Gielen et al. 1972
	10000g S	—	3-MC	—	NS	Poland et al. 1974
		—	TCDD	—	6.3	Poland et al. 1974
	Microsomes	—	PB	—	2.0	Gielen et al. 1972
NZB	Homogenate	—	3-MC	NS	NS	Gielen et al. 1972
		114	BA	11.1	NS	Wiebel et al. 1973
		—	PB	NS	—	Gielen et al. 1972
	10000g S	120	3-MC	2.0	1.4	Poland et al. 1974
		120	TCDD	9.9	5.8	Poland et al. 1974
	Microsomes	—	PB	—	2.2	Gielen et al. 1972
NZW	Homogenate	—	3-MC	NS	NS	Gielen et al. 1972
		57	BA	12.4	1.4	Poland et al. 1974
		—	PB	NS	—	Gielen et al. 1972

	10000g S	317	3-MC	4	NS	Poland et al. 1974
		317	TCDD	15	3.5	Poland et al. 1974
	Microsomes	—	PB	—	1.7	Gielen et al. 1972
AKR	Homogenate	39	BA	10.9	1.6	Wiebel et al. 1973
	9000g S	26	3-MC	1.9	NS	Burki et al. 1973
	10000g S	—	3-MC	—	NS	Poland et al. 1974
		—	TCDD	—	3.8	Poland et al. 1974
A/HeJ	Homogenate	73	β-NF	5.6	1.2	Wattenberg and Leong 1968
		175	β-NF	4.5	1.4	Wattenberg and Leong 1970
		175	QPE	3.4	NS	Wattenberg and Leong 1970
BALB	10000g S	96	3-MC	1.9	3.7	Poland et al. 1974
CBA	1000g S	41	3-MC	1.7	3.3	Poland et al. 1974
	Homogenate	41	TCDD	7.9	5.3	Poland et al. 1974
SOL	9000g	60	BA	7.4	N.S.	Wiebel et al. 1973
Af	10000g S	14.5	3-MC	2.0	3.3	Burki et al. 1973
Swiss		9.6	3-MC	8.3	3.9	Wiebel et al. 1973
		9.6	BA	13.4	3.8	Wiebel et al. 1973
		9.6	BF	13.3	4.3	Wiebel et al. 1973

[a] Abbreviations used: 3-MC = 3-methylcholanthrene, BA = benzanthracene, PB = phenobarbital, TCDD = 2,3,7,8-tetrachlorodibenzo-p-dioxin, β-NF = β-naphthoflavone, QPE = quercetin pentamethyl ether, BF = 5,6-benzoflavone.
[b] NS = not significant.

AHH activity by trace metal (Ni^{2+}, Co^{2+}, Cr^{6+}) contaminants of asbestos also suggests that AHH activity is predominately protective.

Perhaps the evidence suggesting that the carcinogenic properties of polycyclic hydrocarbons result from metabolic activation by MFO enzymes (see review, Heidelberger 1973) can be reconciled with the apparent protective effect of the same metabolic system, if we consider the possibility that induction of pulmonary AHH activity may take place primarily in nontarget cells, cells where the effects of activated metabolites may be minimal. Some cells, such as those of the liver, are resistant to the effects of polycyclic hydrocarbons (Wattenberg 1971), yet they contain high AHH activity. And in vitro experiments have clearly shown that covalent binding of benzpyrene metabolites to DNA can be affected in hepatic microsomal preparations. The induction of AHH activity in nontarget cells could effectively reduce the chances of polycyclic hydrocarbons, reaching target cells where metabolic activation could be of some consequence. Thus, the hypothesis of Dixon et al. (1970) that "the major determinant for carcinogenesis is the residence time of the unmetabolized benzpyrene in the lung" may be true but not because, as they suggest, unmetabolized benzpyrene acts as the carcinogen. The half-life of benzpyrene in the lung may determine whether or not it reaches a target cell and is activated. Induction of AHH activity would effectively lower the half-life of benzpyrene in the lung and inhibition would increase it. In situations of chronic exposure to carcinogens, such as with smokers, high AHH activity may serve to prolong the onset of lung cancer but not prevent it.

B.   Other Pathways of Metabolism

In addition to oxidative metabolism by the mixed-function oxidase system, other metabolic pathways by which foreign compounds are degraded are present in the lung. Table 10 is a partial listing of non-MFO enzymes present in the lung of some species. The reader should consult reviews by Brown (1974) and by Hook and Bend (1976) for additional listings of non-MFO enzymes present in lung tissue. A few of the more important non-MFO enzymes of the lung are discussed here.

Amine Oxidase

The major route of metabolism for secondary and tertiary amines is N-dealkylation via the MFO system. However, secondary and tertiary amines also undergo N-oxidation by a system not inhibited by CO or SKF-525A and therefore not dependent on cytochrome P-450 (Bickel 1969, Hlavica and Kiese 1969). In addition, amine oxidase has been purified and found to be a

TABLE 10 Non-MFO Enzymes in Lung

Enzyme	Species	References
Amine oxidase	Rabbit, rat, pig	Uehleke 1972 Breyer 1971 Machinist et al. 1968 Devereux and Fouts 1974
Reduction of *N*-oxides	Rat	Bickel et al. 1968 Bickel 1972
Gluthathione-S-epoxide transferase	Guinea pig, rat, rabbit	James et al. 1976
Gluthathione-*s*-aryl transferase	Guinea pig, rat, rabbit	James et al. 1976
Epoxide hydrase	Guinea pig, rat, rabbit	James et al. 1976
Glucuronyl transferase	Guinea pig, rat rabbit, human L-132	James et al. 1976 Aitio 1973 Locke et al. 1971
Nitro reductase	Rat	Bartosek et al. 1970
Sulfotransferase	Rabbit	Hook and Bend 1976
N-methyl transferase	Rabbit	Fuller and Roush 1975 Dingell et al. 1964

flavoprotein that utilizes NADPH as a cofactor (Masters and Ziegler 1971, Ziegler et al. 1969). The biochemistry of *N*-oxidation has recently been reviewed by Uehleke (1971) and Bickel (1969).

The rate of *N*-oxide formation appears to be significant in the lung of some species. The rate of oxidation of *N*-methylaniline and *N,N*-dimethylaniline is nearly as great in rabbit lung microsomal preparations as in rabbit liver microsomal preparations (Uehleke 1972).

Species differences in *N*-oxidation by the lung are seen for rabbit, rat, and pig, using perazine as a substrate for the amine oxidase. High rates of parazine *N*-oxidation were observed in rabbit pulmonary microsomes in contrast to the rates observed in pig and rat pulmonary microsomes (Breyer 1971). Pulmonary microsomes from pig were approximately one-fourth as active as hepatic microsomes from pig in the *N*-oxidation of *N*-methylaniline, *N,N*-dimethylaniline, and *N*-ethylaniline (Heinze et al. 1970).

In view of the potential toxicity of *N*-oxide metabolites (Uehleke 1971) formed by the amine oxidase reaction in lung, this enzyme may be important in the elucidation of mechanisms by which certain environmental agents produce toxic effects in the lung.

Metabolism of Epoxides

Epoxides formed from aliphatic and aromatic double bonds by the MFO system appear to be important in the induction of carcinogenesis (Sims and Grover 1974), mutagenesis, and teratogenesis. Epoxides are generally more reactive than their precursors and have been found to bind covalently to macromolecules (see section entitled *Pulmonary Mixed-Function Oxidation of Polycyclic Hydrocarbons*. Epoxides are metabolized to trans-dihydrodiols via a hydration reaction catalyzed by epoxide hydrase (Oesch et al. 1971) and are conjugated with glutathione via glutathione-*S*-epoxide transferase (Boyland and Williams 1968).

Both of these enzymatic conversions result in the inactivation of the epoxide. James and associates (1976) have studied the metabolism of epoxides in the lung, using styrene oxide as a substrate. Lungs of guinea pig, rat, and rabbit contain epoxide hydrase and glutathione-*S*-epoxide transferase, but with activities lower than found in liver. The liver-to-lung ratios for the activities of these enzymes are about 25 and 10 for epoxide hydrase and glutathione-*S*-epoxide transferase, respectively.

Lower epoxide hydrase activity in rat lung as compared to rat liver was reported by Grover (1974), using benz[α]anthracene-5,6-oxide as a substrate. Hayakawa et al. (1974) also found that naphthalene-1,2-oxide was metabolized at one-tenth the rate in sheep lung as compared to sheep liver.

The relatively low rates of epoxide metabolism in pulmonary tissue may be of significant consequence to the overall metabolism of polycyclic hydrocarbons in the lung. This may be of particular importance in polycyclic hydrocarbon-induced lung cancers.

IV. Metabolism of Chemicals by Isolated Perfused Lung

The lung is unique in that chemicals may enter it from either the circulation or from the alveolar space. Of considerable interest and importance is the question of how the lung metabolizes inhaled chemicals. The balance between rates of activation and deactivation of an inhaled pollutant could be a determinate in the induction of lung damage or lung carcinogenesis. The isolated perfused lung is a means of examining the pulmonary metabolism of airborne pollutants. In addition, the IPL allows for the study of the pulmonary metabolism of xenobiotics in the absence of metabolism by other organs and tissues in the body.

A. Metabolism of Chemicals in the Circulation

Metabolism of chemicals by the IPL has received relatively little attention. *N*-dealkylation of *N*-methylaniline, *N*-methyl-*p*-chloroaniline, and aminopyrine have been observed in the isolated perfused rabbit lung (Uehleke 1968). Hydroxylation of *N*-methylaniline has been detected (Uehleke 1968). We have examined the metabolism of a number of chemicals in the isolated perfused rabbit lung (Wilson et al. 1976, Orton et al. 1973, Law et al. 1974). The basic amines, methadone and amphetamine, accumulate in and are extensively degraded by the lung, while imipramine and chlorcyclizine, which also accumulate in the lung, are not degraded. Interestingly, all of these basic amines are degraded by lung tissue homogenates and the pulmonary microsomal fraction. Thus, care must be exercised in extrapolating metabolic data from lung tissue fractions to the intact organ. Methadone appears to be extensively degraded by the IPL (Wilson et al. 1976, Law et al. 1974). Metabolites of methadone detected in the lung and the perfusate are the products of oxidative *N*-demethylation. Pentobarbital, parathion, and aldrin are also degraded by the perfused rabbit lung. Pentobarbital is converted to the d and l diastereoisomers of pentobarbital alcohol (Law et al. 1974), parathion to paraoxon and unidentified water soluble metabolites (Law et al. 1974), and aldrin to the epoxide dieldrin (Mehendale and El-Bassiouni 1976).

Metabolism of the bronchodilator drugs, isoprenaline, isoetharine (catecholamines), and terbutaline was studied in the isolated perfused dog lung (Briant et al. 1973). Isoprenaline and isoetharine were extensively metabolized by *o*-methylation but terbutaline, which is not a catecholamine, was not significantly degraded.

B. Metabolism of Inhaled Chemicals

Metabolism of inhaled chemicals by the lung has not been extensively studied and little information on this subject is available. Briant and associates (1973) have examined the metabolism of inhaled isoprenaline and isoetharine in the isolated perfused dog lung. *O*-Methylation of these catecholamines was noted in a system that employed a recirculating perfusate. In a single pass experiment, 30% of an absorbed dose of isoprenaline was detected in the venous effluent 30 min after the inhalation. This may indicate metabolism during passage from the airways to the vascular system.

Metabolites of inhaled benzpyrene have been found in the perfusate and tissue of isolated perfused rat and rabbit lungs (Niemeyer 1976). In view of the possible relationship between the metabolism of benzpyrene and pulmonary carcinogenesis, this problem needs further examination. An understanding of the pulmonary metabolism of inhaled chemicals, particularly those that may undergo metabolic activation, is vitally important from the standpoint of environmental effects on human health. Refinement and utilization of the IPL technique should greatly increase our knowledge in this area.

References

Aitio, A. (1973). Glucuronide synthesis in the rat and guinea pig lung. *Xenobiotica*, **3**:13–22.

Alvares, A. P., Schilling, G., Levin, W., and Kuntzman, R. (1967). Studies on the induction of CO-binding pigments in liver microsomes by phenobarbital and 3-methylcholanthrene. *Biochem. Biophys. Res. Commun.*, **29**: 521–526.

Anderson, M. W., Orton, T. C., Pickett, R. D., and Eling, T. E. (1974). Accumulation of amines in the isolated perfused rabbit lung. *J. Pharmacol. Exp. Ther.*, **189**:456–466.

Bakhle, Y. S. and Vane, J. R. (1974). Pharmacokinetic function of the pulmonary circulation. *Physiol. Rev.*, **54**:1007–1045.

Baldwin, R. C., Pasi, A., MacGregor, J. T., and Hine, C. H. (1975). The rates of radical formation from the dipyridyium herbicides paraquat, diquat, and morfamquat in homogenates of rat lung, kidney, and liver: An inhibitory effect of carbon monoxide. *Toxicol. Appl. Pharmacol.*, **32**:298–304.

Bartosek, I., Mussini, E., Saroino, C., and Grattini, S. (1970). Studies on nitrazepam reduction in vitro. *Eur. J. Pharmacol.*, **11**:249–253.

Bend, J. R., Hook, G. E. R., Easterling, R. E., Gram, T. E., and Fouts, J. R. (1972). A comparative study of the hepatic and pulmonary microsomal mixed-function oxidase systems in the rabbit. *J. Pharmacol. Exp. Ther.*, **183**:206–217.

Bend, J. R., Hook, G. E. R., and Gram, T. E. (1973). Characterization of lung microsomes as related to drug metabolism. *Drug Metab. Disposition*, **1**: 358–367.

Bickel, M. H. (1969). The pharmacology and biochemistry of N-oxides. *Pharmacol. Rev.*, **21**:325–355.

Bickel, M. H. (1972). Liver metabolic reactions: Tertiary amine *N*-dealkylation, tertiary amine *N*-oxidation, *N*-oxide reduction, and *N*-oxide *N*-dealkylation. *Arch. Biochem. Biophys.*, **148**:54–62.

Bickel, M. H. and Minder, R. (1970). Metabolism and biliary excretion of the lipophilic drug molecules, imipramine and desmethylimipramine in the rat. *Biochem. Pharmacol.*, **19**:2437–2443.

James, M. O., Fouts, J. R., and Bend, J. R. (1976). Hepatic and extrahepatic metabolism, in vitro, of an epoxide (8-^{14}C styrene oxide) in the rabbit. *Biochem. Pharmacol.,* in press.

Jernstrom, B., Capdevila, J., Jakobsson, S., and Orrenius, S. (1975). Solubilization and partial purification of cytochrome P-450 from rat lung microsomes. *Biochem. Biophys. Res. Commun.,* **64**:814–822.

Juchau, M. R., Pedersen, M. G., and Symms, K. G. (1972). Hydroxylation of 3,4-benzpyrene in human fetal tissue homogenates. *Biochem. Pharmacol.,* **21**:2269–2272.

Kiese, M. and Uehleke, H. (1961). Der Ort der N-Oxydation des Anilins im Hoheren Tier. *Naunyn-Schmiedeberg's Arch. Pharmacol.,* **242**:117–129.

Kikkawa, Y. and Suzuki, K. (1972). Alteration of cellular and acellular alveolar and bronchiolar walls produced by hypercholesteremic drug AY9944. *Lab. Invest.,* **26**:441–447.

Klinger, W. (1973). Amidopyrine-N-demethylation by lung 9000 X g supernatant of newborn and adult rats. *Acta Biol. Med. Ger.,* **31**:467–469.

Kuntzman, R., Klutch, A., Tsai, I., and Burns, J. J. (1965). Physiological distribution and metabolic inactivation of chlorcyclizine and cyclizine. *J. Pharmacol. Exp. Ther.,* **149**:29–35.

Kuschner, M., Laskin, S., Cristofano, E., and Nelson, N. (1957). Experimental carcinoma of the lung. In Proceedings of the Third National Cancer Conference. J. B. Lippincott and Co., Philadelphia (1971), pp. 485–495.

La Du, B. N., Mandel, H. G., and Way, E. L. (1971). *Fundamentals of Drug Metabolism and Disposition.* Williams and Wilkins Co., Baltimore.

Law, F. C. P., Wilson, A. G. E., Eling, T. E., and Anderson, M. (1976). Uptake, metabolism, and efflux of methadone in "single pass" isolated perfused rabbit lungs. *J. Pharmacol. Exp. Ther.,* in press.

Locke, R. K., Bastone, V. B., and Baron, R. L. (1971). Studies of carbamate pesticide metabolism utilizing plant and mammalian cells in culture. *J. Agr. Food Chem.,* **19**:1205–1209.

Lu, A. Y. H. and Levin, W. (1974). The resolution and reconstitution of the liver microsomal hydroxylation system. *Biochim. Biophys. Acta,* **344**: 205–240.

Lüllman, H., Lullman-Rauch, R., and Reil, G. H. (1973a). A comparative ultrastructural study of the effects of chlorphentermine and triparanol in rat lung and adrenal gland. *Virchows Arch. B.,* **12**:91–103.

Lüllmann, H., Rossen, E., and Seiler, K. U. (1973b). The pharmacokinetics of phentermine and chlorphentermine in chronically treated rats. *J. Pharm. Pharmacol.,* **25**:239–243.

Lüllmann-Rauch, R., Lullman, H., and Wassermann, O. (1973a). Drug-induced phospholipidosis. *Ger. Med. Month.,* **3**:128–135.

Lüllmann-Rauch, R. and Reil, G. H. (1974). Chlorophentermine-induced lipidosis-like ultrastructural alterations in lungs and adrenal glands of several species. *Toxicol. Appl. Pharmacol.,* **30**:408–421.

Lüllmann-Rauch, R., Reil, G. H., Rosen, E., and Seiler, K. U. (1972). The ultra-structure of rat lung changes induced by an anoretic drug (chlorphentermine). *Virchows Arch. B.,* **11**:167–181.

Lüllmann-Rauch, R., Reil, G. H., and Sceid, D. (1973b). Lipidosis-ahnliche Zellveranderungen bei der Ratte nach Behandlung mit Thymoleptika. *Verh. Dtsch. Ges. Pathol.,* **57**:425.

Machinist, J. M., Dehner, E. W., and Ziegler, D. M. (1968). Microsomal oxidases. III. Comparison of species and organ distribution of dialkylarylamine N-oxide dealkylase and dialkylarylamine *N*-oxidase. *Arch. Biochem. Biophys.,* **125**:858–864.

Marcotte, J. and Witschi, H. P. (1972). Induction of pulmonary aryl hydrocarbon hydroxylase by marijuana. *Res. Commun. Chem. Pathol. Pharm.,* **4**:561–568.

Masters, B. S. and Zeigler, D. M. (1971). The distinct nature and function of NADPH-cytochrome *c* reductase and NADPH-dependent mixed-function amine oxidase of porcine liver microsomes. *Arch. Biochem. Biophys.,* **145**:358–364.

Matsubara, T., Prough, R. A., Burke, M. D., and Estabrook, R. W. (1974). The preparation of microsomal fractions of rodent respiratory tract and their characterization. *Cancer Res.,* **34**:2196–2203.

Matsubara, T. and Tochino, Y. (1971). Electron transport systems of lung microsomes and their physiological functions. I. Intracellular distribution of oxidative enzymes in lung cells. *J. Biochem. Tokyo,* **70**:981–991.

Mehendale, H. M. and El-Bassiouni, E. A. (1976). Uptake and disposition of aldrin and dieldrin by isolated perfused rabbit lung. *Drug Metab. Disposition,* in press.

Minder, R., Schnetzer, F., and Bickel, M. H. (1971). Hepatic and extrahepatic metabolism of the psychotropic drugs, chlorpromazine, imipramine, and imipramine-N-oxide. *Naunyn-Schmiedeberg's Arch. Pharmacol.,* **268**:334–347.

Murray, R. E. and Gibson, J. E. (1972). A comparative study of paraquat intoxication in rats, guinea pigs and monkeys. *Exp. Molec. Pathol.,* **17**:317–325.

Neal, R. A. (1976). A comparison of the in vitro metabolism of parathion in the lung and liver of the rabbit. *Toxicol. Appl. Pharmacol.,* **23**:123–130.

Niemeyer, R. (1976). Isolated perfused lung – A critical appraisal. *Environ. Health Persp.,* in press.

Oesch, F., Jerina, D. M., and Daily, J. W. (1971). A radiometric assay for hepatic epoxide hydrase activity with [7-^{3}H] styrene oxide. *Biochim. Biophys. Acta,* **227**:685–691.

Okamoto, T., Chan, Po-C., and So, B. T. (1972). Effect of tobacco, marijuana, and benzo(a)pyrene on aryl hydrocarbon hydroxylase in hamster lung. *Life Sci.,* **11**:733–741.

Oppelt, W. W., Zange, M., Ross, W. E., and Remmer, H. (1970). Comparison of microsomal drug hydroxylation in lung and liver of various species. *Res. Commun. Chem. Pathol. Pharmacol.,* **1**:43–56.

Orton, T. C., Anderson, M. W., Pickett, R. D., and Eling, T. E. (1973). Xenobiotic accumulation and metabolism by isolated perfused rabbit lung. *J. Pharmacol. Exp. Ther.,* **186**:482–497.

Parke, D. V. (1968). The Biochemistry of Foreign Compounds. Pergamon Press, New York.

Philpot, R. M., Arinc, E., and Fouts, J. R. (1975). Reconstitution of the rabbit pulmonary microsomal mixed-function oxidase system from solubilized components. *Drug Metab. Disposition,* **3**:118–126.

Pickett, R. D., Anderson, M. W., Orton, T. C., and Eling, T. E. (1975). The pharmacodynamics of 5-hydroxytryptamine uptake and metabolism by the isolated perfused rabbit lung. *J. Pharmacol. Exp. Ther.,* **194**:545–553.

Poland, A. P., Glover, E., Robinson, J. R., and Nebert, D. W. (1974). Genetic expression of aryl hydrocarbon hydroxylase activity: Induction of monooxygenase activities and cytochrome P_1-450 formation by 2,3,7,8-tetrachlorodibenzo-*p*-dixoin in mice genetically "nonresponsive" to other aromatic hydrocarbons. *J. Biol. Chem.,* **249**:5599–5606.

Poore, R. E. and Neal, R. A. (1972). Evidence for extrahepatic metabolism of parathion. *Toxicol. Appl. Pharmacol.,* **23**:759–768.

Reid, W. D., Glick, J. M., and Krishna, G. (1972). Metabolism of foreign compounds by alveolar macrophages of rabbits. *Biochem. Biophys. Res. Comm.,* **49**:626–634.

Reid, W. D., Illett, K. F., Glick, M. M., and Krishna, G. (1973). Metabolism and binding of aromatic hydrocarbons in the lung: Relationship to experimental bronchiolar necrosis. *Am. Rev. Resp. Dis.,* **107**:539–551.

Reid, W. D. and Krishna, G. (1973). Centrolobular hepatic necrosis related to covalent binding of metabolites of halogenated aromatic hydrocarbons. *Exp. Molec. Pathol.,* **18**:80–99.

Richards, J. C., Boxer, G. E., and Smith, C. C. (1950). Studies on the distribution and metabolism of methadone in normal and tolerant rats by a new colorimetic method. *J. Pharmacol. Exp. Ther.,* **98**:380–385.

Robertson, B., Enhorning, G., Ivemark, B., Malmqvist, E., and Modee, J. (1971). Experimental respiratory distress induced by paraquat. *J. Pathol.,* **103**:239–244.

Rose, M. S., Smith, L. L., and Wyatt, I. (1974). Evidence for energy-dependent accumulation of paraquat into rat lung. *Nature,* **252**:314–315.

Roth, J. A. and Gillis, C. N. (1974). Inhibition of lung, liver and brain monoamine oxidase by imipramine and desipramine. *Biochem. Pharmacol.,* **23**:1138–1140.

Roth, J. A. and Gillis, C. N. (1975). Inhibition of rabbit mitochondrial oxidase by iprindole. *Biochem. Pharmacol.,* **24**:151–152.

Saffiotti, U., Cefis, F., and Kolb, L. H. (1968). A method for the experimental induction of bronchogenic carcinoma. *Cancer Res.,* **28**:104–124.

Schmien, R., Seiler, K. U., and Wasserman, O. (1974). I. Lipid composition and chlorphentermine content of rat lung tissue and alveolar macrophages after chronic treatment. *Naunyan-Schmiedeberg's Arch. Pharmacol.,* **283**:331–334.

Selkirk, J. K., Huberman, E., and Heidelberger, C. (1971). An epoxide is an intermediate in the microsomal metabolism of the chemical carcinogen, dibenz(a,h)anthracene. *Biochem. Biophys. Res. Commun.*, **43**:1010–1023.

Seydel, J. K. and Wassermann, O. (1973). NMR studies on the molecular basis of drug-induced phospholipidosis. *Naunyn-Schmiedeberg's Arch. Pharmacol.*, **279**:207–210.

Sharp, W. C., Ottolenghi, A., and Posner, H. S. (1972). Correlation of paraquat toxicity with tissue concentrations and weight loss of the rat. *Toxicol. Appl. Pharmacol.*, **22**:241–251.

Sher, S. P. (1971). Drug enzyme induction and drug interactions: literature tabulation. *Toxicol. Appl. Pharmacol.*, **18**:780–834.

Shikata, T., Kanetaka, T., Endo, Y., and Nagashima, K. (1972). Drug-induced generalized phospholipidosis. *Acta Pathol. Jap.*, **22**:517–531.

Sims, P. and Grover, P. L. (1974). Epoxides in polycyclic aromatic hydrocarbon metabolism and carcinogenesis. *Adv. Cancer Res.*, **20**:166–262.

Sorokin, S. P. (1970). In P. Nettesheim, M. G. Hanna, Jr., and J. W. Deatherage, Jr. (eds.): The cells of the lung. *Morphology of Experimental Respiratory Carcinogenesis.* U.S. Atomic Energy Commission, Oak Ridge.

Stock, K. and Westermann, E. (1965). Quantitative estimation and tissue distribution of Ko 592, 1-(3-methylphenoxy)-3 isopropylaminopropanol(2)-hydrochloride, a new sympathetic β-receptor blocking agent. *Biochem. Pharmacol.*, **14**:227–236.

Stripp, B., Menard, R. H., Zampaglione, N. G., Hamrick, M. E., and Gillette, J. R. (1973). Effect of steroids on drug metabolism in male and female rats. *Drug Metab. Disposition*, **1**:216–223.

Theiss, E., Hummler, H., Lengsfeld, H., Staiger, L. R., and Trazger, J. P. (1973). Lipidspeicherung bei Versuchstieren nach Verabreichung trizyklischer Amine. *Schweiz. Med. Wochenschr.*, **103**:424–427.

Thorstrand, C. (1974). Cardiovascular effects of poisoning with tricyclic antidepressants. *Acta Med. Scand.*, **195**:505–514.

Uehleke, H. (1968). Extrahepatic microsomal drug metabolism. In *Proceedings of the European Society for the Study of Drug Toxicity, Xth Meeting.* Oxford, pp. 94–100.

Uehleke, H. (1971). N-hydroxylation. *Xenobiotica*, **1**:327–338.

Uehleke, H. (1972). The Biological Oxidation of Nitrogen in Organic Molecules. J. W. Bridges, J. W. Gorrod, and D. V. Parke (eds.). Taylor and Francis, London, pp. 15–26.

Vijeyaratnam, G. D. and Corrin, B. (1972). Pulmonary histiocytosis simulating desquamative interstitial pneumonia in rats receiving oral iprindole. *J. Pathol.*, **108**:105–113.

Wang, I. Y., Marver, M. S., Rasmussen, R. E., and Crocker, T. T. (1971). Enzymatic conversion of benz(a)pyrene. *Arch. Intern. Med.*, **128**:125–130.

Wattenberg, L. W. (1971). Symposium on Fundamentals of Cancer Research, M. D. Anderson Hospital and Tumor Institute, **24**:241–255.

Wattenberg, L. W. (1972). Dietary modification of intestinal and pulmonary aryl hydrocarbon hydroxylase activity. *Toxicol. Appl. Pharmacol.*, **23**:741–748.

Wattenberg, L. W. and Leong, J. L. (1962). Histochemical demonstration of reduced pyridine nucleotide-dependent polycyclic hydrocarbon metabolizing systems. *J. Histochem. Cytochem.,* **10**:412–420.

Wattenberg, L. W. and Leong, J. L. (1965). Effects of phenothiazines on protective systems against polycyclic hydrocarbons. *Cancer Res.,* **25**:365–370.

Wattenberg, L. W. and Leong, J. L. (1968). Inhibition of the carcinogenic action of 7,12-dimentylbenz(a)anthracene by β-naphthoflavone. *Proc. Soc. Exp. Biol. Med.,* **128**:940–943.

Wattenberg, L. W. and Leong, J. L. (1970). Inhibition of the carcinogenic action of benzo(a)pyrene by flavones. *Cancer Res.,* **30**:1922–1925.

Wattenberg, L. W., Leong, J. L., and Galbraith, A. R. (1968a). Induction of increased benzpyrene hydroxylase activity in pulmonary tissue in vitro. *Proc. Soc. Exp. Biol. Med.,* **127**:467–469.

Wattenberg, L. W., Page, M. A., and Leong, J. L. (1968b). Induction of increased benzpyrene hydroxylase activity by flavones and related compounds. *Cancer Res.,* **28**:934–937.

Wattenberg, L. W., Page, M. A., and Leong, J. L. (1968c). Induction of increased benzpyrene hydroxylase activity by 2-phenylbenzothiazoles and related compounds. *Cancer Res.,* **28**:2539–2544.

Way, E., Leong, J. L., and Dailey, R. E. (1950). Adsorption, distribution and excretion of tripelennamine (pyribenzamine). *Proc. Soc. Exp. Biol. Med.,* **73**:423–427.

Welch, R. M., Cavallito, J., and Loh, A. (1972). Effect of exposure to cigarette smoke on the metabolism of benzo(a)pyrene and acetophenetidin by lung and intestine of rats. *Toxicol. Appl. Pharmacol.,* **23**:749–758.

Welch, R. M., Loh, A., and Conney, A. H. (1971). Cigarette smoke: Stimulatory effect on metabolism of 3,4-benzpyrene by enzymes in rat lung. *Life Sci.,* **10**:215–221.

Wiebel, F. J., Leutz, J. C., Diamond, L., and Gelboin, H. V. (1971). Aryl hydrocarbon (benzo[α]pyrene) hydroxylase in microsomes from rat tissues: differential inhibition and stimulation by benzoflavones and organic solvents. *Arch. Biochem. Biophys.,* **144**:78–86.

Wiebel, F. J., Leutz, J. C. and Gelboin, H. V. (1973). Aryl hydrocarbon (benzo[α]pyrene) hydroxylase: Inducible in extrahepatic tissues of mouse strains not inducible in liver. *Arch. Biochem. Biophys.,* **154**:292–294.

Williams, R. T. (1959). *Detoxication Mechanisms.* John Wiley and Sons, New York.

Wilson, A. G. E., Law, F. C. P., Eling, T. E., and Anderson, M. (1976). Uptake, metabolism, and efflux of methadone in "single pass" isolated perfused rabbit lungs. *J. Pharmacol. Exp. Ther.,* **199**:360–367.

Wynder, E. L. and Hoffman, D. (1968). Experimental tobacco carcinogenesis. *Science,* **162**:862–871.

Ziegler, D. M., Mitchell, C. H., and Jallow, D. (1969). In J. R. Gillette (ed.): *Microsomes and Drug Oxidation.* Academic Press, New York, p. 193.

6

Possible Clinical Implications of Metabolism of Bloodborne Substrates by the Human Lung

C. NORMAN GILLIS and NICHOLAS M. GREENE

Yale University School of Medicine
New Haven, Connecticut

I. Introduction

Many reports in the literature refer to the ability of mammalian lung to clear certain vasoactive hormones from pulmonary blood and to synthesize or activate others, which then enter blood leaving the pulmonary circulation. Unfortunately, few of the published reports refer to study of those processes in human lung. However, if human lungs, like those of other mammalia, can alter systemic arterial blood concentrations of important vasoactive hormones, then apparently these properties might be of significance in cardiopulmonary physiology or pathophysiology (Said 1968, Gillis 1973, Fishman and Pietra 1974, Junod 1975).

In this chapter we will review the limited amount of data that pertains to inactivation of bloodborne substrates by human lung and will direct attention to situations in which such inactivation may be altered. The term

Original investigations by the authors, referred to in this chapter were supported by grants from the U.S. Public Health Service (HL-13315 and HL-05942) and the Connecticut Heart Association.

substrate will be used to describe any bloodborne drug or hormone removed and/or metabolized during its passage through lung. *Removal* of a substrate during its passage through lung describes process(es) that result in movement of substrate into lung. *Removal*, therefore, connotes a net reduction in the concentration of a substrate in pulmonary venous, compared with pulmonary arterial blood. This use of *removal* implies nothing about the nature of the process by which removal is accomplished, for example, whether active transport or lipid solubility are involved, nor does it indicate whether the substrate removed is subsequently inactivated by catabolism or by binding to intrapulmonary storage sites. *Uptake* refers to removal associated with net accumulation of substrate within lung. Although uptake of 5-hydroxytryptamine, noradrenaline, and other substrates is known to occur in lungs of experimental animals (Gillis 1973, 1976, Bakhle and Vane 1974), such has not been proven in man.

Figure 1 is a diagramatic representation of processes known to occur in lungs of other species and which may occur in human lung. While there is little direct evidence to support the existence of these mechanisms in human lung, the diagram serves to identify potential sites for changes induced by drugs or disease. From Figure 1, it can be seen, for example, that physiologically inactive precursors of certain vasoactive hormones, such as angiotensin I or arachidonic acid, or the hormones themselves may be removed from the vascular or extracellular space of human lung by processes of transport and/or diffusion and reach the extravascular space. Here, one or more presumably enzymically catalyzed steps might occur with ultimate formation of active product (or metabolite), which then reaches the extracellular and ultimately reenters the vascular space. Clinically used drugs, for example, propranolol (Hayes and Cooper 1971), imipramine, or desmethylimipramine (Rosenbloom

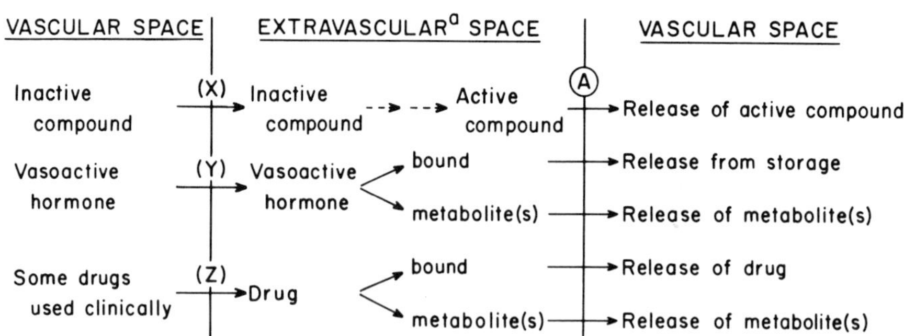

FIGURE 1   Processes of metabolism that may occur in human lung. [a]Intra- or extracellular. (Reprinted from Gillis, C. N. et al. (1974). *Surgery*, **76**:608–616, with permission of C. V. Mosby Company and the authors.)

and Bass 1970), also may be removed and metabolized by lung. X, Y, and Z encompass transport processes as well as physical factors that might be involved in removal, including lipid solubility and diffusion through cell membranes or through interendothelial cell gaps (Aschheim 1974). The *A* symbolizes all processes by which substances, including those synthesized endogenously, are released from lung into the circulation. Accordingly, *A* includes events leading to release of hormones regardless of the nature of the stimulus provoking such release. For example, release of prostaglandins in response to ventilation (Berry et al. 1971) anaphylaxis (Bakhle and Vane 1974) or hypoxia (Said et al. 1974) can be mentioned in this context.

Factors that may influence removal of substrates by lung include:

1. Concentration of substrate in blood.

2. Lipid solubility of the substrate.

3. Diffusional characteristics of the substrate.

4. The pattern of blood flow through the lung, including the presence or absence of anatomic or functional shunting of blood.

5. Degree of protein binding and/or ionization of substrate.

II. 5-Hydroxytryptamine

Removal of 5-hydroxytryptamine (5-HT) by human lung has been studied more extensively than that of other substrates. Interest in pulmonary removal of 5-HT in man stems from the observation (Lembeck 1953, Pernow and Waldenstrom 1954) that patients suffering from carcinoid tumors have elevated blood levels of 5-HT and frequently show cardiac valvular lesions, which are characteristically on the right side of the heart. In 1955 Goble, Hay, and Sandler reported that endogenous plasma and serum levels of 5-HT were 60% lower in brachial arterial than in pulmonary arterial blood simultaneously obtained in a patient with carcinoid. The authors proposed, therefore, that valvular lesions in the right rather than left heart of patients with carcinoid tumors reflect removal of 5-HT from pulmonary arterial blood so that the right side of the heart is exposed to higher concentrations of the amine than is the left. However, the difference between blood 5-HT sampled on the left and right sides of the heart could not be confirmed by Sjoerdsma and Associates (1957).

In 1968 Davis evaluated 5-HT removal in man with a technique (Davis and Wang 1965) in which indocyanine green and [^{14}C] 5-HT were administered as a bolus into the pulmonary artery, following which blood was sampled continuously from the brachial artery for approximately 25 sec. Cardiac output was determined both by the standard indicator dilution technique (Macintyr et al. 1951) and also from the ratio of total counts per minute injected to total counts recovered at the brachial artery. The difference between cardiac output measured with 5-HT and that measured with indocyanine green was taken to reflect removal of 5-HT. With this technique, Davis (1968) examined 5-HT removal in 4 patients with carcinoid disease, 2 with and 2 without cardiac valve lesions. Surprisingly, 1 patient with carcinoid heart disease removed 12% of injected 5-HT; the other removed none. In contrast, the 2 patients without cardiac involvement removed 38% and 66% of injected 5-HT during one passage through the pulmonary vascular bed. The explanation for the difference in the two types of patients is not clear. In both groups over 80% of 5-HT was free in plasma, suggesting that platelet binding was not necessary for pulmonary removal of the amine. Davis (1968) found little correlation between measured endogenous 5-HT concentration and removal of radioactive 5-HT and concluded that pulmonary removal was more efficient in patients without cardiac lesions than in those with such lesions.

Davis (1968) also found that when $[^{14}C]$ 5-HT was administered intravenously to a patient with carcinoid, all radioactivity in brachial arterial plasma was associated with unchanged 5-HT and none represented metabolites of the amine. This indicated that in man 5-HT passes through the lung without being deaminated, an observation later confirmed by Gillis and associates (1974). These findings contrast with data obtained in perfused lungs from the rat (Alabaster and Bakhle 1970, Junod 1972) and the rabbit (Gillis et al. 1975) in which 5-HT is rapidly deaminated. The findings in man may explain the absence of changes in the concentration of 5-hydroxyindolacetic acid (5-HIAA) in urine from patients following surgical removal of one lung (Frick and Virkkula 1961).

Larmi and Heikkinen (1967) studied pulmonary 5-HT removal in man by infusing the amine at a rate of 800 ug/min into the superior vena cava in 7 patients undergoing lobectomy, mainly for carcinoma of the lung. Small blood samples were taken from the common pulmonary artery and vein for fluorimetric determination of 5-HT concentration before, and 10 and 15 min after the infusion was started. In each patient the pulmonary artery to pulmonary vein (PA-PV) gradient was determined and the statistical significance of the mean difference was determined by the t test for paired data. Before infusion of 5-HT, there was no measurable gradient of endogenous 5-HT across the lungs. Ten minutes after the infusion started, pulmonary arterial 5-HT was 0.18 ± 0.02 $\mu g/ml$ and pulmonary venous concentration was 0.16 ± 0.02 $\mu g/ml$, a PA-PV gradient that was statistically significant ($P<0.05$). After 15 min of 5-HT infusion, the PA-PV gradient was 0.06 ± 0.02 $\mu g/ml$ ($P<0.05$). There was no significant change in systemic blood pressure during 5-HT infusion, although pulmonary arterial pressure increased. These data suggest, therefore, that concentrations of 5-HT high enough to permit fluorimetric estimation of the amine in blood may be associated with altered blood flow or intrapulmonary arterial pressure; the effect of such hemodynamic changes on 5-HT removal by human lung is unknown.

We have studied pulmonary removal of 5-HT in patients undergoing cardiac surgery with cardiopulmonary bypass (Gillis et al. 1972, Gillis et al. 1974). A mixture of $[^{14}C]$ 5-HT and either $[^{3}H]$ norepinephrine or, in some cases $[^{3}H]$ inulin or $[^{3}H]$ water was administered as a bolus via a central venous catheter at the level of the superior vena cava. Total doses of amine given were not large enough to affect blood pressure or pulse rate. Blood samples were withdrawn into 3-mm diameter plastic tubing at a constant rate, simultaneously from the pulmonary artery and left atrium, for about 30 sec. Each length of tubing was then divided between clamps into six or eight segments. Total isotope in each segment was measured and expressed per unit weight of blood. A sequential plot of isotope (counts per minute per gram of blood) yielded a *profile* of isotope present in blood entering and leaving the lung during the sampling period (Fig. 2). When breakdown of amine in blood after withdrawal was prevented, over 90% of the radioactivity was associated with unchanged amine. Accordingly, the difference between total isotope entering and leaving the lung during the 30-sec sampling period specifically measured pulmonary removal of 5-HT (Gillis et al. 1972). Percent amine extraction was calculated according to the formula,

$$[1- (I_{LA}/I_{PA})] \times 100$$

where I_{LA} and I_{PA} are total isotope in blood sampled at the left atrium and pulmonary artery, respectively. Before cardiopulmonary bypass, lungs of 9 patients undergoing aortocoronary saphenous vein grafting removed an average of 65% 5-HT in a single circulation; this value increased significantly ($P < 0.05$) to 81% after bypass. Prebypass removal of 5-HT in these patients was about the same as in the 2 carcinoid patients without related cardiac disease, studied by Davis (1968).

· We subsequently observed that the magnitude of 5-HT removal is influenced by pulmonary intravascular pressure (Gillis et al. 1974). In 10 patients with mitral or aortic valvular disease in whom mean pulmonary arterial pressures at the time of catheterization exceeded 22 mm Hg, there was a significantly ($P < 0.05$) greater than normal removal of 5-HT (78%) followed by a decrease to 67% after bypass. We suggested that obstruction of left heart outflow caused by aortic or mitral valvular disease, with resulting increase in back pressure to the venous system and consequent capillary recruitment or distension, might increase *functional* endothelial surface and hence increase the potential for 5-HT removal. This proposal to explain the difference between normotensive and pulmonary hypertensive patients is based upon the fact that

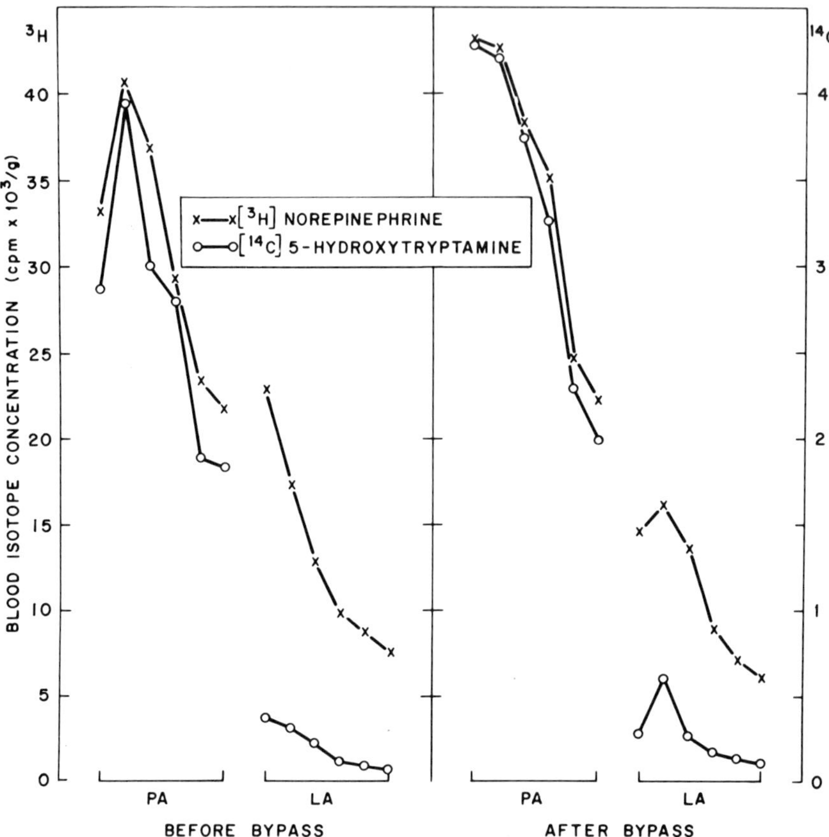

FIGURE 2   Isotope concentrations in blood withdrawn continuously, for approximately 30 sec, from pulmonary artery (PA) and left atrium (LA) both before and after cardiopulmonary bypass. At the start of injection of a mixture of [³H] NE and [¹⁴C] 5-HT, withdrawal of blood was begun. In each isotope concentration profile illustrated, the first point on the left represents isotope concentration in the first blood fraction withdrawn; the last point on the right reflects isotope concentration in the sixth and last sample withdrawn. The same profile was seen in patients with or without pulmonary hypertension. (Reprinted from Gillis, C. N. et al. 1974, *Surgery,* **76**:608–616 with the permission of C. V. Mosby Company and the authors.)

in perfused lungs of rat (Strum and Junod 1972, Cross et al. 1974) and rabbit (Iwasawa et al. 1973, Iwasawa and Gillis 1974, Gillis 1976) capillary and small vessel endothelium apparently plays an important role in removal of amine. However, there is presently no information about specific cells involved in the removal of 5-HT by human lung. Fluorescence microscopy or autoradiography in human lung obtained during surgery would be useful in this regard.

There are limitations in the interpretation of data derived by our technoque (Gillis et al. 1972, 1974), including the fact that movement of small molecules across vascular endothelial cells may be purely passive. We attempted to evaluate this possibility by injecting a mixture of [^{14}C] 5-HT and [^{3}H] water and determining the *apparent* water extraction along with that of 5-HT. Both before and after cardiopulmonary bypass, the direction and quantitative change in apparent extraction of water was unpredictable and apparently unrelated to the behavior of injected 5-HT. Even though the concentrations of 5-HT injected were below those that caused any change in heart rate or blood pressure, we felt it necessary to determine the influence, if any, of altered lung blood flow on removal. Therefore we used an indirect method to compare right ventricular flow among the patients studied. This was the ratio of the total isotope withdrawn at the pulmonary arterial sampling site divided by the total amount injected. There was no relationship between change in this measure and altered 5-HT extraction (Gillis et al. 1972). Therefore we concluded that our method gives a valid estimate of the disappearance of the amine within the pulmonary vascular bed.

Since most bloodborne 5-HT is platelet bound (Maupin 1969), and since platelets have the ability to take up and bind 5-HT, is removal of the amine merely a passive reflection of either platelet trapping in lungs or uptake into platelets that line pulmonary vascular endothelium (Kaufman et al. 1965)? For the following reasons we suggest that it is difficult to accept this as a major explanation: First, one is forced to postulate a much more rapid uptake of 5-HT by either circulating or endothelial-adherent platelets than has actually been observed (Okuda and Nemerson 1971). Since lung removes about 60% of a bolus injection of 5-HT (Davis 1968, Gillis et al. 1974), if removal were due solely to platelet binding, then many more circulating platelets must be trapped during a single pass through the lung circulation than present data indicate. Castro and associates (personal communication 1973) detected no difference between pulmonary arterial and venous blood platelet counts in patients undergoing cardiac catheterization. Davis (1968) also found no relation between platelet uptake of amine and the capacity of human lung to remove 5-HT. Finally, there is ample evidence that removal of 5-HT and other amines occurs effectively and rapidly in lungs of cat, rat, rabbit, and guinea pig perfused in vitro with physiologic saline solutions devoid of platelets. It seems unlikely, therefore, that platelet uptake of 5-HT and subsequent trapping of platelets on the endothelial membrane can explain pulmonary removal. Removal of 5-HT should be considered a function of human lung vasculature per se, at least until definative evidence to the contrary is produced.

If there were extensive pulmonary metabolism then, by analogy with lungs of experimental animals, metabolites might be released rapidly into pulmonary venous blood. By this criteria, the work of Davis (1968) and our own studies (Gillis et al. 1974) indicate that during the transit time of a *bolus* of 5-HT across the lung vasculature there is no intrapulmonary metabolism. To answer this question definitively, however, studies are required in which steady state infusions of labeled 5-HT are given into the pulmonary artery. Unfortunately, in the single published study with this design (Larmi and Heikkinen 1967), only 5-HT in blood was measured and there was no determination of 5-HIAA in pulmonary venous blood.

Pulmonary removal of 5-HT in man might be related to platelet aggregation. A tenfold increase in blood 5-HT promotes, while much higher concentrations of the amine inhibit, platelet aggregation (Baumgartner and Born 1968). In this context, control of plasma 5-HT, possibly by lung, could represent an important element of such homeostatic control, derangement of which may be linked to postoperative venous thrombosis in man (Gruby et al. 1971).

In addition to the link between right-sided heart lesions in patients with intestinal carcinoid tumors (Goble et al. 1955) and pulmonary removal of 5-HT referred to above, Sandler (1968) suggested that certain symptoms of bronchial carcinoid tumors are due to bypassing normal hepatic 5-HT inactivation. However, if the lung, rather than the liver, is the major site of 5-HT inactivation, then these symptoms equally could reflect inefficiency of pulmonary removal of 5-HT.

III.   Catecholamines

A.   Noradrenaline

One of the few studies of noradrenaline (NE) removal by human lung is that carried out by Biron and his collaborators who studied pulmonary inactivation by means of the "systemic pressor response" (Biron et al. 1969a, Boileau et al. 1972a) during cardiac catheterization in patients shown to have no hemodynamic abnormality. Noradrenaline was administered either via the pulmonary artery or via the thoracic aorta. Normally one or two series of four injections (two into the pulmonary artery and two into the aorta) were administered. Percent removal of NE was calculated as:

$$\left(1 - \frac{A}{PA}\right) \times 100$$

where PA and A referred to doses of NE required to cause equipotent pressor effects (20 min of systolic blood pressure) when given into the pulmonary artery and aorta, respectively. On this basis Boileau et al. (1972a) reported a mean removal of 13.0% ± 5.8% (standard error) in 5 patients. However, in these studies intraaortic administration does not permit injected amine to enter the coronary circulation and therefore eliminates the cardiac component of the pressor response. On the other hand, the pressor response to injection of NE into the pulmonary artery may include a direct effect of the amine on myocardial contractility following its entry into the coronary circulation. To evaluate the potential contribution of myocardial stimulation, Boileau et al. (1972a) carried out additional studies in which the left atrium, reached by means of a transseptal approach from the right atrium, was used as the intra-arterial injection site. In this study amine injected into either the pulmonary artery or the left atrium reached the coronary circulation and presumably exerted equal effects on the heart. With this modification, mean pulmonary inactivation in 4 patients was 17.5% ± 6.6% (SE). The authors suggest that the 4% to 5% difference between the mean values reflect the contribution of cardiac stimulation. However, the difference between these estimates was not statistically significant. Also, the authors estimate that the method has an inherent experimental error of 10% to 15% (Boileau et al. 1970). It is difficult, therefore, to accept the conclusion of these investigators that use of left atrium instead of aorta as the postlung injection site for NE adequately assesses the contribution of cardiac effects.

Use of the systemic pressor technique as a means of measuring pulmonary NE is also complicated by the fact that NE (or other substrates) may alter intravascular pressures within the lung, and in so doing stimulate pulmonary reflexes, either directly or indirectly, and thus modify the pressor response observed. Another limitation of this technique is that it cannot be used when sustained infusions of amine are to be given, since even modest elevation of systemic arterial pressure will elicit reflex restoration of control blood pressure levels. Despite these difficulties, however, the technique nevertheless is capable of distinguishing between NE, which is removed by lung, and adrenaline or isoproterenol, which are not removed to any significant degree by human lung (see below).

We have studied NE removal by human lung by a more direct technique, as described above under *5-hydroxytryptamine*. In these experiments we found (Gillis et al. 1974) that isotope in left atrial blood was associated largely with unchanged amine (see also, Stjärne et al. 1975). Therefore, the technique provides a valid measure of NE removal. As with 5-HT (Fig. 2) blood isotope concentration decreased as a function of time to baseline levels prior to recirculation of amine (i.e., within approximately 30 sec). In our first study, (Gillis et al. 1972) removal of NE before cardiopulmonary bypass was 23% and increased to 50% after cardiopulmonary bypass. Prebypass removal of NE measured by our direct technique thus agrees quite closely with the indirect estimate of Boileau et al. (1972). Removal of NE by lung of man appears, therefore, to be quantitatively similar to that reported in other species (Ginn and Vane 1968, Hughes et al. 1969, Alabaster and Bakhle 1973). In each patient we studied, prebypass extraction of NE was significantly lower than that of 5-HT (Gillis et al. 1972), again paralleling observations made in other species. As with 5-HT, removal of NE also was significantly increased in patients with pulmonary hypertension (Gillis et al. 1974), perhaps as a result of increased mean transit time and thus longer contact with endothelial surfaces in the lung vascular bed.

Pulmonary removal of [^{3}H] NE also occurs after bolus intravenous injections of the amine either to healthy subjects (Stjärne et al. 1975) or to patients undergoing cardiac catheterization (J. A. Will, personal communication 1976). Furthermore, Will and his colleagues (personal communication) also find a direct relationship between pulmonary transit time and the magnitude of removal, thus supporting the observation of increased removal accompanying pulmonary hypertension (Gillis et al. 1974).

Removal of about 20% to 25% of a single dose of NE during a single passage through lung does not necessarily imply the existence, normally, of a gradient of this magnitude across the pulmonary vascular bed. Proof of such a gradient depends upon measurement of endogenous NE in pulmonary arterial and left atrial blood. Unfortunately these are lacking, although the availability of highly sensitive enzymic methods for blood NE determination (Roizen et al. 1974) makes such studies in man possible.

While there is no information concerning the transpulmonary gradient of endogenous catecholamine in man, some studies in dogs may be relevant. Lammerant and de Herdt (1965) reported that the fluorimetrically determined endogenous catecholamine content of dog left atrial blood consistently was 50% lower than in pulmonary arterial blood sampled simultaneously. Since there is evidence that dog lung does not remove epinephrine (Ginn and Vane 1968), a 50% decrease in total endogenous catecholamine could reflect a greater removal of NE. A gradient of catecholamine across the lungs was maintained despite a large (50-fold) increase in pulmonary arterial blood levels induced by 2 min of hypoxia, suggesting that the removal process was not saturable. Boileau et al. (1972) infused NE into the femoral vein of dogs at rates from 0.23 to 3.0 μg/kg/min and measured plasma NE both in pulmonary artery and ascending aorta. Pulmonary inactivation in 16 dogs ranged from 5% to 54% (mean, 28.8% ± 3.8%). There was a highly significant negative correlation between the magnitude of infusion rate and percent inactivation, suggesting saturation of NE removal.

Can we attach any physiologic significance to the documented 20% to 25% removal of exogenously administered NE across the human pulmonary vascular bed? Boileau et al. (1972) calculated total peripheral resistance in 3 subjects to whom NE was given successively *via* the pulmonary artery and the aorta. They found that injection into the aorta produced a significantly greater elevation in peripheral resistance than did injection into the pulmonary artery. These data may reflect pulmonary inactivation, which prevented some of the infused NE from reaching the systemic arterial blood.

This demonstration offers some support for the proposal that the lungs may regulate arterial blood concentrations of NE. Also it suggests that increased lung removal of NE in normotensive patients after cardiopulmonary bypass (Gillis et al. 1972) may have clinical consequences. For example, NE is frequently administered as a pressor substance intravenously immediately after the patient is taken off total cardiopulmonary bypass. In this circumstance less NE may reach the peripheral arteriolar bed than anticipated. When and if a vasopressor is indicated at such a time, use of an amine that is not removed by the lung (e.g., epinephrine) may be preferable to administration of NE. Alternatively, left atrial, as opposed to intravenous, administration of pressor amines might be desirable.

There is no information on the effect of drugs on pulmonary removal of NE in man. However, it is instructive to consider several studies in which data may be partly explained by the effects of drugs on the process. In 4 volunteers, Boakes and associates (1973) found that imipramine (25 mg three times daily) caused a four- to eightfold potentiation of the pressor response to intravenous NE infusion. Interpretation of these data is difficult because the response to epinephrine was also potentiated, although to a smaller extent (two- to fourfold). However, imipramine is known to inhibit NE removal by rabbit (Iwasawa and Gillis 1974) and rat (Nicholas et al. 1974) lungs. Should this effect extend to human lung, it is possible that decreased pulmonary removal of NE contributed to the increased concentration of amine that reached the arteriolar vascular bed.

Electrocardiographic abnormalities reflecting arrhythmias of various types after tricyclic drug dosage are well documented in man (Moir 1973, Hong et al. 1974). If tricyclic drugs inhibit pulmonary uptake of NE in man, these arrhythmias may reflect greater than normal concentrations of NE in the coronary circulation during tricyclic drug administration. Some support for this proposal is offered by Eble et al. (1971) who found in dogs, that desmethyl-imipramine significantly potentiated both the systemic pressor response and the vascular resistance of the hind legs to intravenously administered NE. In contrast there was little increased vasoconstrictor action in skeletal muscle of the leg when NE was administered directly into the arterial circulation of this vascular bed.

Also, Kirkendol and Woodbury (1972) observed a sustained pressor response during a 60-min intravenous infusion of NE to dogs on total cardiopulmonary bypass. In contrast, *tolerance* to the same duration and magnitude of infusion in control animals occurred within 15 min. Although not considered by these authors, we believe an explanation for this phenomenon may be that exclusion of lungs during experimental bypass would have eliminated a normally significant extent of NE removal. Thus, increased blood concentrations reached the thoracic aorta during bypass.

An additional potential clinical implication of pulmonary removal of NE is found in studies concerning the effectiveness of α-receptor blockage in restoring cardiac function in patients following cardiopulmonary bypass for open heart surgery. It was reported (Burack et al. 1972) that pretreatment with phenoxybenzamine prevented the low cardiac output normally anticipated following cardiopulmonary bypass in the 7 patients studied. All were functional class IV patients by New York Heart Association criteria. Burack and his colleagues conclude that phenoxybenzamine may exert a *direct inotropic* (sympathomimetic?) effect. While this may be true, another explanation seems possible. Phenoxybenzamine effectively inhibits pulmonary removal of NE in perfused rabbit lungs (Iwasawa and Gillis 1974). If the same effect occurs in man, the concentration of NE in the left heart (and hence reaching the coronary vascular bed) may be significantly increased by phenoxybenzamine and so explain the beneficial effect of pretreatment with this drug.

B.　Adrenaline, Isoprenaline, and Dopamine

Only one group has studied adrenaline removal by human lung. In 3 patients, Boileau and associates (1971) compared pressor responses to pulmonary arterial and left atrial adrenaline administration: there was negligible removal of this amine (0.5%). This conclusion was supported by observations in an additional 3 patients after administration of propranolol to block the cardiac component of the cardiovascular response to adrenaline; in these cases adrenaline was equipotent, whether given by intraaortic or by intravenous (i.e., into the pulmonary artery) routes.

Boileau et al. (1970) examined the intrapulmonary fate of isoprenaline in 2 patients by comparing depressor responses after injections to the left atrium and the pulmonary artery. Depressor potency by the *arterial* route of injection (i.e., *via* the left atrium) was only 5% greater than that by the pulmonary route, implying that isoprenaline is not removed by the pulmonary vascular bed of conscious, sedated patients.

Dopamine also escaped pulmonary inactivation, according to a report (Boileau et al. 1972b) describing observations in 2 patients. On the basis of the limited evidence available, it appears that human lungs, like those of the rat (Nicholas et al. 1974) have little capacity to remove significant quantities of circulating dopamine, adrenaline, or isoprenaline.

IV. Peptides

A. Angiotensin I

In adults angiotensin I, given into the pulmonary artery, often had more pressor activity than similar doses administered by the intraaortic route (Biron et al. 1969, Biron and Campeau 1971). These data were interpreted as demonstrating intrapulmonary conversion of the decapeptide angiotensin I to a more potent vasoconstrictor substance, perhaps angiotensin II. The degree of conversion, was, however, variable. In adults (Biron and Campeau 1971) and children (Friedli et al. 1972) the increase in pressor potency, when pulmonary arterial and intraaortic administration of angiotensin I were compared, ranged from 0 to approximately 40%. Biron and Campeau (1971) suggested that this variability may reflect the existence of extrapulmonary sites for angiotensin I conversion. This proposal is considerably strengthened by the recent direct demonstration of extrapulmonary conversion of angiotensin I to angiotensin II during cardiopulmonary bypass in patients undergoing cardiac surgery (Favre et al. 1974). It should also be recognized, however, that potential sources of error, implicit in comparing pressor responses to pulmonary arterial and aortic administration of NE (referred to above), apply equally to angiotensin I.

Converting enzyme, responsible for hydrolysis of angiotensin I to the octapeptide angiotensin II, has been demonstrated in human lung (Fitz and Overturf 1972, Overturf et al. 1975), although its molecular weight differs from that found in lungs of other species (Fitz and Overturf 1972). Furthermore, Overturf et al. (1975) conclude that, unlike converting enzyme in lungs of other species, the dipeptidase of human lung may be distinct from the enzyme that hydrolyzes bradykinin. However, it is presently unclear whether converting enzyme normally hydrolyzes *circulating* angiotensin I in human lung. The studies of Biron and his collaborators, which demonstrated that patients had greater pressor responses after pulmonary arterial than after intraaortic administration of angiotensin I, do not establish the presence of the hydrolysis product, angiotensin II, in their pulmonary venous blood. Data provided by the systemic pressor response technique do not prove, therefore, that conversion of angiotensin I to angiotensin II normally occurred in human lung.

It has nevertheless generally been assumed, despite the lack of direct evidence, that angiotensin I is converted to angiotensin II in human lung as it is in lungs of experimental animals (Bakhle and Vane 1974) and furthermore, that inhibitors of converting enzyme in lungs of experimental animals act in man also by reducing conversion. One such inhibitor of converting enzyme, a nonapeptide designated SQ 20881, was found in 6 normal subjects to reduce pressor responses to angiotensin I, but to have no effect on the pressor response to angiotensin II (Collier et al. 1973). Recently, the same inhibitor was shown to cause a significant and prolonged reduction of blood pressure in 12 of 13 hypertensive patients (Gavras et al. 1974). However, these data do not necessarily prove that inhibition of human lung converting enzyme is the cause of altered pressor response to angiotensin I. Proof that such does occur in man requires direct demonstration not only that angiotensin II normally occurs in pulmonary venous blood after intravenous injection of angiotensin I, but also that the concentration of the octapeptide in pulmonary venous or peripheral arterial blood is reduced by an inhibitor of converting enzyme, for example SQ 20881. Evidence of this type seems long overdue in view of the importance in pathogenesis of certain forms of human hypertension of angiotensin II and the potential clinical usefulness of drugs that inhibit its production.

B. Angiotensin II

In 2 patients angiotensin II appeared to escape pulmonary removal and inactivation (Biron et al. 1969), as also reported for rat, guinea pig, dog, and cat lungs (Bakhle and Vane 1974).

C. Lysine-Vasopressin

This peptide apparently was unaffected by its passage through lungs of 6 patients undergoing cardiac catheterization (Crexell et al. 1972). In this regard human lung compares with that of cat, dog, and rabbit, which also failed to remove the peptide from the pulmonary circulation (Gilmore and Vane 1970). According to the definition of Vane (1969) vasopressin, therefore, may be regarded as a *circulating hormone.*

V. Prostaglandins

There exists a considerable body of data indicating that nonhuman mammalian lungs remove and inactivate prostaglandins (PG). It is also well established that lungs of experimental animals contain a specific enzyme, 15-hydroxy-prostaglandin dehydrogenase, responsible for the oxidation and inactivation of prostaglandins, especially PGE and PGF compounds; PGA compounds are less susceptible to oxidation (Bakhle and Vane 1974), at least in certain species. 15-Hydroxyprostaglandin dehydrogenase is also present in human lung (Samuelsson et al. 1971). Despite the impressive evidence in experimental animals demonstrating that lung is a major site for inactivation of PGE and PGF compounds, and despite numerous statements in the literature to the effect that the same occurs in man (e.g., Shaw and Moser 1975), direct proof that human lung does indeed biodegrade prostaglandins has become available only within the last year. Golub and associates (1975) studied removal of $[^3H]PGE_1$ (3 patients) and $[^3H]PGA_1$ (7 patients) during 2 continuous intravenous infusions to patients undergoing elective cardiac catheterization. Concentrations of both prostaglandins in pulmonary arterial and left ventricular blood were measured 90, 105, and 120 min after beginning infusion. The mean removal of PGE_1 was 67.8%, whereas that of PGA_1 was only 8.1%. These data establish that in man, as in other species (Bakhle and Vane 1974), circulating PGA_1 largely escapes degradation in lung. Jose and associates (1976) measured immuno-reactive $PGF_{2\alpha}$ in pulmonary arterial and aortic blood of 8 patients during diagnostic cardiac catheterization. During a 10-min infusion of $PGF_{2\alpha}$ they found that the mean transpulmonary $PGF_{2\alpha}$ gradient was 77% in 6 patients who had no evidence of lung disease. Significantly, however, there was no loss of $PGF_{2\alpha}$ in the lung circulation of another patient diagnosed as having primary pulmonary hypertension.

It is unclear in these studies whether removal of prostaglandins reflected uptake or metabolism within lung. Studies in this laboratory, however, have concerned the metabolic fate of a bolus intravenous injection of $[^3H]PGE_1$ or $[^3H]PGA_1$ in anesthetized patients during cardiac surgery (Gillis et al. 1976). We used the technique of pulmonary arterial-left atrial difference described earlier (Gillis et al. 1972, 1974). In 11 patients given $[^3H]PGE_1$, over 90% of tritium in pulmonary arterial blood, withdrawn continuously for 40 sec after PGE_1 injection, was present as unchanged PGE_1. Left atrial blood, withdrawn simultaneously from 10 of these patients, contained only 19% to 22% unchanged PGE_1, reflecting extensive removal of this prostaglandin (cf. Golub et al. 1975). In 1 patient, however, with evidence of poor gas exchange (and likely considerable intrapulmonary shunting), over 50% of the tritium in left atrial blood was unchanged PGE_1, indicating decreased inactivation within the lung circulation. In all other cases the bulk (over 80%) of tritium in left atrial blood was in the form of a metabolite that had the same chromatographic mobility in two solvent systems as did marker 15-keto PGE_1. When similar determinations were made after periods on cardiopulmonary bypass (5 patients), there was a significant ($P < 0.01$) decrease in pulmonary removal of total tritium but no detectable change in the proportion of radioactivity in left atrial blood associated with unchanged PGE_1. In contrast to our observations with PGE_1, we found no chromatographic evidence for metabolic degradation of $[^3H]PGA_1$ after bolus intravenous injections (5 patients).

Additional studies are needed to confirm these observations and also to extend the tentative suggestion (Jose et al. 1976, Gillis et al. 1976) that the presence of lung disease may modify prostaglandin inactivation.

VI. Histamine

Numerous reports indicate that lungs of many mammalian species contain high concentrations of N-methyltransferase, the enzyme involved in catalyzing the biodegradation of histamine. Animal data suggest, however, that pulmonary inactivation of histamine in vivo plays a relatively minor role compared to that of other organs, notably the liver and kidneys (Vane 1969). Whether human lung inactivates histamine in vivo at all or, if it does, the extent to which it does so remain, however, undefined in the absence of direct in vivo studies in man. Indeed, even in vitro data are fragmentary. Lilja et al. (1960) for example, evaluated the metabolism of $[^{14}C]$ histamine by adding it to a minced specimen of lung obtained from a single patient during surgery. After 3 hr of incubation at 37°C, approximately one-third of the radioactivity was associated with methylhistamine and about two-thirds represented unchanged histamine, with trace amounts representing methylimidazole acetic acid and free and conjugated imidazole acetic acid. While Lilja and associates concluded that human lung could inactivate histamine, further data are required to prove the presence, extent, and mechanism of pulmonary biotransformation of bloodborne histamine in man.

VII. Summary and Conclusions

Knowledge of removal or inactivation of bloodborne substrates by human lung is fragmentary. Although 5-HT and NE are removed from the pulmonary circulation, their subsequent intrapulmonary fate is unclear. Both PGE_1 and $PGF_{2\alpha}$ are extensively inactivated in human lung, while PGA_1 appears to be unaffected. Preliminary data suggest that PGE_1 is degraded to a compound with the same chromatographic mobility as 15-keto PGE_1. There is very limited evidence to suggest that isoproterenol, adrenaline, dopamine, and vasopressin apparently are unaffected by their passage through lung. Additional and confirmatory observations of the absence of lung removal of these substances are required. It is clear that conversion of angiotensin I to a more effective pressor substance occurs during transpulmonary movement of this decapeptide; however, whether the substance produced in lung is angiotensin II remains to be proven.

There are many literature references containing extrapolation to human lung of data derived from studies in experimental animals. While human lung may be capable of controlling pulmonary venous blood levels of certain drugs and vasoactive hormones, there are no data that definitely establish this as a physiologic function. Until such evidence is forthcoming, comment concerning modification of these processes by drugs or by disease, therefore, must remain speculative.

References

Alabaster, V. A. and Bakhle, Y. S. (1970). Removal of 5-hydroxytryptamine in the pulmonary circulation of rat isolated lungs. *Br. J. Pharmacol.,* **40**: 468–482.

Alabaster, V. A. and Bakhle, Y. S. (1973). The removal of noradrenaline in the pulmonary circulation of rat isolated lungs. *Br. J. Pharmacol.,* **47**:325–331.

Aschheim, E. (1974). Traffic of metabolites between blood and tissues. *Microvasc. Res.,* **8**:64–69.

Bakhle, Y. S. and Vane, J. R. (1974). Pharmacokinetic function of the pulmonary circulation. *Physiol. Rev.,* **54**:1007–1045.

Baumgartner, H. R. and Born, G. V. R. (1968). Effect of 5-hydroxytryptamine on platelet aggregation. *Nature (Lond.),* **218**:137–141.

Berry, E. M., Edmonds, J. F., and Wyllie, J. H. (1971). Release of prostaglandin E₂ and unidentified factors from ventilated lungs. *Br. J. Surg.,* **58**:189–192.

Biron, P., Boileau, J. C., and Campeau, L. (1969a). Norepinephrine inactivation in the pulmonary circulation of animals and humans. *Clin. Res.,* **17**:230.

Biron, P., Campeau, L., and David, P. (1969b). Fate of angiotensin I and II in the pulmonary circulation. *Am. J. Cardiol.,* **24**:544–547.

Biron, P. and Campeau, L. (1971). Pulmonary and extrapulmonary fate of angiotensin I. *Rev. Can. Biol.,* **30**:27–34.

Boakes, A. J., Laurence, D. R., Teoh, P. C., Barar, F. S. K., Benedikter, L. T., and Prichard, B. N. C. (1973). Interactions between sympathomimetic amines and antidepressants in man. *Br. Med. J.,* **1**:311–315.

Boileau, J. C., Campeau, L., and Biron, P. (1970). Pulmonary fate of histamine, isoproterenol, physalaemin and substance P. *Can. J. Physiol. Pharmacol.,* **48**:681–684.

Boileau, J. C., Campeau, L., and Biron, P. (1971). Comparative pulmonary fate of intravenous epinephrine. *Rev. Can. Biol.,* **30**:281–286.

Boileau, J. C., Campeau, L., and Biron, P. (1972a). Pulmonary fate of intravenous norepinephrine. *Rev. Can. Biol.,* **31**:185–192.

Boileau, J. C., Crexells, C., and Biron, P. (1972b). Free pulmonary passage of dopamine. *Rev. Can. Biol.,* **31**:69–72.

Burack, B., Marcus, D., Miyamoto, A., Escher, D. J. W., and Robinson, G. (1972). Response of Class IV patients to alpha blockade prior to open-heart surgery. *Am. Heart J.*, **84**:456–462.

Collier, J. G., Robinson, B. F., and Vane, J. R. (1973). Reduction of the pressor effects of angiotensin I in man by synthetic nonapeptide (BPP$_{9a}$ or SQ 20881) which inhibits converting enzyme. *Lancet,* **1**:72–74.

Crexell, C., Bourassa, M. G., and Biron, P. (1972). Free passage of lysine-vasopressin through the human pulmonary circulation. *J. Clin. Endocrinol. Metab.*, **34**:592–594.

Cross, S. A. M., Alabaster, V. A., Bakhle, Y. S., and Vane, J. R. (1974). Sites of uptake of ^{3}H-5-hydroxytryptamine in rat isolated lung. *Histochemistry,* **39**:83–91.

Davis, R. B. (1968). Discussion of the role of 5-hydroxyindoles in the carcinoid syndrome. *Adv. Pharmacol.,* **6**, Pt B:146–149.

Davis, R. B. and Wang, Y. (1965). Rapid pulmonary removal of 5-hydroxytryptamine in the intact dog. *Proc. Soc. Exp. Biol. Med.*, **118**:797–803.

Eble, J. N., Gowdey, C. W., and Vane, J. R. (1971). Blood concentration of noradrenaline in the dog after intravenous administration and the effects of desipramine. *Nature,* **231**:181–182.

Favre, L., Vallotton, M. B., and Muller, A. F. (1974). Relationship between plasma concentrations of angiotensin I, angiotensin II and plasma renin activity during cardiopulmonary bypass in man. *Eur. J. Clin. Invest.,* **4**: 135–140.

Fishman, A. P. and Pietra, G. G. (1974). Handling of bioactive materials by the lung. *N. Engl. J. Med.,* **291**:884–890 and 953–959.

Fitz, A. and Overturf, M. (1972). Molecular weight of human angiotensin I. Lung converting enzyme. *J. Biol. Chem.,* **247**:581–584.

Frick, M. H. and Virkkula, L. (1961). 5-Hydroxyindoleacetic acid excretion after penumonectomy. *Ann. Med. Exp. (Biol.) Fenn.,* **39**:101–103.

Friedli, B., Davignon, A., Fouron, J. C., and Biron, P. (1972). Pulmonary contribution to angiotensin I conversion in children. *Rev. Can. Biol.,* **31**: 223–225.

Gavras, H., Brunnet, H. R., Laragh, J. H., Sealey, J. E., Gavras, I., and Vukovich, R. A. (1974). An angiotensin converting-enzyme inhibitor to identify and treat vasoconstrictor and volume factors in hypertensive patients. *N. Engl. J. Med.,* **291**:817–821.

Gillis, C. N. (1973). Metabolism of vasoactive hormones by lung. *Anesthesiology,* **39**:626–632.

Gillis, C. N. (1976). Extraneuronal transport of noradrenaline in the lung. In D. M. Paton (ed.): *The Mechanism of Neuronal and Extraneuronal Transport of Catecholamines.* Raven Press, New York, pp. 281–297.

Gillis, C. N., Greene, N. M., Cronau, L. H., and Hammond, G. L. (1972). Pulmonary extraction of 5-hydroxytryptamine and norepinephrine before and after cardiopulmonary bypass in man. *Circ. Res.,* **30**:666–674.

Gillis, C. N., Cronau, L. H., Greene, N. M., and Hammond, G. L. (1974). Removal of 5-hydroxytryptamine and norepinephrine from the pulmonary vascular space of man: Influence of cardiopulmonary bypass and pulmonary arterial pressure on these processes. *Surgery,* **76**:608–616.

Gillis, C. N., Roth, J. A., and Baker, K. (1975). Evidence for different forms of monoamine oxidase in perfused rabbit lung. *Chest,* **67**:26S–28S.

Gillis, C. N., Hammond, G. L., Cronau, L. H., and Whittaker, D. (1976). Fate of prostaglandins E_1 and A_1 in the human pulmonary circulation. *Surgery.* In press.

Gilmore, N. J. and Vane, J. R. (1970). A sensitive and specific assay for vasopressin in the circulating blood. *Br. J. Pharmacol.,* **38**:633–652.

Ginn, R. and Vane, J. R. (1968). Disappearance of catecholamines from the circulation. *Nature (Lond.),* **219**:740–742.

Goble, A. J., Hay, D. R., and Sandler, M. (1955). 5-Hydroxytryptamine metabolism in acquired heart disease associated with argentaffin carcinoma. *Lancet,* **2**:1016–1017.

Golub, M., Zia, P., Matsumo, M., and Horton, R. (1975). Metabolism of prostaglandins A_1 and E_1 in man. *J. Clin. Invest.,* **56**:1404–1410.

Gruby, L. A., Rowlands, C., Varley, B. Q., and Wyllie, J. H. (1971). The fate of 5-hydroxytryptamine in the lungs. *Br. J. Surg.,* **58**:525–532.

Hayes, A. and Cooper, R. G. (1971). Studies of the absorption, distribution and excretion of propranolol in rat, dog and monkey. *J. Pharmacol. Exp. Ther.,* **176**:302–311.

Hong, W. K., Mauer, P., Hochman, R., Caslowitz, J. G., and Paraskos, J. A. (1974). Amitriptyline cardiotoxicity. *Chest,* **66**:304–306.

Hughes, J., Gillis, C. N., and Bloom, F. E. (1969). The uptake and disposition of dl-noradrenaline in perfused rat lung. *J. Pharmacol. Exp. Ther.,* **169**: 237–248.

Iwasawa, Y., Gillis, C. N., and Aghajanian, G. (1973). Hypothermic inhibition of 5-hydroxytryptamine and norepinephrine uptake by lung: cellular location of amine after uptake. *J. Pharmacol. Exp. Ther.,* **186**:498–507.

Iwasawa, Y. and Gillis, C. N. (1974). Pharmacological analysis of norepinephrine and 5-hydroxytryptamine removal from the pulmonary circulation: Differentiation of uptake sites for each amine. *J. Pharmacol.,* **188**:386–393.

Jose, P., Niederhauser, U., Piper, P. J., Robinson, C., and Smith, A. P. (1976). Inactivation of prostaglandin $F_{2\alpha}$ in the human pulmonary circulation. *Br. J. Clin. Pharmacol.,* **3**:342P–343P.

Junod, A. F. (1972). Uptake, metabolism and efflux of ^{14}C-5-hydroxytryptamine in isolated perfused rat lungs. *J. Pharmacol. Exp. Ther.,* **183**:341–355.

Junod, A. F. (1975). Metabolism, production and release of hormones and mediators in the lung. *Am. Rev. Resp. Dis.,* **112**:93–108.

Kaufman, R. M., Airo, R., Pollock, S., and Crosby, W. H. (1965). Circulating megakaryocytes and platelet release in the lung. *Blood,* **26**:720–731.

Kirkendol, P. L. and Woodbury, R. A. (1972). Hemodynamic effects of infused norepinephrine in dogs on cardiopulmonary bypass. *J. Pharmacol. Exp. Ther.,* **181**:369–376.

Lammerant, J. and deHerdt, P. (1965). Catecholamine plasma levels in the pulmonary artery, the pulmonary vein and the arterial tree of open-chest dogs during ambient air breathing and during acute anoxia. *Arch. Int. Physiol. Biochim.*, **73**:81–96.

Larmi, T. K. I. and Heikkinen, E. (1967). Pulmonary degradation and cardio-vascular effects of intracavally infused 5-hydroxytryptamine in man. *Scand. J. Thorac. Cardiovasc. Surg.*, **1**:123–126.

Lembeck, F. (1953). 5-Hydroxytryptamine in a carcinoid tumor. *Nature*, **172**: 910–911.

Lilja, B., Lindell, S. E., and Saldeen, T. (1960). Formation and destruction of C^{14}-histamine in human lung tissue in vitro. *J. Allergy*, **31**:492–496.

MacIntyre, W. J., Prichard, W. H., Eckstein, R. W., and Friedell, H. L. (1951). The determination of cardiac output by a continuous recording system utilizing iodinated (I) human serum albumin. 1. Animal studies. *Circulation*, **4**:552–556.

Maupin, B. (1969). In *Blood Platelets in Man and Animals*, vol. 1. Pergamon Press, New York, pp. 273–292.

Moir, D. C. (1973). Tricyclic antidepressants and cardiac disease. *Am. Heart J.*, **86**:841–842.

Nicholas, T. E., Strum, J. M., Angelo, L. S., and Junod, A. F. (1974). Site and mechanism of uptake of ^{3}H-l-norepinephrine by isolated perfused rat lungs. *Circ. Res.*, **35**:670–680.

Okuda, M. and Nemerson, Y. (1971). Transport of serotonin by blood platelets: a pump-leak system. *Am. J. Physiol.*, **220**:283–288.

Overturf, M., Wyatt, S., Boaz, D., and Fitz, A. (1975). Angiotensin I (Phe^{8}-His^{9}) hydrolase and bradykininase from human lung. *Life Sci.*, **16**:1669–1682.

Pernow, B. and Waldenstrom, J. (1954). Paroxysmal flushing and other symptoms caused by 5-hydroxytryptamine and histamine in patients with malignant tumors. *Lancet*, **2**:951.

Roizen, M. F., Moss, J., Henry, D. P., and Kopin, I. J. (1974). Effects of halothane on plasma catecholamines. *Anesthesiology*, **41**:432–439.

Rosenbloom, P. M. and Bass, A. D. (1970). A lung perfusion preparation for the study of drug metabolism. *J. Appl. Physiol.*, **29**:138–144.

Said, S. I. (1968). The lung as a metabolic organ. *N. Engl. J. Med.*, **279**:1330–1334.

Said, S. I., Yoshida, T., Katamura, S., and Vreim, C. (1974). Pulmonary alveolar hypoxia: release of prostaglandins and other humoral mediators. *Science*, **185**:1181–1183.

Samuelsson, B., Granstrom, E., Green, K., and Hamberg, M. (1971). Metabolism of prostaglandins. *Ann. N.Y. Acad. Sci.*, **180**:138–161.

Sandler, M. (1968). Role of 5-hydroxyindoles in the cardinoid syndrome. *Adv. Pharmacol.*, **6**, Pt B:127–142.

Shaw, J. O. and Moser, K. M. (1975). The current status of prostaglandins and the lung. *Chest*, **68**:75–80.

Sjoerdsma, A., Weissbach, H., Terry, L. L., and Udenfriend, S. (1957). Further observations on patients with malignant carcinoid. *Am. J. Med.*, **23**:5–15.

Stjärne, L., Kaijser, L., Mathé, A., and Birke, G. (1975). Specific and unspecific removal of circulating noradrenaline in pulmonary and systemic vascular beds in man. *Acta Physiol. Scand.*, **95**:46–53.

Strum, J. M. and Junod, A. F. (1972). Radioautographic demonstration of 5-hydroxytryptamine-^{3}H uptake by pulmonary endothelial cells. *J. Cell Biol.*, **54**:456–467.

Vane, J. R. (1969). Release and fate of vasoactive hormones in the circulation. *Br. J. Pharmacol.*, **35**:209–242.

Part II

CORRELATIONS OF STRUCTURE WITH METABOLIC FUNCTION

7

Correlations Between the Fine Structure of the Alveolar-Capillary Unit and its Metabolic Activities

UNA S. RYAN and JAMES W. RYAN

Papanicolaou Cancer Research Institute
and the University of Miami School of Medicine
Miami, Florida

I.   Introduction

The cellular nature of the alveolar capillary unit was not recognized until the lungs were examined with the electron microscope. Indeed, it was thought that blood and air were separated at the level of the terminal airspace by a simple membrane (Fig. 1). The concept of a membrane sufficed for early biophysical studies of gas exchange. However, even at its narrowest, the boundary separating blood from air is composed of at least two cell-types (the type I alveolar cell and the endothelial cell) (Figs. 2 and 3) and extracellular material, namely the surfactant lining layer, the basement membranes and the so-called *endothelial fuzz,* a surface coating thought to be composed of mucopolysaccharides (Luft 1966).

The thinness of the cellular boundary between blood and air suggests correctly that the two major cell types are remarkable largely for their flatness and their paucity of intracellular organelles. Thus, while the type I alveolar cells and endothelial cells do not contain the subcellular machinery ordinarily

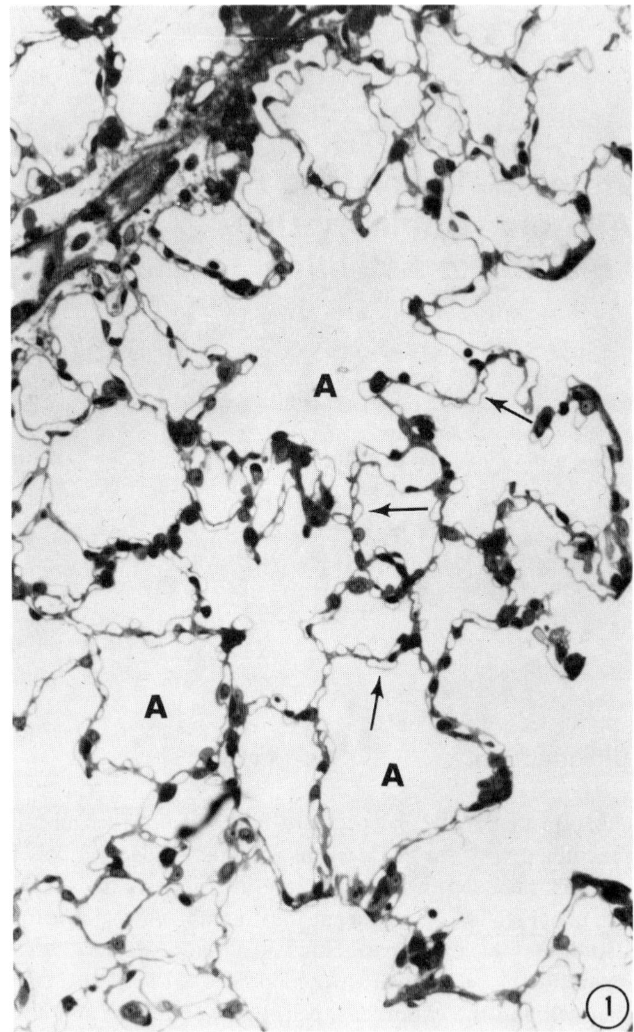

FIGURE 1   Light micrograph of thick section (1 μm) of capillary bed of rat lung. Tissue fixed by vascular perfusion with glutaraldehyde and embedded in Spurr's epoxy resin, as for electron microscopy. Air spaces (A) are surrounded by network of capillaries (arrows). In the light microscope it is not possible to resolve cellular components of the alveolar-capillary wall, which appears to be a simple membrane (compare with Fig. 2) (X168).

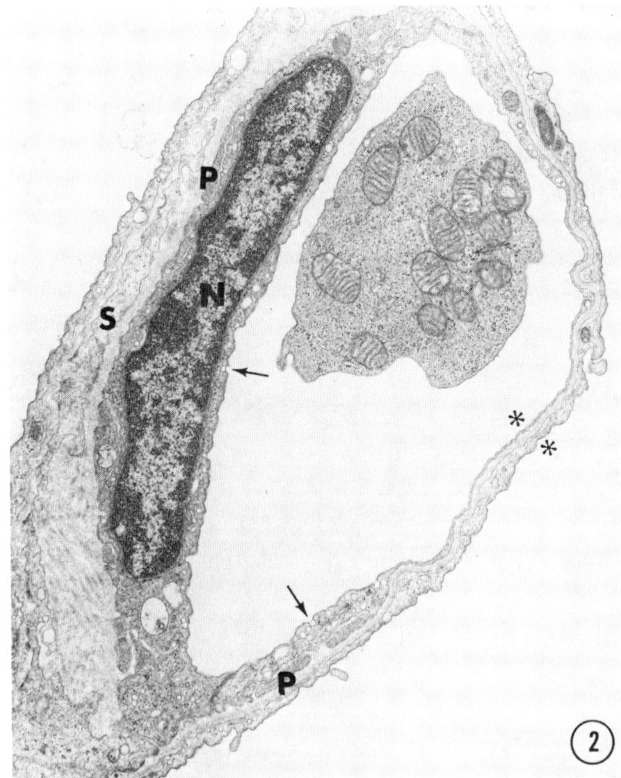

FIGURE 2   Electron micrograph of rat pulmonary capillary illustrating that the alveolar capillary unit, even at its thinnest (e.g., between asterisks), is composed of endothelium and epithelium with intervening basement membranes. Where the endothelial cell is extremely thin, it is little more than two apposing plasma membranes. In other areas, such as in the region of the endothelial nucleus (N), the alveolar capillary unit is considerably thicker and may contain processes of septal cells (s), pericytes (p) and increased amounts of extracellular material. Apart from scattered organelles, such as mitochondria and multivesicular bodies, the predominant feature of the endothelial cells is the large numbers of caveolae intracellulares (pinocytotic vesicles), many of which open directly to the vascular lumen (arrows). This is illustrated at higher magnification in Figure 5. The surfactant lining layer and the endothelial fuzz are not illustrated in this figure (×10,000).

associated with secretory activities, they present enormous surface areas to air on one side and blood on the other. *A priori* these cells must play no less than a passive role in all physical and metabolic events involving airborne or bloodborne substrates. The type I cellular layer is remarkably impermeable to salt-containing solutions (Perl et al. 1976), but little is known about specific metabolic activities of type I alveolar cells. We shall focus on active metabolite events conducted by endothelial cells at the level of the alveolar capillary unit. Type II alveolar cells and macrophages will be discussed in other volumes of this series.

The pulmonary capillary bed is remarkable, not only because of its position in the general circulation, dividing venous from arterial blood, but also because of its vastness, the large quantities of blood processed per unit time, and because of the delicate balance that must be maintained to provide the

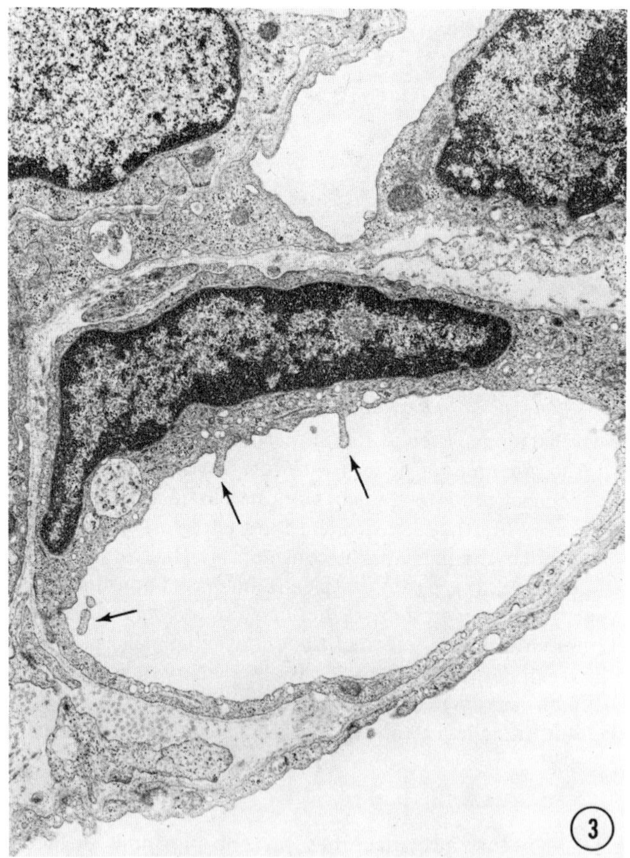

FIGURE 3   Capillary similar to that shown in Figure 2 but also showing endothelial projections (arrows) (×11,000).

lungs with their hormonal and metabolic requirements while limiting the transport of salts and water into and out of the vascular space. In addition, one might suppose that the lungs, perhaps to a greater degree than other tissues, must make provision for the free, unhindered passage of some hormones and excitatory substances from the venous to the systemic arterial circulation.

It has been known since 1925 that the lungs eliminate vasoactive substances and do so in a highly efficient way (Starling and Verney 1925). The efficiency of metabolism might have suggested a role for the alveolar-capillary unit because it is at this level that circulating substances have their greatest exposure to lung cells. However, during the interval from 1925 to approximately 1968, most observations on the ability of the lungs to process circulating excitatory substances focused on the substances themselves rather than on the lungs. Nonetheless, it is evident from early studies that the lungs are capable of processing selectively a large number of substances of very different chemical types, including biogenic amines, adenine nucleotides, prostaglandins, polypeptides, drugs, and lipids. In addition, it is well recognized that blood components, volatile at about 37°C, pass from blood to air presumably at the level of the alveolar-capillary unit. Furthermore, the lungs, possibly at the level of the alveolar-capillary unit, contain enzymes and other agents active in coagulation and anticoagulation reactions. The limits of the ability of the lungs to process lipids, hormones, hormone precursors, and drugs are not known. However, for the purposes of this chapter, we plan to focus on interactions of the lungs with circulating substances known or thought to be processed actively by endothelial cells. The metabolism of drugs will be considered elsewhere in this volume (Philpot et al.).

It has been estimated that in man, alveolar blood vessels (primarily capillaries) have a luminal surface area on the order of 70 m^2 (Fishman 1963). However, early calculations of surface area assumed a more or less regular ellipsoidal shape of capillaries having smooth luminal surfaces. It is now evident that the surfaces are not smooth but are covered with irregular complex projections (Smith et al. 1971). The projections are approximately 300 nm in diameter and may extend in length to 3,000 nm. Some projections come to blunt ends, while others bud, branch, or reflect back on the main body of the cell. At present, the functional significance of the endothelial projections is not known. However, the projections cannot fail to affect fluid dynamics at the cell body. Their size and the density of the meshwork is such that one can anticipate an eddy flow of cell-free plasma along the main body of the cell. This feature could well have implications for the exchange of metabolites between endothelium and blood. Although the surface projections shown in Figure 4 are of the main stem pulmonary artery, there is ample evidence, from examination of thin sections of endothelial cells of smaller vessels, including capillaries and venules, to indicate that surface projections are a common

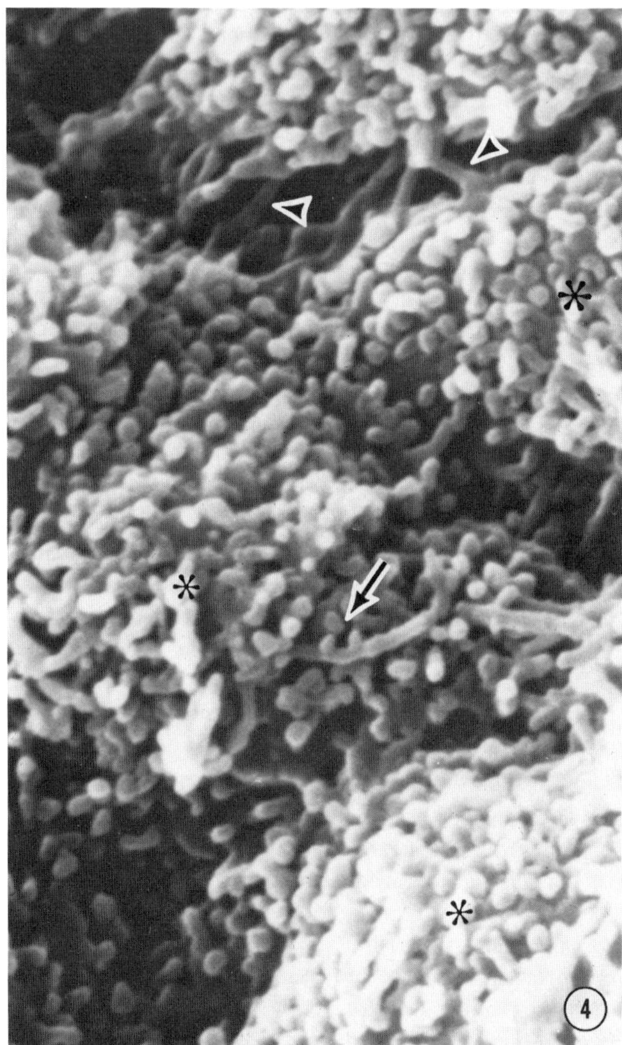

FIGURE 4   Scanning electron micrograph of luminal surface of pulmonary artery of the dog. Endothelial cells are covered by projections, some of which end bluntly while others bud and branch (arrow). They are most dense over the main body of the cells (asterisks) but also stretch between cells (arrowheads). Projections are approximately 250 to 350 nm in diameter and range from 300 to 3000 nm in length. Endothelial projections can be readily identified in thin sections by transmission electron microscopy. They also occur in smaller vessels, such as venules and capillaries (e.g., Fig. 3) (×9,000). (Reprinted by permission from Smith, U. et al. (1971). *Science,* **173**:925–927.)

feature (Fig. 3). In addition to the surface projections, it is evident from Figure 5 that pulmonary capillary endothelial cells contain enormous numbers of

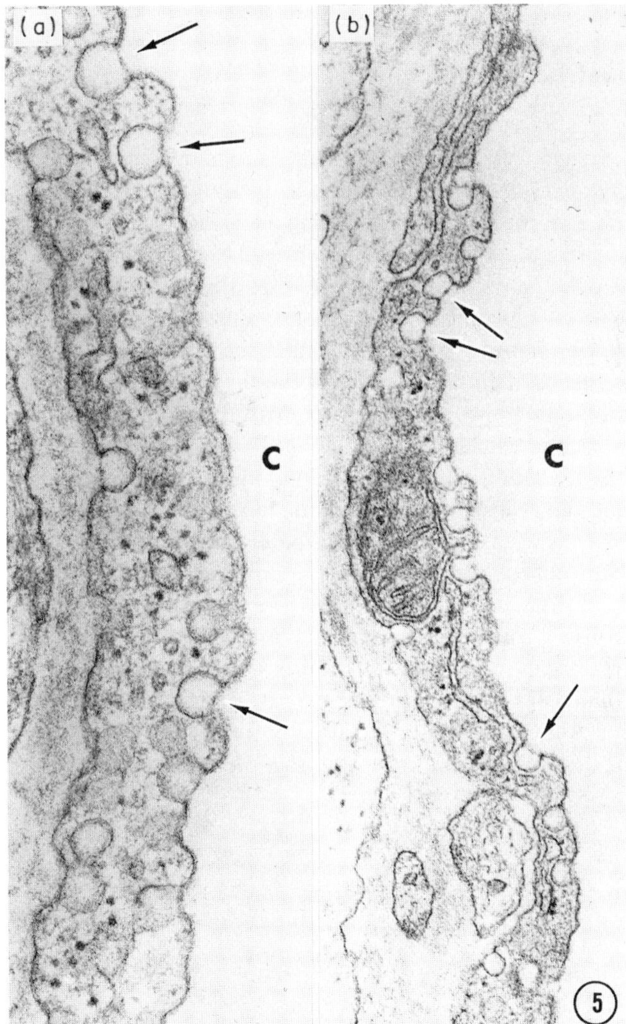

FIGURE 5 (a and b) Portions of two capillary endothelial cells illustrating the large numbers of caveolae intracellulares many of which directly face the vascular lumen (C). The luminal stoma of the caveola is spanned by a delicate diaphragm composed of a single lamella (arrows), in contrast to the unit membrane construction of endothelial plasma membranes and caveolae membranes (a)X68,000, (b)X44,000.

caveolae intracellulares (pinocytotic vesicles), a large proportion of which appear to communicate directly with the vascular lumen (Smith and Ryan 1970, 1972a). Therefore, it would appear that the true surface area of capillary endothelial cells is very much larger than previous estimates.

II. Metabolism of Lipids

Schoefl and French (1968) have described morphologic features of the processing of chylomicrons by endothelial cells of lactating mammary glands and of lungs. The endothelial cells of lactating mammary glands are very much more active in this process, but it is notable that chylomicrons can be processed in the pulmonary circulation as well, possibly via a lipoprotein lipase thought to be located on or near the luminal surface. Indeed, there may be some physiologic importance to the fact that the lymphatic drainage of the gut proceeds first to the lungs via the subclavian vein and not to the liver (Fishman and Pietra 1974). Furthermore, Vatter and coworkers (1968) have provided evidence of esterase activity along the luminal surface of pulmonary endothelial cells, although the relationship of this esterase activity to the processing of lipids and, in particular, chylomicrons is not yet known. It may be of interest that these authors mention unpublished data that show one of their substrates (*p*-nitrophenylthiol acetate) is hydrolyzed by glycerolester hydrolase enzymes. It remains to be seen whether the enzyme systems suggested by these studies play a role in prostaglandin synthesis (e.g., in the mobilization of free arachidonic acid). A number of studies on the origin of surfactant (e.g., Askin and Kuhn 1971), have followed the fate of [^{3}H] palmitic acid injected intravenously. These studies have focused on type II alveolar cells and not on endothelium, thus little is known on the role of endothelium in the uptake of palmitate.

III. Processing of Biogenic Amines

Pharmacologic data on the fates of the catecholamines, 5-hydroxytryptamine (serotonin, 5-HT) and histamine are presented in other chapters of this volume. Suffice it to say that 5-HT and noradrenaline are to greater or lesser degrees eliminated as they pass through the lungs while adrenaline and histamine are allowed unhindered passage. In addition, it is becoming clear that the pulmonary endothelium plays an active role in the removal of noradrenaline and 5-HT from the circulation.

Hughes and associates (1969) have shown, by combined autoradiographic and biochemical techniques, that endothelial cells of isolated rat lungs actively take up tritiated dl-noradrenaline. Under control conditions, the noradrenaline is rapidly metabolized by O-methylation and deamination. The uptake process is saturable and is blocked by cocaine. Nicholas and associates (1974), using [^{3}H]l-noradrenaline, have confirmed and extended these findings. Uptake of noradrenaline is inhibited by cocaine, imipramine, ouabain, potassium-free medium, low temperature, and by decreasing the concentration of sodium in the medium. Nicholas and associates postulated that the uptake of noradrenaline is a sodium-dependent, carrier-mediated transport. Both Hughes and collaborators and Nicholas and associates noted from their autoradiograph experiments that the distribution of silver grains was not uniform. Some capillary beds were heavily labeled and others not at all, a point raising the possibility that the endothelial cells of the lungs are not a homogeneous population.

Strum and Junod (1972) have described similar findings on the pulmonary processing of 5-HT. The elimination of 5-HT is more efficient than that of noradrenaline. There are, as yet, few data on the chemical form of the radioactive material accumulated by endothelial cells exposed to [^{3}H] 5-HT, although one assumes an early exposure to monoamine oxidase enzymes, a possibility consistent with the efflux of 5-HIAA (Eiseman et al. 1964). Possibly, a question such as this will be answerable through the use of isolated pulmonary endothelial cells.

IV.　Metabolism of Nucleotides

Binet and Burstein (1950) showed that adenosine 5′-triphosphate (ATP) does not pass from the pulmonary artery to the pulmonary vein. Recently, we had occasion to reinvestigate the fate of ATP and its lower homolog, adenosine 5′-monophosphate (AMP) using combined biochemical and cytochemical techniques (Smith and Ryan 1970, Ryan and Smith 1971a). When ATP or AMP (labeled intrinsically with ^{3}H, ^{14}C or ^{32}P) is perfused through isolated lungs, all of the radioactivity entering the pulmonary artery is recoverable in the venous effluent, yet none of the radioactivity remains in the form of the original adenine nucleotide. In addition, it was noted that the apparent mean transit time and volume of distribution of radioactivity of either ATP or AMP were virtually identical to those of an intravascular marker, blue dextran (mol. wt. approximately 2,000,000). As will be discussed under Section V, these peculiar features are not unique to the metabolism of adenine nucleotides by the lungs but appear to be features of the fate of substances metabolized by enzymes on the luminal surface of pulmonary endothelial cells.

The metabolism of adenine nucleotides by the lungs via phosphate esterase enzymes provides an excellent opportunity for examining the subcellular localization of the enzymes themselves. Using methods adapted from those described by Wachstein and Meisel (1959) and Marchesi and Barrnett (1963), we examined ATPase and 5'-nucleotidase activities by trapping released inorganic phosphate with lead to form insoluble, electron-dense, lead phosphate precipitates (Fig. 6). When blocks of fixed lung tissue were incubated with ATP and $Pb(NO_3)_2$, lead phosphate deposits were detectable in caveolae across the endothelium (Smith and Ryan 1970, 1971). However, when intact lungs were perfused with 5'-AMP and $Pb(NO_3)_2$, the lead phosphate deposits were restricted to those caveolae and incipient caveolae open to the vascular lumen (Ryan and Smith 1971a). These data suggest that although a large number of cell types and organelles have phosphate esterase enzymes, it is only those enzymes facing the vascular lumen that are exposed to, and react with, circulating nucleotides. The apparent localization of ATPase and 5'-nucleotidase along the vascular lumen and associated caveolae very likely explains how the metabolic products of the adenine nucleotides are returned to the circulation with no apparent delay nor uptake by tissue.

The physiologic significance of the processing of ATP and AMP during passage through the lungs is not yet evident. However, one of their metabolic products is adenosine, a compound thought to play a role in functional vasodilation (Haddy and Scott 1968). Mentzer and associates (1974) have suggested that adenosine is a pulmonary vasodilator. Should this be the case, then the metabolism of adenine nucleotides by the lungs might represent an activation reaction. On the other hand, the pathophysiologic significance may be easier to conceive, as adenine nucleotides have strong pharmacologic effects of their own (Green and Stoner 1950) and are known to be released by trauma to large muscle masses (e.g., in crush injury). In addition, adenine nucleotides may be released during strenuous exercise (Boyd and Forrester 1968).

V. Metabolism of Polypeptide Hormones

The first efforts to examine endothelial cells for a possible role in the active metabolism of bloodborne substrates, primarily vasoactive hormones, were prompted by a series of observations made by Vane and colleagues in 1967. For example, Ferreira and Vane (1967a) found that relatively little bradykinin survives circulation through the lungs. In contrast, Hodge et al. (1967), confirming previous observations by Goffinet and Mulrow (1963), found that the biologic activity of angiotensin II is not lost during passage through the lungs.

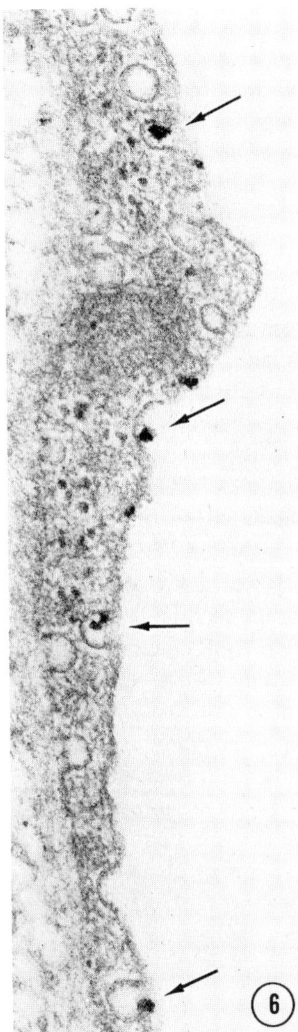

FIGURE 6 Cytochemical localization of 5'-nucleotidase. Endothelial cell is from rat lung, which had been perfused with 5'-AMP and lead nitrate. At the site of hydrolysis of the phosphate ester bond, insoluble, electron-dense lead phosphate is precipitated. The reaction product, indicating sites of 5'nucleotidase activity, is specifically localized in those caveolae facing the vascular lumen (arrows) ($\times$203,000). (Reprinted by permission from Smith, U. and Ryan, J. W. (1971). *Chest*, **59**, 13S.)

In addition, Ng and Vane (1967) found that the venous effluent of lungs perfused with angiotensin I contains more angiotensin-like activity than can be accounted for by the amount of angiotensin I used for infusion; a result that was interpreted to mean that angiotensin I is converted to angiotensin II during a single passage through the lungs. Verification of their hypothesis was provided 3 years later (Ryan et al. 1970b).

A. Bradykinin

The first suggestion of a role of endothelial cells in the processing of vasoactive polypeptides arose from an examination of the fate of radioactive bradykinin ($[^{14}C]Pro^2$-bradykinin) in isolated perfused lungs (Ryan et al. 1968). In this and subsequent studies it was found that bradykinin is hydrolyzed in no fewer than 5 peptide bonds during the 3 to 5 sec required to pass from the pulmonary artery to the left atrium of the heart (Ryan et al. 1969, 1970a). None of the radioactivity is taken up by the lungs. In fact, there is a quantitative recovery of radioactivity in the pulmonary venous effluent. The apparent mean transit time and volume of distribution of radioactivity are virtually identical to those of blue dextran, an intravascular marker. It was also noted that the lungs do not secrete enzymes, having either the activity or the specificity to account for the metabolic products obtained. As the isolated lungs used in these studies were pumped free of blood, blood enzymes could be ruled out. It was also observed, on incubation of radioactive bradykinin with homogenized lung, that bradykinin was broken down to its free amino acids, metabolic products different from those produced by intact lungs. These results were interpreted to mean that not all of the hydrolase enzymes of intact lungs have access to circulating substrates. In addition, it was found that the apparent kinetics of metabolism of bradykinin by intact lungs are virtually identical to those of the adenine nucleotides, substances known to be metabolized by enzymes on the luminal surface of pulmonary endothelial cells.

B. Angiotensin I

When intrinsically-labeled angiotensin I became available, it was used in perfusions of isolated intact lungs (Ryan et al. 1970b, 1971, 1972b). In brief, angiotensin I is processed similarly to bradykinin and the adenine nucleotides; namely, blood enzymes are not required, radioactivity is not taken up by the lungs but is recovered immediately in the pulmonary venous effluent, and the apparent mean transit time and volume of distribution of radioactivity are identical to those of an intravascular marker. In addition, whole lung homogenates are capable of degrading angiotensin I and angiotensin II to their component amino acids, whereas intact lungs perfused with $[^{14}C]Leu^{10}$-angiotensin I produce primarily the dipeptide, His-Leu and angiotensin II. Similarly, we found that $[^{14}C]Ile^5$-angiotensin II is not degraded by more than 10% to 15% during passage through intact lungs (W. P. Leary and J. W. Ryan, unpublished observations).

C. Mechanisms of Metabolism

From such results, we postulated that bradykinin and angiotensin I are metabolized by enzymes on the luminal surface of pulmonary endothelial cells (Ryan et al. 1968, 1970a,b, 1971, 1972a,b, Smith and Ryan 1970, 1971). Because of the apparent efficiencies of their metabolism, it was further postulated that the reactions probably occur at the level of the alveolar-capillary unit, at which level bloodborne substrates would have their greatest exposure to endothelial cells. The hypothesis had testable aspects. For example, the plasma membrane fraction of lung homogenate (Fig. 10c) should be capable of metabolizing bradykinin and angiotensin I to provide metabolites like those produced by intact lungs. Such was found to be the case: $[^{14}C]Pro^{2,3}$-bradykinin is metabolized by a plasma membrane fraction to yield the radioactive dipeptide, Pro-Pro, a metabolite produced by intact lungs (Ryan and Smith 1971a,b, Ryan et al. 1972b, Smith and Ryan 1972b). Similarly, $[^{14}C]Phe^8$-angiotensin I is converted to $[^{14}C]Phe^8$-angiotensin II. Furthermore, if the hypothesis were correct, then isolated pulmonary endothelial cells should be capable of forming the same products as produced by intact lungs. We found that endothelial cells of the mainstem pulmonary artery, isolated on cellulose acetate paper (Pugatch and Saunders 1968) could be used in a system analogous to descending chromatography, such that when $[^{14}C]Phe^8$-angiotensin I was applied to the top of the paper, $[^{14}C]Phe^8$-angiotensin II could be collected from the bottom (Ryan and Smith 1973, Smith and Ryan 1973a).

Recently, it has been possible to examine the pulmonary capillary bed more directly. In 1972, Dorer and coworkers succeeded in isolating angiotensin converting enzyme in homogeneous form. They subsequently showed that the enzyme is also capable of degrading bradykinin (Dorer et al. 1974) in a way analogous to that of an enzyme known previously as kininase II (Yang et al. 1971). In fact, bradykinin appears to be the preferred substrate. The enzyme converts angiotensin I to angiotensin II by removing the C-terminal dipeptide, His-Leu; a finding consistent with the observation that intact lungs metabolize $[^{14}C]Leu^{10}$-angiotensin I to yield radioactive His-Leu (Ryan et al. 1970b). Bradykinin is inactivated by the enzyme in a similar manner, but can be degraded in two steps: the C-terminal dipeptide, Phe-Arg, is released and

then the new C-terminal dipeptide, Ser-Pro, is removed. Again, these findings
are consistent with results of experiments using intact lungs: the venous effluent of lungs perfused with $[^3H]Phe^8$-bradykinin contains a single radioactive
metabolite, namely Phe-Arg (Ryan et al. 1969, 1970a).

In collaborative studies, we prepared antibodies to hog lung angiotensin
converting enzyme (Ryan et al. 1975b). The antiserum (goat) was purified by
$(NH_4)_2SO_4$ precipitation and by chromatography on DEAE-cellulose. The
final antibody fraction was coupled to microperoxidase, a heme-undecapeptide
moiety of cytochrome C (Feder 1971). Coupling was effected by the method
of Avrameas (1969). The antibody-microperoxidase conjugate was reacted
with very small blocks of rat lung tissue, which previously had been fixed with
paraformaldehyde-picric acid and preincubated with nonimmune goat serum.
Antibody localization was achieved by reacting the microperoxidase moiety
with H_2O_2 and 3,3'-diaminobenzidine. Results are shown in Figures 7 and 8.
The luminal surface of the pulmonary endothelial cells reacted with the antibody-microperoxidase reagent as expected. The reaction product, oxidized
diaminobenzidine, was most abundant on the surface of the endothelial cells
of capillaries and venules. Using a new marker, 8-microperoxidase, a heme-
octapeptide of cytochrome C (Kraehenbuhl et al. 1974), coupled to anti-pig
lung angiotensin converting enzyme via a bifunctional active ester (Ryan et
al. 1976a), a similar localization was obtained on pig lung endothelial cells in
situ and in tissue culture (Ryan et al. 1976b).

The developing picture is that of an enzyme in solid phase washed
with its substrates, angiotensin I and bradykinin, in a continuously flowing
liquid phase. At the level of the capillary bed, 1.0 ml of blood may occupy
more than 10 miles of capillary length, a circumstance that could favor efficient metabolism by relatively small amounts of enzyme. The ability of the
lungs to inactivate bradykinin, a substance that lowers blood pressure, and to
activate angiotensin I by converting it to angiotensin II, a substance that raises
blood pressure, suggests a role of the lungs in blood pressure homeostasis. If,
as appears to be the case, both reactions are catalyzed by a single enzyme, the
role of the lungs in blood pressure homeostasis may become understandable at
the molecular level.

The situation of angiotensin converting enzyme within an organ that receives the entire cardiac output and that drains to the systemic arterial circulation poses interesting physiologic and pathologic possibilities. For example,
the lungs have a number of ways in which they may influence the quantities
of endothelial enzymes exposed to circulating substrates. The numbers of
capillaries open at any given time and the rate and volume of blood flow
through them are complex functions of posture, exercise, depth of ventilation,
the composition of inhalants, and several other factors, not the least of which

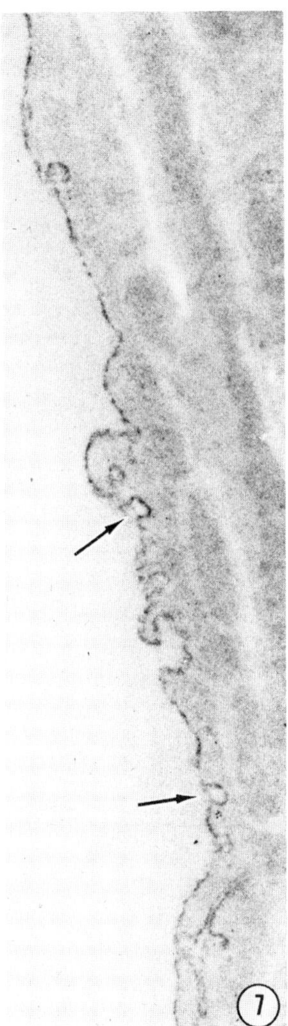

FIGURE 7 Endothelial cell from rat lung tissue, which had been incubated with antibodies to angiotensin converting enzyme coupled to microperoxidase. The peroxidase moiety was then reacted with 3,3'-diaminobenzidine and H_2O_2. The reaction product is localized along the luminal plasma membrane of the endothelial cell and in caveolae (arrows). The section was not stained ($\times$47,000). (Reprinted by permission from Ryan, U. S. et al., 1976: *Tissue and Cell*, 8:125–145.)

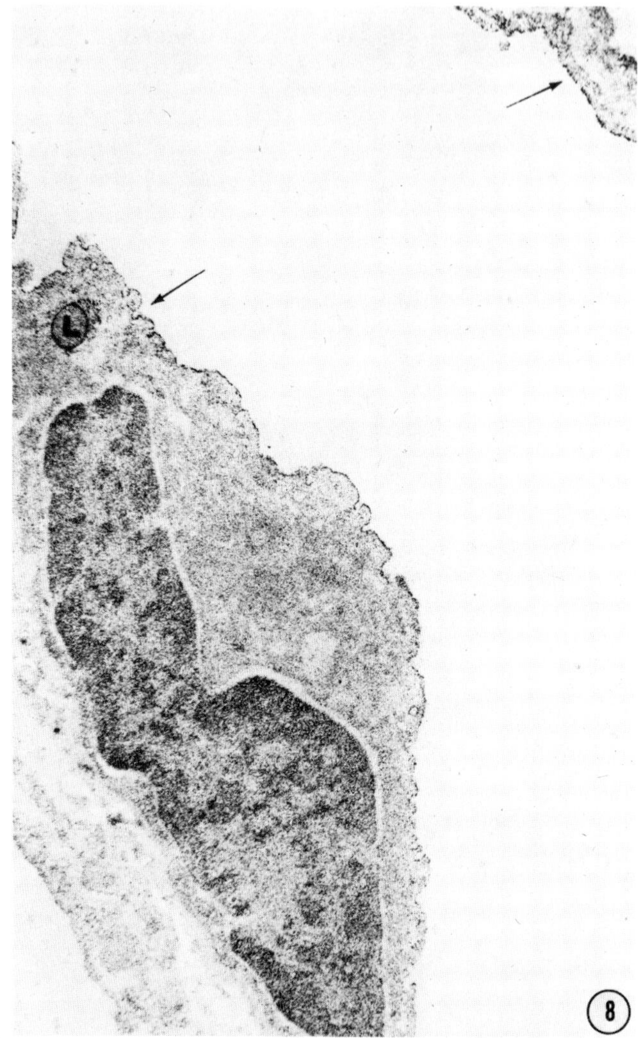

FIGURE 8   Low power field of an unstained section showing immunocyto-
chemical localization of angiotensin converting enzyme. The material was incubated as described in the text and in Figure 7. The reaction product is
specifically localized on the luminal surface of the endothelial cells (arrows).
The reaction product surrounding the lipid droplet (L) may be due to the reaction of lipid peroxides with diaminobenzidine (X20,000). (Reprinted by permission from Ryan, U. S. et al., 1976: *Tissue and Cell,* 8:125–145.)

is the structural integrity of the lungs themselves. One might expect that factors, which significantly increase or decrease mean transit time of blood through the lungs, could affect the quantities of angiotensin II and bradykinin delivered to the systemic arterial circulation and hence to target organs. Recently, Fanburg and Glazier (1973) reported evidence of increased angiotensin II-like immunoreactivity in the venous effluent of dog lungs manipulated to increase pulmonary vascular surface area. Similar increases were found in lungs with full vascular distention when the mean transit time was increased. However, the increased efflux of angiotensin II-like immunoreactivity occurred only when large quantities (0.5 to 1.0 mg) of angiotensin I were used for perfusion, a point suggesting that the ability of normal lungs to metabolize angiotensin I may greatly exceed the amounts of angiotensin I likely to be found in central venous blood. However, bradykinin is an excellent inhibitor of the conversion of angiotensin I by angiotensin converting enzyme (Sander et al. 1971, Dorer et al. 1974), and it remains to be determined whether the simultaneous presence of bradykinin, angiotensin I, and other possible substrates in central venous blood can modulate the net quantities of bradykinin and angiotensin II entering the systemic arterial circulation. At present, it appears entirely possible that the physical changes of the lungs associated with ventilation and respiration may affect the processing of vasoactive polypeptides.

D. Substructural Specializations of Endothelial Plasma Membrane

It may become feasible to visualize angiotensin converting enzyme (kininase II) as it exists on the surface of endothelial cells. Towards this end, we have examined an homogeneous preparation of the enzyme by negative staining (Fig. 9). The enzyme appears to exist as a tetrameric or hexameric structure having a diameter of about 60 Å. Endothelial surface structures of this size can be seen in thin sections (Smith and Ryan 1972a, 1973b), and on replicas of freeze-fractured lung tissue (Smith et al. 1973; Figs. 10, 11, and 12). Estimations of size from the replicas assume that the thickness of the shadowing material (carbon-platinum) is about 20 Å. The globular particles seen on replicas of freeze-fractured endothelium are randomly distributed over the plasma membrane but are organized into rings and plaques in association with caveolae. The globular particles seen on thin sections of caveola membranes may correspond to those seen in replicas of freeze-fractured material. However, it is not yet known which, if any, of these particles are converting enzyme. Some of the particles may well have enzymatic activity, as some bind lead phosphate formed on reaction of 5'-nucleotidase with 5'-AMP in the presence of lead nitrate (Smith and Ryan 1971, 1972a,b, Ryan and Smith 1971; Fig. 10d).

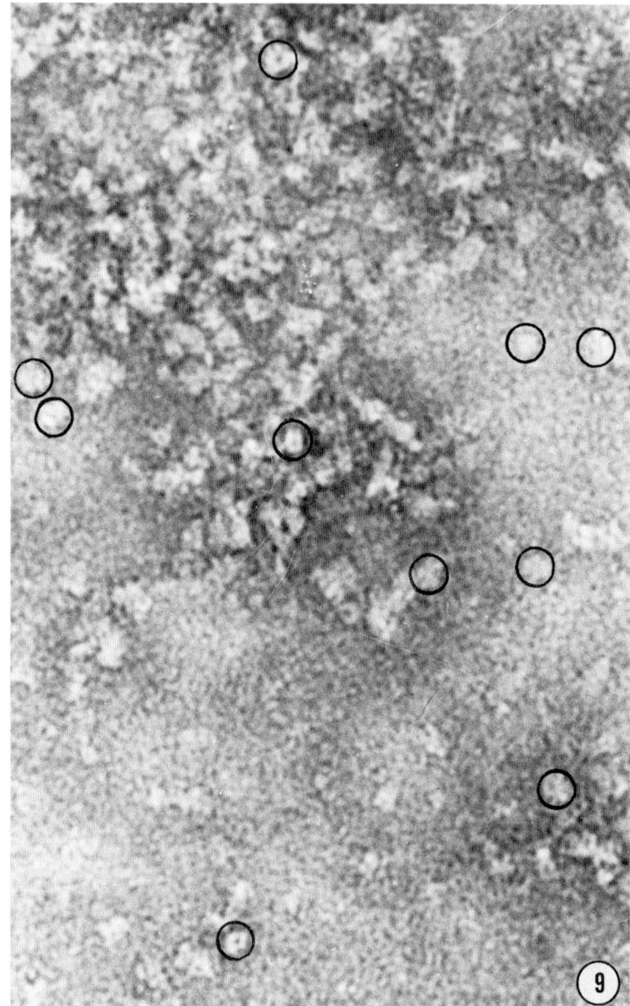

FIGURE 9 Preparation of hog lung angiotensin converting enzyme negatively stained with 1% phosphomolybdic acid. The enzyme appears to exist in clusters of four or six subunits, the clusters (encircled) have a diameter of approximately 60 Å. Globular substructures of this size can be seen in thin sections and on replicas of freeze-fracture endothelial plasma membranes (compare with Figs. 10, 11, and 12) (×371,000). (Reprinted by permission from Ryan, U. S. et al., 1976: *Tissue and Cell,* 8:125–145.)

FIGURE 10 (continued)
(×108,000). (Reprinted by permission from Smith, U. and Ryan, J. W. *Tissue Cell,* **4,** 51. (d) Plasma membrane-caveolae fraction prepared as in (c) showing discrete deposition of reaction product along caveolae membranes (arrows), suggesting preferential binding sites or enzyme clusters (×151,000). (Reprinted by permission from Smith, U. and Ryan, J. W., 1972. *Tissue Cell,* **4:**49–54.)

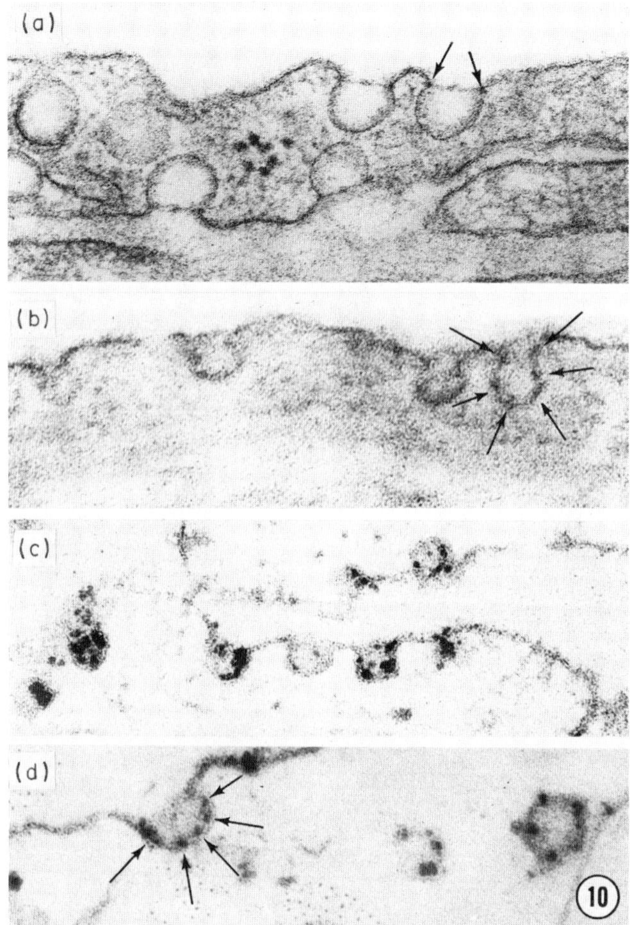

FIGURE 10 (a) Part of capillary endothelial cell of a rat lung prepared for electron microscopy by standard techniques. Caveola membranes appear to be of unit membrane construction while diaphragm is composed of a single lamella. Dense knobs at junction of diaphragm with caveola membrane and plasma membrane (arrows) may represent skeletal rim or ring of beads, which could help to maintain patency of stoma and integrity of diaphragm. Some substructural beading of caveolae membranes can be seen (×90,000). (b) Portion of luminal plasma membrane of capillary endothelial cell showing localization of pulmonary angiotensin converting enzyme. Localization of reaction product (oxidized diaminobenzidine) shows preferential deposition, which may be associated with substructural specialization of caveola membrane (arrows) (×120,000). (Reprinted from Ryan, J. W. et al. (1975). *Biochem J.,* **146**, 499. (c) Plasma membrane-caveolae fraction of rat lung homogenate incubated with 5′-AMP and lead nitrate. Deposition of lead phosphate within caveolae allows collection of long strands of plasma membrane with attached caveolae. Caveolae maintain their characteristic shape even after homogenization and centrifugation. This structural stability may be conferred, in part, by stomal ring (Figs. 10a, 11, and 12)

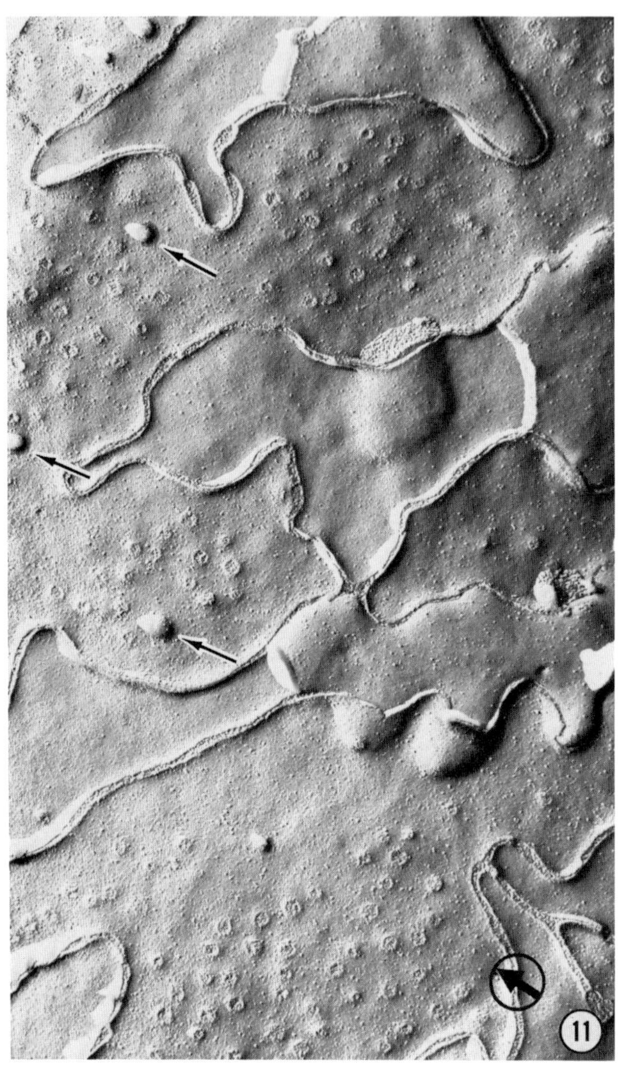

FIGURE 11   Replica of freeze-fractured rat lung exposing the OFF (outer fracture face, A face, intracellular aspect of the outer leaflet) of several endothelial cells. Caveolae appear as domes (arrows) where the plane of fracture followed their contours. Where caveolae were avulsed by the plane of fracture, their position is marked by a ring or plaque of intramembranous particles. Particles in association with caveolae may represent stomal ring (Fig. 10a) and are shown at higher magnification in Figure 12. Direction of shadowing (carbon and platinum) indicated by encircled arrow (×145,000).

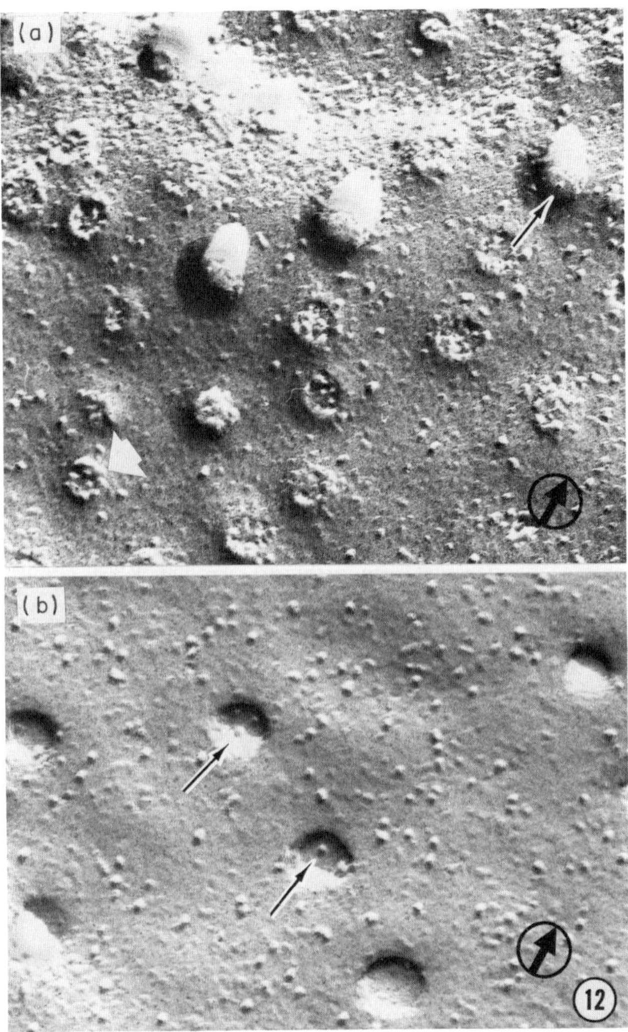

FIGURE 12   (a) OFF (outer fracture face) of endothelial plasma membrane from freeze fractured rat lung. Intramembranous particles (approximately 85 Å in diameter) are grouped in rings at base of caveolae which have been avulsed during fracture (white arrow) and, where shadow angle is appropriate, over bulb of caveolae (arrow). Disposition of intramembranous particles in freeze fracture replicas corresponds with substructural specializations of endothelial caveolae in thin sections (X102,000). (b) IFF (inner fracture face, B face, extracellular aspect of inner leaflet) of endothelial plasma membrane. Caveolae appear as pits at base of which intramembranous particles can be seen. In both (a) and (b), encircled arrow indicates direction of shadowing (X148,000). (Reprinted by permission from Smith, U. et al. (1973). *J. Cell Biol.*, **56**, 492–499.)

E.   Other Polypeptide Hormones

Rubenstein, Swi, and Miller (1968) have reported that insulin may be metabolized during circulation through the lungs. In 6 patients, without demonstrable shunts, blood samples were drawn simultaneously from the right atrium or pulmonary artery and from the aorta or iliac artery. Insulin-like material was measured by radioimmunoassay (double antibody precipitation). In 5 of the 6 patients, systemic arterial blood contained 10% to 19% less insulin-like material, and the sixth patient showed a slight positive gradient (13.0 μU/ml in right ventricular blood and 14.0 μU/ml in arterial blood). Although these changes are probably within the experimental error of radioimmunoassay, further interest in the processing of insulin by the lungs arose when Erdös and colleagues (Igic et al. 1972) reported that hog lung angiotensin converting enzyme can metabolize the B-chain of insulin.

Recently, an effort was begun to confirm these observations (F. E. Dorer and J. W. Ryan, unpublished). In a survey on insulin-like immunoreactivity in arterial and central venous blood (samples drawn simultaneously) no consistent evidence was found for the uptake or degradation of insulin by the lungs. Of 8 patient samples, 3 showed negative venous-arterial gradients, 1 showed a positive gradient, and the remaining 4 showed no changes. Similar results were obtained on assay of blood samples from 3 dogs (six assays) and 5 rabbits (38 assays). It is conceivable that insulin could have undergone limited hydrolysis, e.g., by angiotensin converting enzyme, such that its metabolic products were still reactive with antibody. However it was found that the B-chain of bovine insulin is not detectably hydrolyzed by hog lung angiotensin converting enzyme in vitro, under conditions in which the hydrolyses of bradykinin and angiotensin I are rapid. Although the B-chain was derived from cow, the primary amino acid sequence is the same as that of pig.

Thus, at present, it is not clear whether insulin is metabolized by the lungs. If metabolism occurs, it probably does not proceed through degradation of the B-chain by angiotensin converting enzyme. Possibly, determination of clearance rates, especially using an assay technique as nonspecific and imprecise as radioimmunoassay, will not suffice for measurement of pulmonary uptake. Where the uptake is relatively low, as is the case with glucose, even precise assays cannot reliably detect clearances (e.g., Tierney 1974).

The fates of other polypeptide hormones (e.g., substance P, vasopressin, gastrin, and oxytocin) are discussed in previous chapters of this volume.

VI. Metabolism of Prostaglandins

A. Degradation

As discussed in previous chapters of this volume, prostaglandins of the E and F series are eliminated during passage through the lungs (Ferreira and Vane 1967b). Prostaglandins of the A series are spared in some species, but not in others (McGiff et al. 1969, Horton and Jones 1969, Piper et al. 1970). At present, the role of endothelial cells in the elimination of prostaglandins is not known; although for reasons discussed in Section I, it seems likely that these cells must play at least a passive role. When $[^3H]PGF_{1\alpha}$ or $[^3H]PGE_1$ is perfused with an intravascular marker, the emergence of radioactivity into the pulmonary venous effluent is delayed, and up to 30% of the radioactivity is retained by the lungs, points indicating that cellular uptake occurs (Ryan and Smith 1971a, Ryan et al. 1972a, 1975a).

Degradation of prostaglandins $F_{1\alpha}$ and E_1 by intact rat lungs appears to occur by oxidation of the C-15 secondary hydroxyl group and by reduction of the C-13 double bond. Although the structures of the metabolites produced by intact lungs have not been proved, the formation of the 15-keto-prostanoic acid derivatives of $PGF_{1\alpha}$ and PGE_1 would be consistent with the report by Anggard and Samuelsson (1967) that the particle-free supernatant of guinea pig lung homogenate contains a 15-hydroxydehydrogenase and C-13 reductase. An equivalent supernatant of pig lung homogenate does not contain a C-13 reductase, but we are not aware of studies on the prostaglandin metabolites produced by pig lung.

As was found to be the case in studies of the metabolism of bradykinin by intact versus homogenized lungs (Ryan 1970a) it is conceivable that lungs contain prostaglandin catabolic enzymes which do not have access to circulating substrates. On this point, it may be relevant that prostaglandins of the A series are spared during passage through the lungs but are good substrates for 15-hydroxydehydrogenase in vitro (Anggard and Samuelsson 1967). Whether the formation of 15-ketoprostanoic acid derivatives of $PGF_{1\alpha}$ and PGE_1 eliminates biologic activities is not known. However, it is conceivable that their spectra of activities are changed.

At present the cell types involved in the degradation of prostaglandins are not known. However, in view of the efficiency of the elimination of prostaglandins E_1 and $F_{1\alpha}$, it is conceivable that the relevant cell types occur at the level of the alveolar-capillary unit. If, as existing data indicate, degradation occurs by oxidation of the C-15 hydroxyl group, cytochemical studies at the level of the electron microscope may be feasible. Insoluble formazans detectable by light and electron microscopy are formed by reduction of tetrazolium salts by dehydrogenase enzymes (Barrnett 1959). The prostaglandin 15-hydroxydehydrogenase requires NAD (Anggard and Samuelsson 1967), a point exploited in histochemical studies by Nissen and Andersen (1968). These authors found formazan deposits on frozen sections of kidney, most prominently in the thick ascending limb of the loop of Henle and in the distal tubule. Lesser activity was found in the collecting tubules of the inner medulla, in the interstitial cells of the medulla, in the epithelial cells of the pelvis, in the tunica media of the cortical arteries and arterioles, and in the visceral epithelium of the renal corpuscles. If their approach can be adapted for electron microscopy, it should be possible not only to identify the cell types but also the specific organelles involved, as has been achieved in localizations of succinic dehydrogenase (Ogawa and Barrnett 1965).

B.   Synthesis

The lungs, like virtually all other tissues, are capable of synthesizing prostaglandins and related substances, in particular, thromboxanes A_2 and B_2 (Anggard and Samuelsson 1965, Hamberg et al. 1975), some of which emerge in the pulmonary venous effluent (Piper and Vane 1971). Pharmacologic aspects, including interactions of bradykinin with pulmonary prostaglandin synthetase systems, are described in previous chapters of this volume.

Little is known of the tissue localization of prostaglandin synthetase. In the tissues studied biochemically, the synthetase has been associated with microsomal fractions (Hamberg and Samuelsson 1973, Hamberg et al. 1974). However, the origins of the cellular elements that become microsomes during homogenization are not clear (Amar-Costesec et al. 1974).

We have begun to attempt to localize the enzyme at the level of electron microscopy. Our approach was based on that of Janszen and Nugteren (1973), who examined sections of the urinary tract by light microscopy. Their tissues were incubated with dihomo-γ-linolenic acid. Diaminobenzidine was oxidized presumably by the peroxide precursor(s). The oxidized diaminobenzidine was used as the histochemical stain. Heavy reactions were discernable in collecting ducts of the renal medulla, papillary epithelium, interstitial cells, and basal cells of the transitional epithelium of the urinary drainage system.

In our experiments, lung tissue was fixed briefly with glutaraldehyde and then incubated with arachidonic acid and 3,3′-diaminobenzidine. Faint deposits of oxidized diaminobenzidine were detectable on the membranes surrounding lipid droplets in lung perivascular (or interstitial) cells. Similar deposits were evident in lipid droplets of macrophages and in lamellar bodies of type II alveolar epithelial cells.

Following the findings of Hamberg and Samuelsson (1973) and Hamberg et al. (1974), we then attempted to preserve the endoperoxide precursors formed from arachidonic acid by adding the sulfhydryl enzyme inhibitor, *p*-chloromercuribenzoate (*p*-CMB). This reagent, as well as *N*-ethyl maleimide, apparently blocks the isomerase leading to PGE_2 and the reductase leading to $PGF_{2\alpha}$ (Hamberg et al. 1974). Under these conditions, the results were striking (Fig. 13). Localization of reaction product appeared to be restricted at the level of the alveolar-capillary unit to the perivascular cells, type II alveolar cells, and macrophages.

At present, we cannot conclude that we have definitely localized prostaglandin synthetase. The 3,3′-diaminobenzidine is not specific for endo- and hydroperoxy precursors of prostaglandins. Other lipid peroxides may oxidize the substrate. Similarly, in the presence of H_2O_2, peroxidase enzymes of macrophages and red and white blood cells would be expected to oxidize diaminobenzidine (e.g., Huber et al. 1974). Furthermore, supporting biochemical and pharmacologic experiments are yet to be carried out; in particular, the effects of prostaglandin synthetase inhibitors, such as aspirin and indomethacin, must be examined for their effects on the cytochemical reaction.

Nonetheless, our results suggest that a peroxide has been formed and that the quantity formed or accumulated can be increased by adding *p*-CMB, a compound known to cause the accumulation of the endoperoxides PGG_2 and PGH_2. In addition, the subcellular localization of the oxidized diaminobenzidine deposits is consistent with the presence of prostaglandin synthetase in membrane systems likely to form microsomes on homogenization.

The localization of a possible prostaglandin synthetase system in cells adjacent to the capillary endothelium suggests easy access of products of the system to the circulation. Endothelial cells themselves occasionally contain lipid droplets. However, we have not observed endothelial lipid droplets in

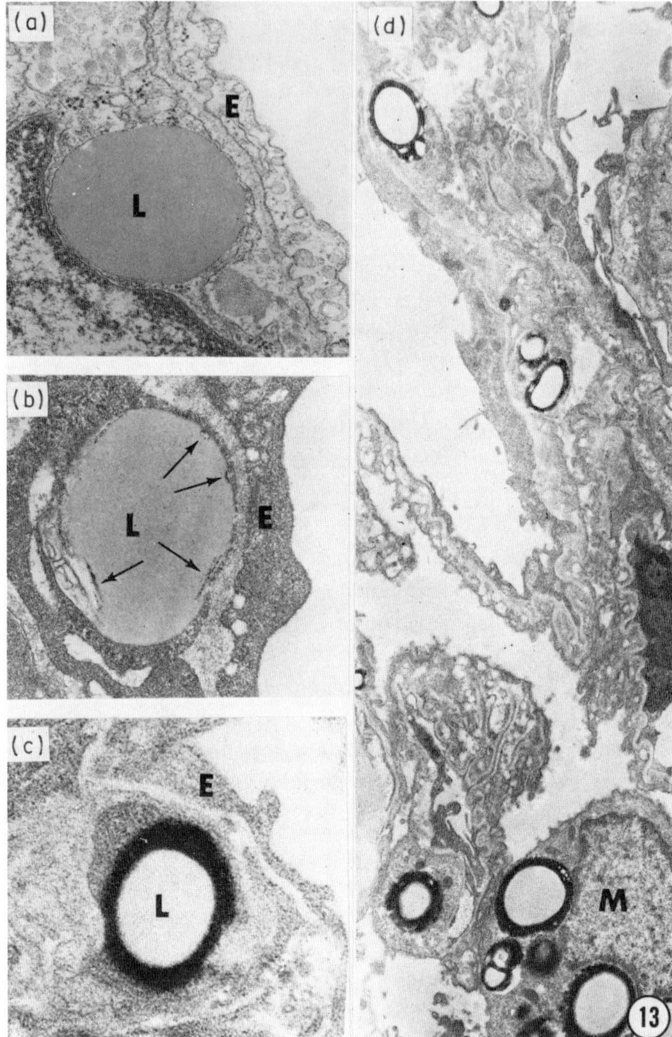

FIGURE 13   (a) Lipid droplet (L) in interstitial cell immediately adjacent to capillary endothelial cell (E). Rat lung tissue illustrated in this figure was prepared for electron microscopy by standard techniques. Section stained with uranyl acetate and lead nitrate (×26,000). (b) Lipid droplet in similar position to that in (a) but from lung tissue incubated with arachidonic acid and 3,3′-diaminobenzidine. Faint deposits of reaction product, possibly indicating sites of prostaglandin synthesis, discernible around lipid droplet (arrows). Section unstained (×30,000). (c) Heavy deposits of reaction product seen when lung tissue

this study and do not know if they react with diaminobenzidine, as do the lipid droplets of the perivascular cells.

The ability of the lungs to eliminate, at once, prostaglandins of the E and F series and to form similar prostaglandins and prostaglandin precursors, which pass into the systemic circulation, presents a paradox. At present, there is little evidence indicating that prostaglandins and their precursors are released under physiologic conditions. However, the ability of lungs to eliminate prostaglandins is such that one can assume that degradative metabolism occurs under physiologic conditions, if prostaglandins of the E and F series occur in central venous blood. Possibly the synthesis and release of prostaglandins by the lungs do not occur physiologically but occur under pathologic circumstances, e.g., following embolism or anaphylaxis (Piper and Vane 1969, 1971, Palmer et al. 1973). Said and associates (1974) have reported evidence indicating release of prostaglandins in association with extreme hyper ventilation, a point suggesting that the effects of vigorous physical exercise and continuous positive pressure ventilation should be examined. To our knowledge, physiologic manipulations known to influence pulmonary blood flow and volume, e.g., Valsalva's and Muller's maneuvers, have not been examined for their effects on prostaglandin release.

The ability of the lungs to release both $PGF_{2\alpha}$ and PGE_2 presents another paradox, as the former tends to raise blood pressure and contract tracheal smooth muscle while the latter tends to lower blood pressure and relax tracheal smooth muscle (e.g., Puglisi 1973). It is not clear whether the two are released simultaneously, nor is much known of the relative quantities released. However, the formation of PGE_2 and $PGF_{2\alpha}$ from common precursors occurs through different enzyme systems (Hamberg et al. 1974), raising the possibility of selective synthesis.

FIGURE 13 (continued)

was incubated with arachidonic acid and 3,3'-diaminobenzidine in presence of *p*-chloromercuribenzoate (*p*-CMB), which favors accumulation of hydroxy- and endoperoxide precursors of prostaglandin synthesis. Section unstained ($\times 18,000$). (d) Low power survey micrograph from capillary bed of rat lung incubated with arachidonic acid and DAB in presence of *p*-CMB. Reaction product chiefly localized on lipid droplets of interstitial (septal) cells but also found in macrophages (M) ($\times 5,000$). [(a),(b), and (c) Reprinted from Ryan, J. W. and Ryan, U. S. (1976). *Lung Metabolism.* Edited by Junod and de Haller, with the permission of Academic Press and the authors.]

VII. Metabolism of Steroid
and Thyroid Hormones

The lungs, like other tissues, undoubtedly take up hormones for their own use. As will be discussed in other volumes of this series, glucocorticoids hasten the production of surfactant by fetal lungs (Torday et al. 1975). Several investigators (e.g., Toft and Chytil 1973) have shown that homogenates of adult and fetal rat lung contain macromolecules, possibly receptors, capable of binding natural and synthetic glucocorticoids with high affinity and some specificity. Others (e.g., Wang et al. 1971) have shown that glucocorticoids accelerate the appearance of osmiophilic bodies in type II alveolar cells, the likely origin of the surfactant lining layer. Redding and associates (1972) have reported that the morphology of type II alveolar cells and the content of surface-active material in lung lavage fluid of adult rats can be profoundly influenced by thyroid hormones: thyroidectomy was associated with reduced surfactant and type II cells appeared to be immature (decreased cell size and fewer and smaller osmiophilic bodies). Thyroxine treatment had the opposite effects.

The disposition of metabolites following uptake of glucocorticoids and thyroxine has not been studied but may present a fruitful line of inquiry. Only part of the triiodothyronine of serum originates in the thyroid gland. Thus the triiodothyronine (T-3) that originates elsewhere has become a matter of concern, especially in view of so-called *T-3 hyperthyroidism*. Rabinowitz and Hercker (1971) have reported that isolated rat hearts perfused with thyroxine may release up to 5% of the original thyroxine as triiodothyronine. We are unaware of studies on the amounts of thyroxine taken up by the lungs; but in view of the large volume of blood processed by the lungs [especially during exercise, a condition in which T-3 utilization may be increased (Middlesworth 1974)], and their strategic position within the circulation, such studies may be indicated. Similarly, the disposition of the metabolites of glucocorticoids may be of interest, as Giannopoulos (1974) has shown that fetal lungs can convert cortisone to its more active analog, cortisol. Recently, Nicholas and Kim (1975) have shown that isolated lungs perfused with [³H] cortisone contain [³H] cortisol in their venous effluent. Subcellular fractions of rabbit, dog, and rat lungs metabolize testosterone (Hartiala 1974). However, the disposition of the metabolites is not known.

VIII. Coagulation and Fibrinolysis

Todd (1959, 1964) has shown that endothelial cells of veins, venules, capillaries, and pulmonary artery, but not arteries of the systemic circulation, contain a factor, plasminogen activator, capable of initiating fibrinolysis. Warren (1963) confirmed and extended Todd's findings. Of the tissues studied, the vessels of lung, heart, and brain were most active. Whether the lungs are a source of circulating plasminogen activator is not known. Similarly, the precise location of plasminogen activator within endothelial cells is not known.

Williams (1964) has reported that lung microsomes, like an extract of Russell's viper venom, can function enzymically in initiating coagulation. Although the cellular origins of membrane systems which become microsomes during or following homogenization, are not fully elucidated (e.g., Amar-Costesec et al. 1974) plasma membrane fragments undoubtedly contribute. Recently, Zeldis et al. (1972), using peroxidase-conjugated antibodies to bovine lung thromboplastin, showed that thromboplastin or tissue factor antigen occurs on plasma membranes of several cell-types but is particularly prominent on endothelial cells of the pulmonary artery and its vasa vasorum. Simmons and coworkers (1974), using a similar preparation of lung thromboplastin (Nemerson and Pitlick 1970), have reported that in vitro, thromboplastin degrades angiotensin I, angiotensin II, bradykinin, Lys-bradykinin, Met-Lys-bradykinin, and substance P. In view of the apparent localization of thromboplastin on the plasma membrane of pulmonary endothelial cells, Simmons and colleagues suggested that thromboplastin may act to metabolize circulating vasoactive peptides in addition to its function as an initiator of the extrinsic clotting system. However, the number of polypeptides hydrolyzed by thromboplastin in vitro and the types of products formed are not consistent with data obtained in experiments using intact lungs (see Section V). Further evaluation of a possible role of thromboplastin in the metabolism of circulating polypeptides requires further data on the rapidity of hydrolytic reactions, as the mean transit time of blood through the pulmonary capillary bed is probably less than 1 sec. Similarly, it would be useful to know whether thromboplastin occurs at the level of the alveolar-capillary unit and whether it is active under physiologic conditions or requires activation or cofactors not ordinarily present. Recently, Maynard and associates (1975) have shown that tissue factor exists in a dormant state on cells in culture but can be activated by prolonged digestion with trypsin.

Antihemophilic factor (factor VIII), without procoagulant activity, has been found in association with endothelial cells in culture (from umbilical vein; Jaffe et al. 1973). Whether factor VIII occurs in association with endothelial cells of lung remains to be investigated. However, Hoyer and associates (1973) have reported that factor VIII occurs on endothelial cells of a number of other tissues.

Acknowledgments

It is a pleasure to acknowledge support by grants from the John A. Hartford Foundation, Inc., the Council for Tobacco Research—U.S.A., Inc., the National Institutes of Health (HL15691, HL16407 and contract NO1 HR3-3015). This work was also supported by an Established Investigatorship award to Dr. Una S. Ryan from the American Heart Association and with funds contributed by the Heart Association of Palm Beach County, Florida.

We would like to thank Mrs. Sue Lucas and Mrs. Judy Ashford for typing this chapter.

Note Added in Proof

Freeze-etching Nomenclature

In an attempt to standardize freeze-etching nomenclature, Branton et al., *Science,* **190**:54–56, 1975, have proposed the following terms to describe and label fracture faces and surfaces: The protoplasmic half (P) of a split membrane is that closest to the cytoplasm and the extracellular half (E) is that closest to the extracellular space. These designations can be applied to fracture faces or to true membrane surfaces. Thus, in this chapter (e.g., in Figs. 11 and 12), the outer fracture face corresponds to the E face and the inner fracture face corresponds to the P face.

References

Amar-Costesec, A., Wibo, M., Thines-Sempoux, D., Beaufay, H., and Berthet, J. (1974). Analytical study of microsomes and isolated subcellular membranes from rat liver. IV. Biochemical, physical, and morphological modifications of microsomal components induced by digitonin, EDTA, and pyrophosphate. *J. Cell Biol.,* **62**:717–745.

Änggård, E. and Samuelsson, B. (1965). Biosynthesis of prostaglandins from arachidonic acid in guinea pig lung. *J. Biol. Chem.,* **240**:3518–3521.

Änggård, E. and Samuelsson, B. (1967). The metabolism of prostaglandins in lung tissue. In S. Bergstrom and B. Samuelsson (eds.): *Prostaglandins.* Interscience Publishers, London, pp. 97–105.

Askin, F. B. and Kuhn, C. (1971). The cellular origin of pulmonary surfactant. *Lab. Invest.,* **25**:260–268.

Avrameas, S. (1969). Coupling of enzymes to proteins with glutaraldehyde. *Immunocytochemistry,* **6**:43–52.

Barrnett, R. J. (1959). The demonstration with the electron microscope of the end-products of histochemical reactions in relation to the fine structure of cells. *Exp. Cell Res. Suppl.*, 7:65–89.

Binet, L. and Burstein, M. (1950). Poumon et action vasculaire de l'adenosine-triphosphate (A.T.P.). *Presse Med.*, 58:1201–1203.

Boyd, I. A. and Forrester, T. (1968). The release of adenosine triphosphate from frog skeletal muscle in vitro. *J. Physiol.*, 199:115–135.

Dorer, F. E., Kahn, J. R., Lentz, K. E., Levine, M., and Skeggs, L. T. (1972). Purification and properties of angiotensin-converting enzyme from hog lung. *Circ. Res.*, 31:356–366.

Dorer, F. E., Kahn, J. R., Lentz, K. E., Levine, M., and Skeggs, L. T. (1974). Hydrolysis of bradykinin by angiotensin-converting enzyme. *Circ. Res.*, 34:824–827.

Eiseman, B., Bryant, L., and Waltuch, T. (1964). Metabolism of vasomotor agents by the isolated perfused lung. *J. Thorac. Cardiovasc. Surg.*, 48: 798–806.

Fanburg, B. L. and Glazier, J. B. (1973). Conversion of angiotensin I to angiotensin II in the isolated perfused dog lung. *J. Appl. Physiol.*, 35:325–331.

Feder, N. (1971). Microperoxidase. An ultrastructural tracer of low molecular weight. *J. Cell Biol.*, 51:339–343.

Ferreira, S. H. and Vane, J. R. (1967a). The disappearance of bradykinin and eledoisin in the circulation and vascular beds of the cat. *Br. J. Pharmacol.*, 30:417–424.

Ferreira, S. H. and Vane, J. R. (1967b). Prostaglandins: Their disappearance and release into the circulation. *Nature (Lond.)*, 216868–873.

Fishman, A. P. (1963). Dynamics of the pulmonary circulation. In W. F. Hamilton and P. Dow (eds.): *Handbook of Physiology*, Vol. 2, Sect. 2, *Circulation*. American Physiological Society, Washington, D. C., pp. 1167–1743.

Fishman, A. P. and Pietra, G. G. (1974). Handling of bioactive materials by the lung. *N. Engl. J. Med.*, 291:Pt 1, 884–890, Pt 2, 953–959.

Giannopoulos, G. (1974). Uptake and metabolism of cortisone and cortisol by the fetal rabbit lung. *Steroids*, 23:845–853.

Goffinet, J. A. and Mulrow, P. J. (1963). Estimation of angiotensin clearance by an in vivo assay. *Clin. Res.*, 2:408.

Green, H. N. and Stoner, H. B. (1950). *Biological Actions of the Adenine Nucleotides*, H. K. Lewis, London.

Haddy, F. J. and Scott, J. B. (1968). Metabolically linked vasoactive chemicals in local regulation of blood flow. *Physiol. Rev.*, 48:688–707.

Hamberg, M. and Samuelsson, B. (1973). Detection and isolation of an endoperoxide intermediate in prostaglandin biosynthesis. *Proc. Natl. Acad. Sci. USA*, 70:899–903.

Hamberg, M., Svensson, J., Wakabayashi, T., and Samuelsson, B. (1974). Isolation and structure of two prostaglandin endoperoxides that cause platelet aggregation. *Proc. Natl. Acad. Sci. USA*, 71:345–349.

Hamberg, M., Svensson, J., and Samuelsson, B. (1975). Thromboxanes: A new group of biologically active compounds derived from prostaglandin endoperoxides. *Proc. Natl. Acad. Sci. USA*, 72:2994–2998.

Hartiala, J. (1974). Testosterone metabolism in rabbit lung in vitro. *Steroids Lipids Res.*, 5:91–95.

Hodge, R. L., Ng, K. K. F., and Vane, J. R. (1967). Disappearance of angiotensin from the circulation of the dog. *Nature*, 215:138–141.

Horton, E. W. and Jones, R. L. (1969). Prostaglandins A_1, A_2 and 19-hydroxy A_1, their actions on smooth muscle and their inactivation on passage through the pulmonary and hepatic portal vascular beds. *Br. J. Pharmacol.*, 37:705–722.

Hoyer, L. W., De Los Santos, R. P., and Hoyer, J. R. (1973). Antihemophilic factor antigen. Localization in endothelial cells by immunofluorescent microscopy. *J. Clin. Invest.*, 52:2737–2744.

Huber, G., Pereira, W., Nunnemacher, G., Laguarda, R., and Widmann, J. (1974). Comparative localization of catalase and peroxidase activity in pulmonary alveolar macrophages by ultrastructural histochemistry. *Clin. Res.*, 22:703A.

Hughes, J., Gillis, C. N., and Bloom, F. E. (1969). The uptake and disposition of dl-norepinephrine in perfused rat lung. *J. Pharmacol. Exp. Ther.*, 169:237–248.

Igic, R., Sorrell, K., Nakajima, T., and Erdös, E. G. (1972). Identity of kininase II with an angiotensin I converting enzyme. *Adv. Exp. Biol. Med.*, 21:149–153.

Jaffe, E. A., Hoyer, L. W., and Nachman, R. L. (1973). Synthesis of antihemophilic factor antigen by cultured human endothelial cells. *J. Clin. Invest.*, 52:2757–2764.

Janszen, F. H. A. and Nugteren, D. H. (1973). A histochemical study of the prostaglandin biosynthesis in the urinary system of the rabbit, guinea pig, goldhamster, and rat. *Adv. Biosci.*, 9:287–292.

Kraehenbuhl, J. P., Galardy, R. E., and Jamieson, J. D. (1974). Preparation and characterization of an immunoelectron microscope tracer consisting of a heme-octapeptide coupled to Fab. *J. Exp. Med.*, 139:208–223.

Luft, J. H. (1966). Fine structure of capillary and endocapillary layer as revealed by ruthenium red. *Fed. Proc.*, 25:1773–1783.

Marchesi, V. T. and Barrnett, R. J. (1963). The demonstration of enzymatic activity in pinocytotic vesicles of blood capillaries with the electron microscope. *J. Cell Biol.*, 17:547–556.

Maynard, J. R., Heckman, C. A., Pitlick, F. A., and Nemerson, Y. (1975). Association of tissue activity with the surface of cultured cells. *J. Clin. Invest.*, 55:814–824.

McGiff, J. C., Terragno, N. A., Strand, J. C., Lee, J. B., Lonigro, A. J., and Ng, K. K. F. (1969). Selective passage of prostaglandins across the lung. *Nature*, 223:742–745.

Mentzer, R. M., Rubio, R., and Berne, R. M. (1974). The effects of adenosine on the pulmonary circulation. *Circulation*, 50:Suppl. 3:48 (abstr).

Middlesworth, L. B. (1974). Metabolism and excretion of thyroid hormone, chap. 14. In M. H. Greer and D. H. Solomon (eds.): *Handbook of Phys-*

iology, Vol. 3, Sect 7, *Thyroid.* American Physiological Society, Washington, D.C., pp. 215-231.

Nemerson, Y. and Pitlick, F. A. (1970). Binding of the protein component of tissue factor to phospholipids. *Biochemistry,* **9**:5105-5113.

Ng, K. K. F. and Vane, J. R. (1967). The conversion of angiotensin I to angiotensin II. *Nature,* **216**:762-766.

Nicholas, T. E. and Kim, P. A. (1975). The metabolism of ^{3}H-cortisone and ^{3}H-cortisol by the isolated perfused rat and guinea pig lungs. *Steroids,* **25**: 387-402.

Nicholas, T. E., Strum, J. M., Angelo, L. S., and Junod, A. F. (1974). Site and mechanism of uptake of ^{3}H-1-norepinephrine by isolated perfused rat lungs. *Circ. Res.,* **35**:670-680.

Nissen, H. M. and Andersen, H. (1968). On the localization of a prostaglandin-dehydrogenase activity in the kidney. *Histochemie,* **14**:189-200.

Ogawa, K. and Barrnett, R. J. (1965). Electron cytochemical studies of succinic dehydrogenase and dihydronicotinamide-adenine dinucleotide diaphorase activities. *J. Ultrastruc. Res.,* **12**:488-508.

Palmer, M. A., Piper, P. J., and Vane, J. R. (1973). Release of rabbit aorta contracting substance (RCS) and prostaglandins induced by chemical or mechanical stimulation of guinea pig lungs. *Br. J. Pharmacol.,* **49**:226-242.

Perl, W., Silverman, F., Delea, A. C., and Chinard, F. P. (1976). Permeability of dog lung endothelium to sodium, diols, amides, and water. *Am. J. Physiol.,* **230**:1708-1721.

Piper, P. J. and Vane, J. R. (1969). Release of additional factors in anaphylaxis and its antagonism by anti-inflammatory drugs. *Nature,* **223**:29-35.

Piper, P. J. and Vane, J. R. (1971). The release of prostaglandins from lung and other tissues. *Ann. N. Y. Acad. Sci.,* **180**:363-385.

Piper, P. J., Vane, J. R., and Wyllie, H. J. (1970). Inactivation of prostaglandins by the lungs. *Nature,* **225**:600-604.

Puglisi, L. (1973). Opposite effects of prostaglandins E and F on tracheal smooth muscles. *Adv. Biosci.,* **9**:219.

Pugatch, E. M. J. and Saunders, A. M. (1968). A new technique for making Hautchen preparations of unfixed aortic endothelium. *J. Atheroscler. Res.,* **8**:735-738.

Rabinowitz, J. L. and Hercker, E. S. (1971). Thyroxine: conversion to tri-iodothyronine by isolated perfused rat heart. *Science,* **173**:1242-1243.

Redding, R. A., Douglas, W. H. J., and Stein, M. (1972). Thyroid hormone influence upon lung surfactant metabolism. *Science,* **175**:994-996.

Rubenstein, A. H., Zwi, S., and Miller, K. (1968). Insulin and the lung. *Diabetologia,* **4**:236-238.

Ryan, J. W., Day, A. R., Ryan, U. S., Chung, A., Marlborough, D. I., and Dorer, F. E. (1976a). Localization of angiotensin converting enzyme (kininase II). I. Preparation of antibody-heme-octapeptide conjugates. *Tissue and Cell,* **8**:111-124.

Ryan, J. W., Niemeyer, R. S., and Goodwin, D. W. (1972a). Metabolic fates of bradykinin, angiotensin I, adenine nucleotides and prostaglandins E_1 and $F_{1\alpha}$ in the pulmonary circulation. In N. Back and F. Sicuteri (eds.): Advances in Experimental Medicine and Biology, Vol. 21, Plenum Press, New York, pp. 259–266.

Ryan, J. W., Niemeyer, R. S., Goodwin, D. W., Smith, U., and Stewart, J. M. (1971). Metabolism of (8-L-[^{14}C] phenylalanine)-angiotensin I in the pulmonary circulation. *Biochem. J.*, **125**:921–923.

Ryan, J. W., Niemeyer, R. S., and Ryan, U. (1975a). Metabolism of prostaglandin $F_{1\alpha}$ in the pulmonary circulation. *Prostaglandins,* **10**:101–108.

Ryan, J. W., Roblero, J., and Stewart, J. M. (1968). Inactivation of bradykinin in the pulmonary circulation. *Biochem. J.*, **110**:795–797.

Ryan, J. W., Roblero, J., and Stewart, J. M. (1969). Inactivation of bradykinin in rat lung. *Pharmacol. Res. Commun.,* **1**:192.

Ryan, J. W., Roblero, J., and Stewart, J. M. (1970a). Inactivation of bradykinin in rat lung. In N. Back, F. Sicuteri, and M. Rocha e Silva (eds.): Advances in Experimental Medicine and Biology, Vol. 8, *Bradykinin and Related Kinins.* Plenum Press, New York, pp. 263–272.

Ryan, J. W., Ryan, U. S., Schultz, D. R., Whitaker, C., Chung, A., and Dorer, F. E. (1975b). Subcellular localization of pulmonary angiotensin-converting enzyme (kininase II). *Biochem. J.*, **146**:497–499.

Ryan, J. W. and Smith, U. (1971a). Metabolism of adenosine-5′-monophosphate during circulation through the lungs. *Trans. Assoc. Am. Physicians,* **84**: 297–306.

Ryan, J. W. and Smith, U. (1971b). A rapid, simple method for isolating pinocytotic vesicles and plasma membrane of lung. *Biochim. Biophys. Acta,* **249**:177–180.

Ryan, J. W. and Smith, U. (1973). The metabolism of angiotensin I by endothelial cells. In H. Peeters (eds.): *Protides of the Biological Fluids,* Vol. 20. Pergamon Press, Oxford, England, pp. 379–384.

Ryan, J. W., Smith, U., and Niemeyer, R. S. (1972b). Angiotensin I: Metabolism by plasma membrane of lung. *Science,* **176**:64–66.

Ryan, J. W., Stewart, J. M., Leary, W. P., and Ledingham, J. G. (1970). Metabolism of angiotensin I in the pulmonary circulation. *Biochem. J.*, **120**: 221–223.

Ryan, U. S., Ryan, J. W., Whitaker, C., and Chiu, A. (1976b). Localization of angiotensin converting enzyme (kininase II). II. Immunocytochemistry and immunofluorescence. *Tissue and Cell,* **8**:125–145.

Said, S. I., Kitamura, S., Yoshida, T., Preskitt, J., and Holden, D. L. (1974). Humoral Control of Airways. *N. Y. Acad. Sci. USA,* **221**:103–114.

Sander, G. E., West, D. W., and Huggins, C. G. (1971). Peptide inhibitors of pulmonary angiotensin I converting enzyme. *Biochim. Biophys. Acta,* **242**:662–667.

Schoefl, G. I. and French, J. E. (1968). Vascular permeability to particulate fat: Morphological observations on vessels of lactating mammary gland and of lung. *Proc. Roy. Soc. B.,* **169**:153–165.

Simmons, W. H., Burkholder, D. E., and Brecher, A. S. (1974). Effect of bovine lung thromboplastin on vasoactive polypeptides. *Fed. Proc.,* **33**:291 (abstr.).

Smith, U. and Ryan, J. W. (1970). An electron microscopic study of the vascular endothelium as a site for bradykinin and ATP inactivation in rat lung. In N. Back, F. Sicuteri, and M. Rocha e Silva (eds.): Advances in Experimental Medicine Biology, Vol. 8, *Bradykinin and Related Kinins.* Plenum Press, New York, pp. 249–262.

Smith, U. and Ryan, J. W. (1971). Pinocytotic vesicles of the pulmonary endothelial cell. *Chest,* **59**:12S–15S.

Smith, U. and Ryan, J. W. (1972a). Substructural features of pulmonary endothelial caveolae. *Tissue and Cell,* **4**:49–54.

Smith, U. and Ryan, J. W. (1972b). Pulmonary endothelial cells and metabolism of adenine nucleotides, kinins and angiotensin I. In N. Back and F. Sicuteri (eds.): Advances in Experimental Medicine and Biology, Vol. 21, *Vasopeptides.* Plenum Press, New York, pp. 267–276.

Smith, U. and Ryan, J. W. (1973a). Electron microscopy of endothelial cells collected on cellulose acetate paper. *Tissue and Cell,* **5**:333–336.

Smith, U. and Ryan, J. W. (1973b). Electron microscopy of endothelial components of the lungs: Correlations of structure and function. *Fed. Proc.,* **32**:1957–1966.

Smith, U., Ryan, J. W., Michie, D. D., and Smith, D. S. (1971). Endothelial projections: As revealed by scanning electron microscopy. *Science,* **173**:925–927.

Smith, U., Ryan, J. W., and Smith, D. S. (1973). Freeze-etch studies of the plasma membrane of pulmonary endothelial cells. *J. Cell Biol.,* **55**:492–499.

Starling, E. H. and Verney, E. B. (1925). The secretion of urine as studied on the isolated kidney. *Proc. R. Soc. B.,* **97**:321–363.

Strum, J. M. and Junod, A. F. (1972). Radioautographic demonstration of 5-hydroxytryptamine-^{3}H uptake by pulmonary endothelial cells. *J. Cell Biol.,* **54**:456–467.

Tierney, D. F. (1974). Lung metabolism and biochemistry. *Annu. Rev. Physiol.,* **36**:209–231.

Todd, A. S. (1959). The histological localization of fibrinolysin activator. *J. Pathol. Bacteriol.,* **78**:281–283.

Todd, A. S. (1964). Some topographical observations on fibrinolysis. *J. Clin. Pathol.,* **17**:324–327.

Toft, D. and Chytil, F. (1973). Receptors for glucocorticords in lung tissue. *Arch. Biochem. Biophys.,* **157**:464–469.

Torday, J. S., Smith, B. T., and Giroud, C. J. P. (1975). The rabbit fetal lung as a glucocorticoid target tissue. *Endocrinology,* **96**:1462.

Vatter, A. E., Reiss, O. K., Newman, J. K., Lindquist, K., and Groenboer, E. (1968). Enzymes of the lung. I. Detection of esterase with a new cytochemical method. *J. Cell Biol.,* **38**:80–98.

Wachstein, M. and Meisel, E. (1959). Histochemistry of hepatic phosphatases at a physiologic pH. *J. Biophys. Biochem. Cytol.,* **6**:119–120.

Wang, N. S., Kotas, R. V., Avery, M. E., and Thurlbeck, W. M. (1971). Accelerated appearance of osmiophilic bodies in fetal lungs following steroid injection. *J. Appl. Physiol.,* **30**:362–365.

Warren, B. A. (1963). Fibrinolytic properties of vascular endothelium. *Br. J. Exp. Pathol.,* **44**:365–372.

Williams, W. J. (1964). The activity of lung microsomes in blood coagulation. *J. Biol. Chem.,* **239**:933–942.

Yang, H. Y. T., Erdös, E. G., and Levine, Y. (1971). Characterization of a dipeptide hydrolase (kininase II: Angiotensin I converting enzyme). *J. Pharmacol. Exp. Ther.,* **177**:291–300.

Zeldis, S. M., Nemerson, Y., and Pitlick, F. A. (1972). Tissue factor (thromboplastin): localization to plasma membranes by peroxidase-conjugated antibodies. *Science,* **175**:766–768.

8

Enzyme Histochemistry of the Lung

JOHN E. ETHERTON and DAVID M. CONNING

Imperial Chemical Industries, Ltd.
Alderley Park, Macclesfield,
Cheshire, England

I. Introduction

Studies on the chemistry of tissues began during the 19th century. Most of the early work was based on destructive techniques, such as the removal of nuclei and the isolation of elastic fibers (Stirling 1875) for subsequent study. The subject then suffered a gradual dichotomy, part becoming attached to physiology and part remaining as biologic chemistry. In the latter, increasing importance was attached to the use of tissue sections, particularly with the advent of aniline dyes just before the turn of the century. However, the search for new dyes to assist studies in morphology precluded attempts to relate their staining properties to the chemistry of the tissues being studied, and little scientific progress was made during this period.

By the late 1930s, the gradual evolution of a broad spectrum of admittedly largely empirical techniques for the differential staining of tissue components had given rise to an independent branch of histology termed *histochemistry*. This was confirmed in the literature as a scientific entity with the appearance of a major treatise by Lison, who announced the new science of *histochemistry without* (the previously employed method of) *tissue destruction* in his *Histochimie Animale* (1936). Emphasis on the localization of specific tissue components has become much less empirical in approach with the growth of enzyme histochemistry during the last 35 years. The very considerable progress that has taken place has been admirably summarized in the relevant sections of Pearse's standard textbook, *Histochemistry: Theoretical and Applied* (1960, 1968, 1972), reference to which is made in most of the literature in this field. It is often possible today to design a technique for the demonstration of the relative activity of a particular enzyme among cells of a tissue section fairly easily, but the limitations of histochemistry, discussed in the next section, must be borne in mind. An example of this is the presumptive localization of mouse lung prostaglandin E_2 and $F_{2\alpha}$ dehydrogenases, reported for the first time in this chapter.

II. Enzyme Histochemical Technique

A. Advantages

The histochemical approach presents two main advantages over other disciplines that may be used in the study of a particular enzyme. First, it indicates qualitatively which cell types are responsible for the enzyme's activity in a given tissue, and may even suggest in which organelle the activity is located. Second, quantitative studies may be performed at specific sites in an organ without the cellular disruption necessitated by most biochemical techniques. Advances in the design of scanning microdensitometers and of image analyzing computers have allowed relative enzyme kinetics to be studied in individual cells on a routine basis (Barry 1972, Etherton et al. 1974). The study of absolute enzyme kinetics has been made possible by the development of sophisticated microspectrofluorimetric techniques, which have permitted the Michaelis constant (K_m) to be calculated for certain enzymes (Pearse and Rost 1969). The K_m values obtained by biochemical techniques for the extracted, purified enzymes came within the experimental error of the apparent K_m values obtained by microspectrofluorimetry for the enzymes in situ (Rost et al. 1970). Other quantitative histochemical assays depend on elution of the insoluble endproducts from the tissue section followed by spectrophotometric estimation of the amount formed (Jones 1969b).

B. Limitations

Biochemical methods used in the study of enzyme kinetics usually employ optimum conditions for the enzyme under investigation, while the effect of just one variable is followed. Inhibitors are only included in the assay system when it is specifically desired to examine their effects on rate. Measurements can normally be made by watching the disappearance of natural substrate or the appearance of natural products in the reaction vessel; very low levels of activity may be detected, and minute changes in rate can be monitored under different conditions.

On the other hand, the conditions in a histochemical assay are not so easily controlled because the use of tissue sections releases a variable amount of endogenous material into the incubation medium. These materials may include substrates, allosteric activators or inhibitors, or other enzymes capable of acting on the substrate that the investigator is using. The essence of most histochemical methods is the exploitation of the enzyme's natural activity in order to produce an insoluble colored precipitate as close as possible to the intracellular site of the enzyme in a tissue section. This often includes a second or third step, which may introduce errors of localization. A degree of inhibition is almost always present because these coupling reactions frequently employ heavy metal ions or organic dyes, which inhibit most enzymes to some extent. There are two other common causes of inhibition. First, to demonstrate soluble enzymes it is necessary to use small amounts of histologic fixative to prevent diffusion of enzyme away from its cell of origin. Prolonged fixation inhibits all enzymes to some extent, particularly the dehydrogenases. Second, a degree of steric hindrance may be produced by the accumulation of insoluble reaction products in the vicinity of the active site of the enzyme.

Two further limitations must be mentioned: First, some enzymes can only be demonstrated by the use of highly artificial substrates consisting of a natural substrate bound to a complex organic radical. The action of the enzyme releases the organic moiety, which then takes part in the secondary precipitation step. Second, the activity and distribution of enzymes in tissues may be estimated either subjectively or with instruments, but in each case the amount of color available for measurement is limited primarily by the thickness of the section. Low levels of activity and subtle changes in rate are therefore not easily detected. Prolonging the incubation time usually results in a proportional increase in stain density, provided that the enzyme does not become inactivated and that nonenzymic deposition of stain does not take place.

III. Pulmonary Enzyme Histochemistry

A.   Review of Reported
Enzyme Localizations

The total number of histochemically demonstrable enzymes from a variety of mammalian tissues accounts for less than 10% of the number of known enzymes. Groups of enzymes, which are well represented, include the acid and alkaline phosphatases, the carboxylic ester hydrolases, the glycoside hydrolases and glycosyltransferases, the oxidases and peroxidases, the dehydrogenases and diaphorases, and the peptidases. Techniques have not been published for any of the isomerases, ligases, or decarboxylases, while the carbon-oxygen lyases are represented only by carbonic anhydrase, and the aldehyde lyases only by aldolase. Furthermore, in comparison with studies on other tissues, enzyme histochemistry of the mammalian lung has received little attention. No enzyme studies on the upper respiratory tract have been reported. Studies in this region have usually centered on the histochemistry of mucosubstances and glycoproteins (Ellefsen and Tos 1972, Jones et al. 1973). Enzyme histochemical studies on the more distal regions of the lung have been undertaken in three main fields: (a) the cytopathology of pulmonary irritants, (b) the phagocytic properties of the alveolar parenchyma, and (c) the secretory route of pulmonary surfactant. No enzyme histochemical work has been reported on the metabolism of materials brought systemically to or released endogenously by the lung. Where the literature includes discussions of the metabolic functions of lung, these have centered almost exclusively on either pulmonary surfactant secretion or the disposal of inhaled irritants.

Papers have frequently appeared describing the localization of a particular type of enzyme, and most of the more recent ones have been ultrastructural studies designed to adduce evidence for the secretory route of pulmonary surfactant. Fewer papers have appeared in which a broad spectrum of enzymes has been studied in order to gain insight into the metabolic roles of the different cells of the lung (Sorokin et al. 1959, Klika and Petrik 1965, Tyler and Pearse 1965, Tyler et al. 1965, Azzopardi and Thurlbeck 1969, Barry and Robinson 1969b). The information given in this type of report has been used as the basis for Table 1, in which is listed all pulmonary enzymes that have been studied by histochemical techniques to date, together with an indication of the relative activity of each in the most common types of cell found in the primary lobules of the lung. A widely accepted terminology for the suborders of lobulation of the lung has yet to be devised. For our purposes, the primary lobule is a functional unit of respiratory exchange connected to the tracheobronchial tree via one terminal (i.e., nonrespiratory) bronchiole. The enzymes are listed in order according to their Enzyme Commission number allocation

(EC number), and are given their trivial names. In some cases there were minor discrepancies in the relative activity and distribution of certain enzymes between one report and another. This was assumed to be due to differences in (a) the strain or the species used (mouse, rat, cat, horse, and man); (b) the method of killing the animals; (c) the nature of the medium used to inflate the lungs when this was done, and (d) some of the histochemical techniques used to study a given enzyme. However, these differences were not sufficiently serious to warrant separate conclusions about the metabolic function of the various cell types present in the lung.

Compilation of Table 1 was further hindered by the fact that some reports did not include some or all of the following categories of information: (a) enzyme reactions in the bronchiolar epithelium; (b) separate activities of ciliated and nonciliated bronchiolar (Clara) cells; (c) attempts to distinguish between the activities of endothelial cells, interstitial cells, and type I epithelial cells, which together comprise the alveolar wall; (d) whether certain dehydrogenases were NAD- or NADP-dependent; (e) whether or not fixatives, inhibitors, or control incubation media were used; and (f) in some of the ultrastructural studies what activity, if any, was seen in pulmonary cells other than those that were the prime object of study. In view of the general paucity of information it is not surprising that newly discovered cell types, such as the type III cell (Meyrick and Reid 1968) and the contractile interstitial cell (Kapanci et al. 1974), are not yet mentioned in the histochemical literature.

Most of the enzymes listed have been studied in our own laboratories, using a variety of histochemical techniques, on the lungs of mice and rats. Some of the results obtained were used to complete gaps in Table 1, which could not be filled by reference to the literature. That which does appear correlates well with our own results, and representative staining patterns for some of the main enzyme groups are given in Plates 1 and 2, following page 240.

In order to obtain further information about the localization of enzymes concerned with the metabolism of biologically active compounds brought to or released by the lung, the demonstration of mouse lung prostaglandin dehydrogenase (PGDH) and aniline hydroxylase was attempted. The technique for PGDH was based on the method of Nissen and Anderson (1968), but a 10 mM substrate (prostaglandin E_2 or $F_{2\alpha}$), an incubation time of up to 3 hr, and a pH of 7.5 instead of 8.0, were used to avoid enhancing the activity of *nothing dehydrogenase* referred to later on. The PGDH demonstrated with the two different substrates was probably 15-hydroxyprostanoate dehydrogenase in both cases. Aniline hydroxylase, which is closely similar to aryl hydrocarbon hydroxylase, was demonstrated by the method of Grasso and coworkers (1971). Control preparations were made by omitting the substrate alone from

TABLE 1 Summary of the Presumptive Histochemical Localization and Relative Activity of Some Pulmonary Enzymes[a]

| Enzyme and EC number[b,c] | | Alveolar cell type | | | | | Bronchiolar cell type | | Reference[d] |
		Endo-thelial	Inter-stitial	type I	type II	Macro-phage	Ciliated	Non-ciliated	
1.1.1.1	Alcohol dehydrogenase	−	−	−	±	−	+	+	[1,3]
1.1.1.27	Lactate dehydrogenase	±	+	±	++	+	+++	++++	[1,2,3,10]
1.1.1.30	3-Hydroxybutyrate dehydrogenase	−	−	−	±	−	±	++	[1,2,3,10]
1.1.1.38	Malate dehydrogenase	±	±	±	++	−	++	+++	[1,2,3,10]
1.1.1.41	Isocitrate dehydrogenase	±	±	±	++	±	++	+++	[1,2,10]
1.1.1.47	Glucose dehydrogenase	−	−	−	±	−	±	+	[2,3]
1.1.1.49	Glucose 6 phosphate dehydrogenase	±	±	±	++	±	++	+++	[1,2,3,10]
1.1.1.141	Prostaglandin dehydrogenase	±	++++	±	+++	−	+	++	−
1.1.2.1	Glycerol 3 phosphate dehydrogenase	±	±	±	++	±	+	++	[1,3,10]
1.2.1.12	Glyceraldehyde 3 phosphate dehydrogenase	+	+	+	++	+	+++	++++	[1]
1.3.99.1	Succinate dehydrogenase	−	−	−	±	−	+	++	[1,2,3,10]
1.4.1.2	Glutamate dehydrogenase	−	−	−	+	−	+	++	[1,2]
−	Ubiquinones	+	+	+	+++	+	±	±	[3,10]
1.4.3.4	Monoamine oxidase	−	−	−	±	−	±	+	[3,10]
1.6.99.3	NADH$_2$ diaphorase	±	±	±	++	−	++	+++	[1,2,3,10]
1.6.99.1	NADPH$_2$ diaphorase	+	+	+	+++	±	+++	++++	[1,2,10]
1.9.3.1	Cytochrome oxidase	++	++	+	+++	−	+	++	[1,2,3,10]
1.11.1.7	Peroxidase	+	+	+	++	+	+	++	[3]
−	DOPA oxidase	−	+	−	−	−	−	±	[3]

2.4.1.1	α-Glucan phosphorylase	−	−	−	−	−	−	−	[3]
—	Nonspecific esterase	−	−	−	++	−	−	+++	[2,3,8]
3.1.1.3	Lipase	−	+	+	++	−	++	+++	[3]
3.1.3.1	Alkaline phosphatase	−	−	±	++	±		++	[2,3,5,8]
3.1.3.2	Acid phosphatase	±	+	±	++	++++	±	+	[2,3,6]
3.1.3.4	Phosphatidic acid phosphatase	−	−	−	++	+	−	+	[9]
3.1.3.5	5′-Nucleotidase	−	−	−	+	±	−	+	[3]
3.1.3.9	Glucose-6-phosphatase	−	−	−	++	−	−	+	[2,3]
	Aniline hydroxylase	±	±	±	+	−	±	+	[7]
3.1.6.1	Arylsulphatase	−	−	−	+	++	−	−	[6]
3.2.1.23	β-Galactosidase	−	−	−	+	++	−	−	−
3.2.1.31	β-Glucuronidase	−	±	−	+	++	−	−	[2,3,6]
3.2.1.30	N-Acetyl β-glucosaminidase	−	−	−	+	++	−	−	[6]
3.4.11.1	Leucine amino peptidase	−	−	−	±	−	−	±	[3]
3.6.1.4	ATPase	−	−	−	±	±	±	±	[3]
—	'Proteinase'	−	+	−	+	−	−	−	[4]

aThis table is included in a thesis for the Ph.D. degree submitted to the Council for National Academic Awards by one of the present authors (J.E.E.).
bSome histochemically demonstrable enzymes do not have an EC equivalent due to the curious nature of their substrate.
cIn cases where the results published on a given enzyme did not contain any reference to some of the cell types listed above, the missing information was obtained either by examining the authors' photomicrographs or by repeating some of their experiments.
dReferences in brackets: [1] Azzopardi and Thurlbeck (1969), [2] Barry and Robinson (1969b), [3] Caulet et al. (1968), [4] Esterly (1972), [5] Fredricsson (1956), [6] Goldfischer et al. (1968), [7] Grasso et al. (1971), [8] Klika and Petrik (1965), [9] Meban (1972), [10] Tyler et al. (1965).

the incubation medium. The results are included in Table 1, and are illustrated in Plate 1(a–c), and Plate 2(d). Of the 40 or so different types of cells that have been recorded in the alveolar parenchyma, the seven most common are given in Table 1. All types of blood cells are excluded, but it should be noted that the column headed *interstitial cells* may include blood monocytes that have lodged in the interalveolar septum for a period of acclimatization prior to assuming the role of a free alveolar macrophage (Bowden and Adamson 1972). Ciliated cells, Clara cells, and alveolar macrophages are readily identified in frozen sections. The identification of interstitial cells and type II alveolar epithelial cells is more difficult and is based on a combination of their observed position in the alveolar wall, their known shape provided by previous ultrastructural studies, and their overall enzyme staining characteristics. The identification of capillary endothelial cells and type I alveolar epithelial cells is almost impossible because the thickness of their cytoplasm is often below the limit of resolution of the light microscope, and frozen sections always suffer morphologic damage due to the freezing process and the incubation procedure. Some authors claim to have seen a difference in the enzyme activities of these two types of cell, and this is reflected in Table 1. Where our own results have been used to complete the table, no distinction has been made between them.

With these limitations in mind, the metabolic roles of the seven main types of cell will now be discussed.

B. Metabolic Roles of Endothelial Cells and Type I Cells

Both types exhibited a consistently low activity for most of the enzymes studied. These included representatives of three major metabolic pathways: glycolysis, the Krebs cycle, and the hexose monophosphate shunt. Hydrolytic enzyme activity was generally absent. The most active enzyme was cytochrome oxidase in endothelial cells. This is the terminal oxidase of the respiratory chain and it transfers electrons to molecular oxygen. Its activity is directly correlated with oxygen requirement. The overall results agree with the scanty distribution of organelles seen in these cells with the electron microscope, and they suggest that there is enough activity for their own metabolic requirements but that there is no marked additional metabolic function.

C. Metabolic Role of Interstitial Cells

The general level of activity in this cell was slightly higher than in the neighboring endothelial and type I cells, and more enzymes were demonstrable. Apart from satisfying its own metabolic needs, the enzyme profile indicates two extra metabolic roles, the second of which demands a discussion of the results obtained for prostaglandin dehydrogenase.

First, the slightly elevated acid hydrolase activity indicates that it may play a minor role in the lysosomal breakdown of unwanted materials originating either from the interalveolar septum or from the alveolar lining. Support for the latter suggestion is found in the literature. When finely divided particulate matter, such as colloidal thorium or carbon, is caused to enter the alveoli, it often appears in small amounts in vacuoles in the interstitial cells (e.g., Corrin 1969, Heppleston and Young 1973). Second, tobacco smoking is associated with the appearance of electron-dense droplets in these cells (Etherton and Conning 1971). The vacuoles and the droplets are probably the same type of organelle, and since the droplets show weak acid phosphatase activity in the electron microscope, they may be secondary lysosomes. It is possible that foreign materials on the alveolar lining, such as colloidal particles of thorium, carbon, or condensed tobacco tar, are transported to the interstitial cells for storage and subsequent degradation. Transport may be effected by a pinocytotic shunt operated by the pinocytotically active type I cells. This catabolic function would supplement the major role played by the free macrophages. Furthermore, chronic inhalation of particulates is accompanied by an increase in the number of free macrophages that probably derive from the interstitial cells (Bowden and Adamson 1972, Etherton 1977).

Second, the histochemical assay for prostaglandin dehydrogenase (PGE_2 DH and $PGF_{2\alpha}$DH) produced a staining pattern that did not resemble that for NAD diaphorase. The staining caused by *nothing dehydrogenase* in the control tissue sections incubated without substrate was weak everywhere except in the type II cells and the supranuclear region of the Clara cells, which were slightly darker (Plate 1(a). In the experimental sections the type II cells and both types of bronchiolar epithelial cell were usually covered with a haze of diffuse precipitate of formazan, whereas the interstitial cells had darker and precisely localized deposits in their cytoplasm. Differentiation between type II cells and interstitial cells, both with heavily stained cytoplasm, was made on the following basis. First, depending on the plane of sectioning, the sliced type II cell is roughly circular and has the appearance of a ring or horseshoe of stained cytoplasm around its nucleus. This is because it is a cuboidal cell. On the other hand, the shape of the interstitial cell approximates that of a biconvex hand lens. In section, therefore, it usually appears elongated and has

PLATES 1 and 2 depict the presumptive cellular localization of various enzymes in 10 μm frozen sections of mouse lung. The tetrazolium salts used were NBT, nitroblue tetrazolium (2,2′-di-p-nitrophenyl-5,5′-diphenyl-3,3′-(3,3′-dimethoxy-4,4′-biphenylene) ditetrazolium chloride (Tsou et al. 1956); MTT (3-(4,5-dimethyl-thiazolyl-2)-2,5-diphenyl tetrazolium bromide (Pearse 1957); and YT, yellow tetrazolium (2,2′-di-(3-nitrophenyl)-5,5′-dimethyl-3,3′-(4,4′-biphenylene) ditetrazolium chloride (Jones 1969a). The section in Plate 2(c) was counterstained with Mayer's haemalum; the rest with carmalum. Some of the photographs were taken with a blue filter to enhance the contrast of weak deposits of formazan.

PLATE 1

(a)   Staining pattern of NBT formazan in a control preparation for NAD-dependent dehydrogenases in expanded lung ($\times$64). Incubation was for 3 hr., and activity of "nothing dehydrogenase" produced weak staining of type II cells and bronchiolar epithelium.

(b)   Staining pattern of NBT formazan resulting from activity of prostaglandin E_2 dehydrogenase in expanded lung ($\times$160). Elongated interstitial cells are stained heavily (e.g., left of center). Cuboidal type II cells are covered with diffuse precipitate (e.g., center and lower right).

(c)   Same as in Plate 1(b), but using prostaglandin $F_{2\alpha}$ as the substrate. Three diffusely stained type II cells form a central triangle. Heavily stained interstitial cells show no diffusion of color.

(d)   Staining pattern of MTT formazan resulting from activity of glycerol-3-phosphate dehydrogenase in collapsed lung ($\times$64). Distribution of heavily stained type II cells in deflated tissue clearly seen. Ciliated cells and lower half of Clara cells also stained.

(e)   Staining pattern of YT formazan resulting from activity of lactate dehydrogenase in collapsed lung ($\times$100). Type II and bronchiolar cells heavily stained.

(f)   Staining pattern of NBT formazan resulting from activity of isocitrate dehydrogenase in expanded lung ($\times$64). Type II and bronchiolar cells heavily stained.

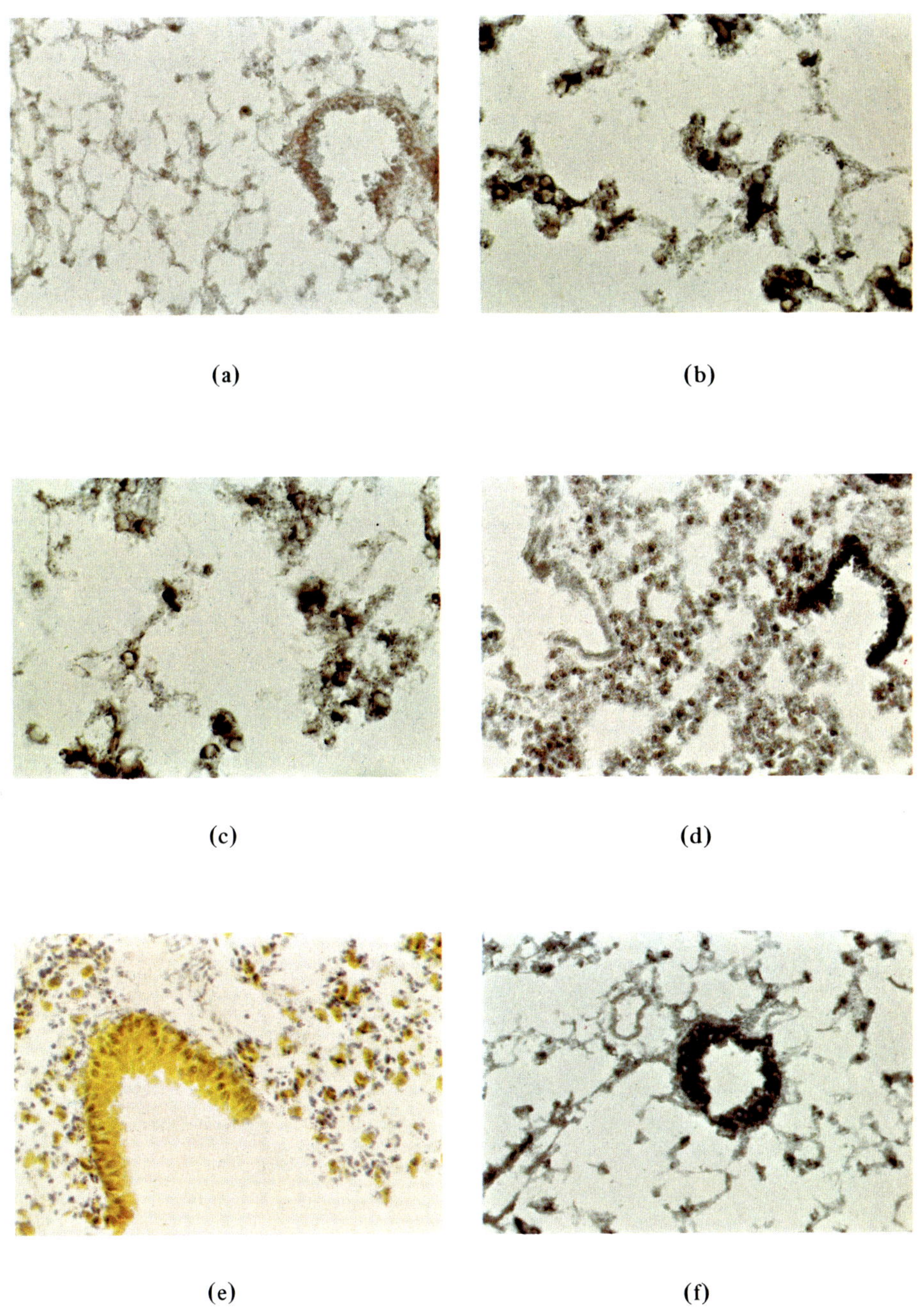

PLATE 2

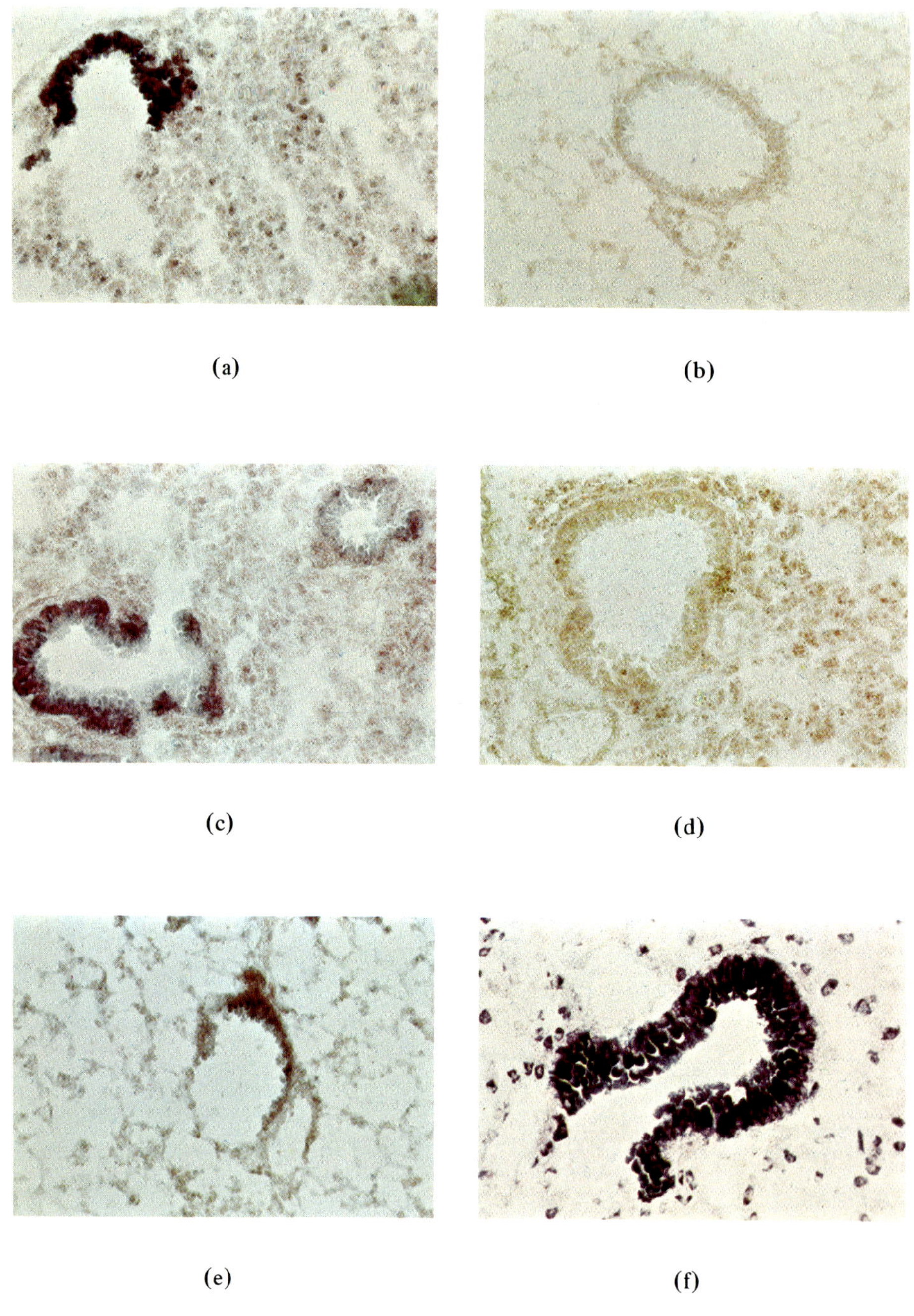

(a)
(b)
(c)
(d)
(e)
(f)

PLATE 2

(a)   Staining pattern of NBT formazan resulting from activity of glucose-6-phosphate dehydrogenase in collapsed lung ($\times$64). Type II cells moderately stained and bronchiolar epithelium heavily stained.

(b)   Same as in Plate 1(a) but using expanded lung. Staining negligible.

(c)   Staining pattern of NBT formazan resulting from activity of 3-hydroxybutyrate dehydrogenase in collapsed lung ($\times$64). Staining significant only in lower half of Clara cells of bronchiolar epithelium.

(d)   Staining pattern of Fast Blue RR resulting from activity of aniline hydroxylase in collapsed lung ($\times$64). All cells weakly stained pale brown, with slightly denser staining of type II cells and bronchiolar epithelium.

(e)   Staining pattern of NBT formazan resulting from activity of succinic dehydrogenase in expanded lung ($\times$64). Staining negligible except in lower half of Clara cells.

(f)   Staining pattern of MTT formazan resulting from activity of NAD diaphorase in expanded lung ($\times$100). Type II cells strongly stained and bronchiolar epithelium intensely stained.

two lateral cytoplasmic projections on either side of the nucleus, which occasionally results in an eye-shaped appearance. Second, the type II cell tends to project into the alveolus, whereas the interstitial cell lies within and in the plane of the alveolar wall. The endothelial cells, type I cells, and macrophages were barely stained. Under identical conditions the distribution of PGE_2DH and of $PGF_{2\alpha}DH$ were the same, but PGE_2DH produced a darker stain (Plate 1(b) and (c).

The results may be interpreted in either or both of the following ways: First, high levels of activity are present in the interstitial cells, and almost as much activity is present in a more soluble and therefore more diffusible form in the type II cells and in the bronchiolar epithelium. Second, the activity is primarily located in the interstitial cells, but due to (a) the rapid production of NADH in the incubation medium, (b) the high levels of NBT reductase activity in type II cells and bronchiolar epithelium, and (c) the long incubation time used, diffuse formazan deposits accumulated in the region of type II cells and bronchiolar epithelium. NBT reductase does not normally produce a diffuse stain because the source of NADH is usually extremely close. In this case, the source is often several cells away, and NBT reductase, which has diffused out of the cell, therefore produces a halo of formazan. The second interpretation, that of primary localization in the interstitial cells, is favored.

The lung inactivates a number of hormones, such as bradykinin, 5-hydroxytryptamine (5-HT), angiotensin I, and the prostaglandins (Vane 1969). If the activity of PGE_2DH and $PGF_{2\alpha}DH$ in the interstitial cell is genuinely high, and if these enzymes may be considered to be markers for cells responsible for the inactivation of this group of hormones, then the pulmonary interstitial cell plays an important role in their metabolism. In partial support of this a *proteinase* has been tentatively identified in pulmonary interstitial cells (Esterly 1972). On the other hand, monoamine oxidase (MAO), which is involved in the metabolism of amines, such as adrenaline and 5-HT, appears to be almost absent from alveolar cells in the histochemical assay. This contradicts the finding of high levels of MAO activity in whole perfused lung for some substrates and in lung homogenates for all substrates.

The efficiency of the histochemical assay of MAO activity in sections of lung is probably suspect, because it works well in liver.

D. Metabolic Role of Type II Cells

With the exception of the acid hydrolases, the activity of all enzyme groups listed was greater in type II cells than in any other cell except the Clara cell. Furthermore, the total number of demonstrable enzymes exceeded that for any other cell type in the lung. The dense staining produced by certain enzymes indicates a very active glycolytic sequence [(glycerol-3-phosphate dehydrogenase (G3PDH), Plate 1(d)]; LDH, Plate 1(e)]; Krebs cycle [(malate dehydrogenase; isocitrate dehydrogenase (IDH), Plate 1(f)]; hexose monophosphate shunt [(Gluc 6 PDH), Plate 2(a)]; an active lysomal system [(lipase, acid phosphatase (AcP), phosphatidic acid phosphatase, aryl sulphatase)]; and an active transport system on the alveolar edge of the cell [(alkaline phosphatase)]. This diverse and elevated metabolic activity would enable the cell to perform any of a number of roles. The most popular function mentioned in the publications referred to so far is the synthesis and secretion of pulmonary surfactant. The presence of lysosomal activity is accounted for by the need for rupture of the cell membrane during the secretory process. A less popular theoretical role is the uptake and metabolism of surfactant (Niden 1967, Etherton 1977), and possibly of other materials. It is not yet possible to decide whether the type II cell concentrates on anabolic or catabolic processes in metabolism.

E.   Metabolic Role of Macrophages

This cell exhibited low levels of activity in the main metabolic pathways, judged by the results obtained for the marker enzymes in Table 1, but it had extremely active lysosomal activity. The various acid hydrolases were more active in the macrophage than in any other cell type, consistent with its accepted role in the phagocytosis of unwanted materials for degradation. No other role was indicated by the results obtained.

F.   Metabolic Role of Bronchiolar Cells

The activity of the three main metabolic pathways was greater in the Clara cell than in any other cell type in the lung, and the presence of 3-hydroxybutyrate dehydrogenase (3HBDH), Plate 2(c) almost exclusively in this cell indicates that it is the only cell type in which fatty acid metabolism is important. This is supported by the finding that its incorporation and turnover of fatty acids are faster than that of any other cell type in the lung (Conning and Etherton 1971). It does, however, contain very low levels of lysosomal activity. It is therefore clearly endowed with extremely active energy-producing mechanisms able to meet the demands of any synthetic process. It is probably more suited to anabolic tasks in metabolism, such as the secretion of surfactant (Etherton et al. 1973a, Smith et al. 1974), than to the catabolic type of activity, such as that seen in the macrophage and, possibly, in the interstitial cell.

The enzyme profile of the ciliated cell reflected that of the Clara cell but with lower levels of activity; as discussed earlier, some enzymes may appear to be present due to the artefactual diffusion of intermediate reactants from the adjacent Clara cells during the assay. The low level of 3HBDII activity suggests that it has no major role in fatty acid metabolism, and it probably carries out no metabolic function additional to its own requirements.

In view of the architecture of the pulmonary vasculature and the relatively low numbers of bronchiolar cells, the Clara cell and the ciliated cell probably play no significant part in the metabolism of vasoactive substances.

IV.   Discussion

A.   Anomalous Results

Three anomalies seen in the results are the unexpectedly low levels of aniline hydroxylase, monoamine oxidase, and succinic dehydrogenase.

Aniline hydroxylase, Plate 2(d), activity was uniformly low and was absent from the alveolar macrophages, and there was no staining of control sections. The photomicrographs published by Grasso et al. (1971) show a fairly dense stain in their lung sections, but the morphology does not appear as well preserved as in other tissues that they describe. The technique may well require special investigation into optimal conditions for its use in the lung, in order to decide which cell type exhibits the greatest activity under optimal conditions. This may also apply to monoamine oxidase.

Succinic dehydrogenase (SDH) was present with high activity in the cardiac type of musculature around the main branches of the pulmonary arteries, with low activity in the bronchioles, and was absent elsewhere in the alveolar parenchyma, Plate 2(e). Its activity was not as great as that of other enzymes of the Krebs cycle, such as IDH, Plate 1(f). This unexpected finding was in agreement with the literature on the subject (e.g., Barry and Robinson 1969b, Tyler et al. 1965). However, biochemical assays for SDH show that it is present in the lung (Wolfe et al. 1968). The finding of low levels of activity in the bronchioles is in accord with the observation that the mitochondria of the Clara cell have poorly developed cristae (Etherton et al. 1973a). Succinic dehydrogenase is bound to the cristae, hence the low activity. But since other pulmonary cells have conventional mitochondria, their absence of SDH in the histochemical assay suggests that optimal conditions for localization of the enzyme in normal mitochondria have not yet been defined.

The conclusions drawn in Section III B to F about the metabolic roles of the various cell types should be regarded as only tentative. This is due to the limitations outlined in Section II B, which will now be amplified.

B.   Preparation of Lung Tissue Sections

The two main decisions to be made are whether to use collapsed or inflated lung, and whether to employ chemical fixatives before using a tissue section for histochemical enzyme assay.

Barry and Robinson (1969a) tested several different aqueous media for use in inflating the lungs before cutting fresh frozen sections in a cryostat. The least amount of enzyme inhibition was produced by inflation with 0.5% polyethylene glycol. In our hands 5% glucose produced marginally less inhibition. The use of expanded rather than collapsed lung allows more confidence to be placed in the identification of cell types. For most enzymes, the degree of inflation makes no difference to the apparent enzyme activity in terms of stain density per unit area of tissue. However, nonspecific esterase activity drops markedly in sections of inflated lung (Barry and Robinson 1969a). Even more striking is the complete loss of demonstrable activity of glucose-6-phosphate dehydrogenase (Gluc-6PDH) in sections of inflated lung [compare Plate 2(a) and (b)].

Fixation presents a number of problems. The use of fresh frozen sections rather than sections cut from blocks of embedded tissue is generally considered to be the best technique for the preparation of material for enzyme histochemical studies because no tissue components are lost, and the only type of inactivation produced is the 5% to 15% loss of enzyme activity caused by the freezing process. It should be noted that the most common method of handling a frozen section is to attach it to a coverslip or slide. This involves melting and refreezing the section, causing a further drop in enzyme activity. It can be avoided by the much more difficult technique of floating the newly cut section directly on the surface of the first solution to be used in the histochemical assay. However, if the frozen section remains unfixed, as soon as it comes into contact with water some tissue components, particularly the soluble enzymes, diffuse into the solution and may give rise to false localization. Very few enzymes are tightly bound to a tissue section. Even an organelle-specific enzyme, such as acid phosphatase, a recognized marker for lysosomes (de Duve 1963), has a soluble component accounting for 52% of its activity (Nachlas et al. 1956, Hannibal and Nachlas 1959). It has been shown that most of the protein in a tissue section may be lost into the medium in this way, and a microcell has been devised in order to monitor constituents of the incubation medium (Kalina et al. 1965). The most common fixatives are acetone or aldehydes, such as formaldehyde or glutaric dialdehyde (glutaraldehyde). Fixation reduces these protein losses and also lessens the histologic damage caused by incubation, but a significant improvement in protein retention is usually accompanied by a significant drop in enzyme activity due to denaturation. A successful compromise developed by Holt and Hicks (1961a, b) was to include 1% formaldehyde in the incubation medium. Another method that lessens the inhibition that results from preincubation fixation procedures is to include, in the fixative, a quantity of substrate equal to the K_m for the enzyme being studied (Etherton, unpublished finding). A thorough review of the role of fixation in enzyme histochemistry has been made by Pearse (1968, 1972).

Most of the results listed in Table 1 were obtained from light microscopic studies of unfixed frozen sections of lung, and for this reason most of the supplementary studies undertaken to complete the table were done in the same way. A small part of the information was gathered from published ultrastructural studies. These invariably used prefixation to preserve the fine structure of the cells. Another source of difficulty in ultrastructural studies is that techniques developed using one tissue are not always successful in a different tissue. For example, the problems encountered when the established lead capture method for the localization of rat liver acid phosphatase (Holt and Hicks 1961b) was applied directly to the rat lung, led to the development of a new technique (Etherton and Botham 1970).

C. Problems in Hydrolytic Enzyme Histochemistry

The two main staining procedures in hydrolytic enzyme histochemistry are (a) simultaneous capture, in which an insoluble precipitate is produced instantaneously, and (b) postincubation coupling, in which the primary reaction product is sufficiently insoluble to remain in place until the secondary reaction can be performed. Although the latter technique avoids having to include inhibitory compounds in the primary incubation medium in most cases, it can give rise to diffusion artefacts, and has been criticized (Burton and Pearse 1952, Defendi 1957).

All hydrolytic enzymes in Table 1 were demonstrated by simultaneous capture methods. Even so, emphasis must be placed on the caution necessary when interpreting the results, because two closely related techniques may still give different staining patterns. An example of this is the two popular simultaneous capture azo-dye methods for the localization of acid phosphatase. That devised by Pearse (1960) uses sodium α-naphthol phosphate as substrate, and that devised by Barka and Anderson (1962) uses substituted naphthol AS phosphates. While both methods show intense activity in alveolar macrophages, the former indicates low levels of activity in the alveolar and bronchiolar epithelia, whereas the latter indicates no activity at all. Control experiments show that the staining produced by the former method is due partly to enzyme activity and partly to the affinity of the azo dye (Fast Garnet GBC salt) for tissue components, especially fat. The different enzyme activities shown by the two methods are probably explained in terms of the different activities of isoenzymes of acid phosphatase towards the two artificial substrates used (Meany et al. 1967).

D. Problems in Oxidoreductase Histochemistry

Most of the enzymes in Table 1 are either hydrolases or oxidoreductases. Some of the more important difficulties that arise in trying to localize the former group of enzymes have been discussed in the preceding section. These apply in general to this section, which includes cytochrome oxidase, peroxidase, DOPA oxidase, monoamine oxidase, the pyridine nucleotide diaphorases, and a large group of dehydrogenases. The chief difference between methods for the oxidoreductases and those for the group of hydrolytic enzymes is that the former nearly always use natural substrates, particularly diaphorases and dehydrogenases. This advantage is offset by serious problems with the validity of localization. The following brief discussion will outline the nature of these difficulties, with special emphasis on dehydrogenase histochemistry.

The hydrolytic enzymes are often organelle-specific and the results obtained are generally considered to be a reliable indicator of their activities in different types of cell. The dehydrogenases, on the other hand, usually employ a second enzyme to produce the staining pattern, as shown by the following simplified scheme.

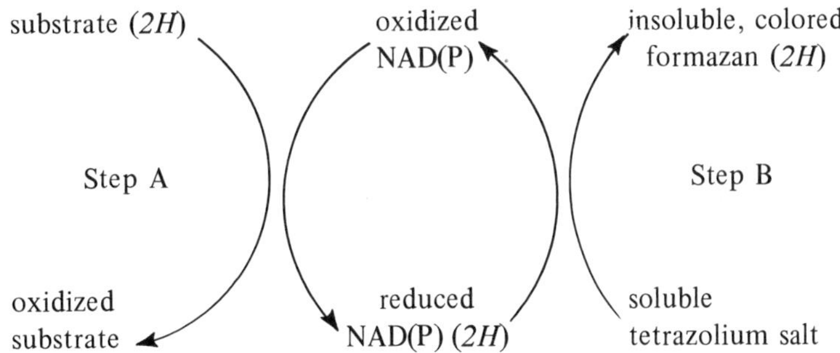

The fate of the hydrogen removed from the substrate is shown by the position of (*2H*). Step A is catalyzed by the primary dehydrogenase, which takes its name from the substrate used; and step B involves the secondary dehydrogenase, an NAD or NADP diaphorase, which is responsible for precipitation of the colored formazan in the tissue section. The diaphorases in this system are often more correctly referred to as tetrazolium reductases. The resultant staining pattern is usually loosely referred to as the localization of a given dehydrogenase. This is not necessarily so. We shall take, as an example, the standard technique for the presumptive localization of lactate dehydrogenase (LDH), using sodium lactate as substrate and nitro-blue tetrazolium (NBT) as the tetrazolium salt (Pearse 1972).

The incubation medium for LDH contains several important constituents in addition to substrate and tetrazole:

1. The coenzyme NAD must be included because there is never enough endogenous NAD to satisfy requirements of the histochemical reaction, and that which is present diffuses away very rapidly from the freeze-damaged tissue. An excess is provided to prevent it from being rate limiting.

2. The use of hypertonic nonelectrolyte media is desirable for the accurate localization of dehydrogenases, particularly for soluble enzymes, such as LDH. This is done by including in the medium polyvinylpyrrolidone (PVP) (7.5% w/v) of molecular weight 10,000. Polyvinylpyrrolidone inhibits protein diffusion and stabilizes cell organelles. Since LDH is magnesium dependent, a trace of magnesium chloride is added; this also helps to stabilize the mitochondria.

3. Cyanide ions are added for two reasons: (a) The direct action of a dehydrogenase is to produce an aldehyde or a ketone. By removing this with a carbonyl-trapping agent, such as cyanide, the equilibrium of the reaction is kept to the right of the equation. (b) The second function of the cyanide is to block the natural electron-transport system of the cell, thereby increasing the efficiency of the tetrazolium reductase step.

4. The incubation medium is kept very slightly acidic at about pH 6.8. This is not the optimum pH for most dehydrogenases, but above pH 7.5 the activity of nothing dehydrogenase (Pearse 1960, Andersen 1965) rises steeply and produces formazan deposits in the absence of primary substrate. This gives a staining pattern after prolonged incubation of sections in control incubation media, (Plate 1(a); incubated for 3 hr at pH 7.5).

Even after these precautions, the resultant staining pattern is not the localization of LDH but strictly the demonstration of an enzyme system termed *mouse lung lactate-NBT reductase* and the color itself is the direct result of NBT reductase (step B). For this reason, the staining pattern of many dehydrogenases is identical with that of a single enzyme, NAD or NADP diaphorase. This was first noticed by Farber and associates as early as 1956. These investigators claimed that the staining patterns for all dehydrogenases fell into three groups: that for NAD diaphorase, that for NADP diaphorase, and that for succinic dehydrogenase (SDH). Succinic dehydrogenase has a tightly bound coenzyme that does not require the addition of exogenous supplies, and it is one of the few dehydrogenases whose staining pattern is considered to represent the accurate localization of the enzyme in the cell (de Fanchiotti et al. 1971). Plate 2(f) is the staining pattern for mouse lung NAD diaphorase, which, therefore, is the pattern produced by most of the NAD-dependent dehydrogenases. This statement is strengthened by the observation that when a single section is used to demonstrate LDH by means of a yellow formazan and NAD diaphorase by means of a blue formazan, the resultant yellow and blue stains are superimposed exactly on each other to give a uniform green staining pattern (Etherton et al. 1973b).

The interpretation of dehydrogenase staining patterns clearly requires caution. As explained above, the SDH stain gives reliable localization because steps A and B occur at the same site. For the other dehydrogenases, the question of whether the stain produced by step B represents the actual distribution of the primary dehydrogenase responsible for step A can be answered by a combination of fixation studies, careful preparation, and observation of the rate of staining in different cell types. The cells in the bronchiole of Plate 2(f) are uniformly heavily stained after the 30-min incubation period, but Azzopardi and Thurlbeck (1969) noticed that during the first few minutes of incubation for certain enzymes, the Clara cells were becoming stained more rapidly than the adjacent ciliated cells. By 30 min all bronchiolar cells were stained equally. It is possible, therefore, that most of the activity of these enzymes lies in the nonciliated cells, but the release of NADH over a half-hour period is sufficient to enable the tetrazolium reductase (step B) in the neighboring ciliated cells to deposit as much formazan as there is in the nonciliated cells. Second, some NAD-dependent enzymes do show different localization to NAD diaphorase, even after the 30-min incubation of an unfixed section. Three examples are the localization of 3-hydroxybutyrate dehydrogenase (3HBDH) in the Clara cells, Plate 2(c); the simultaneous localization in these same cells of LDH and 3-glycerophosphate dehydrogenase (3GPDH, Etherton et al. 1973b); and the localization of prostaglandin dehydrogenases primarily in the large interstitial cells of the alveolar wall, Plate 1(b) and (c).

V. Conclusions

In general, therefore, conservative interpretation of the results from enzyme histochemical assays, combined with results from studies in other disciplines, allows fairly accurate conclusions to be drawn about the relative enzyme activities in different cell types of a tissue section. Further conclusions may then be drawn about the metabolic functions of the cells. The results suggest that the network of pulmonary endothelial and interstitial cells are primarily involved in the metabolism of pharmacologically active substances in the lung. Some processes, such as the conversion of angiotensin I to angiotensin II, may be carried out on the luminal aspect of endothelial cells (Ryan et al. 1972). Other substances, which are actually removed from the circulation, must pass into the endothelial cells. For example, 5-HT appears to be stored in these cells (Strum and Junod 1972, Cross et al. 1974). However, it is reasonable to suppose that if these compounds are to be degraded, they would be transferred to the larger and more suitably equipped interstitial cells. Additional histochemical studies required to test this hypothesis fall into the following categories:

1. Many enzyme histochemical techniques have been devised but not yet used in studies on lung metabolism. Results from some of these, such as the steroid dehydrogenases (Pearse 1972), would provide valuable information.

2. Electron microscopic studies on lung allow accurate identification of cell types. Reports on the successful ultrastructural localization of dehydrogenases (e.g., Seligman et al. 1967, Tsou et al. 1968, de Fanchiotti et al. 1971, Hanker et al. 1973) should be followed up in the lung to test the validity of enzyme localizations reported in the interstitial cell. These should then be compared with results from autoradiographic and biochemical studies to try to define the ultrastructural route by which vasoactive substances are degraded in the lung. It is anticipated that conflicting results would be obtained at first, for the following reason: the use of marker enzymes to test the purity of cell fractions is commonplace. An accepted marker for the soluble fraction is LDH, but Pearse and his colleagues have developed a method for the direct localization of LDH and other enzymes, which confirms a mitochondrial localization for LDH (Hanker et al. 1973). Apart from the enzyme studies, there is room for application to the lung of electron microscopic techniques for the demonstration of biogenic amines (Tranzer et al. 1969).

3. The literature contains no methods for the demonstration of some enzymes. A great deal of work is potentially available for the study of these in order to define more closely which pathways are operative in which cells of the interalveolar septum. The type I cell, for instance, appears to have an extremely active pinocytotic function, but no enzyme studies on this have been reported. Similarly, it should be possible to examine the transport mechanisms across the endothelial cell.

4. Fluorescence microscopy offers a potentially important technique for the localization of biogenic amines in the lung. Formaldehyde-induced fluorescence has so far been used to demonstrate 5-HT, tryptamine, tyramine, noradrenaline, adrenaline, dopamine, leptodactyline, and histamine in various tissues. For a review of this, see Pearse (1972). Results from such studies would either substantiate or disprove any conclusions drawn from (1) to (3) above. Other fluorescence studies could include the use of fluorescent antibodies to specific catabolic enzymes to test the postulated localization of such enzymes in tissue sections. This would, of course, demand the biochemical preparation of enough purified enzyme to be able to raise antibodies to it. It would depend on the electrophoretic mobility or particle size of the enzyme, and on the amount of enzyme normally present in the lung. Low or unsuitable values of these parameters could prevent this idea from being followed (Nairn 1969).

5. Further application of raising antibodies to enzymes concerned with the degradation of vasoactive hormones lies in the preparation of peroxidase-labeled antibody, which could be used to localize enzymes in the electron microscope. This would offer a considerable advantage over other methods in attempts to pinpoint ultrastructural sites of hormone catabolism (Nakane 1968, Kawarai and Nakane 1970).

6. The influence of age, sex, killing technique, and hormone treatment are not covered in the literature on enzyme histochemistry of the interalveolar septum. In our hands the activity of the acid hydrolases appears to increase with age; the sex of the species used has no effect on the results obtained; the mode of death only affects the morphology of small bronchioles, and studies on the effects of hormone administration have not been carried out. There is evidently room for further work on these topics. Nevertheless, we have found an increase in the size and apparent activity of pulmonary interstitial cells following chronic inhalation of tobacco smoke. Using acid

phosphatase as a marker in ultrastructural histochemical studies in rats and mice, it was found that after 3 months daily inhalation of cigarette smoke, there was a marked rise in the numbers of lysosomes in pulmonary interstitial cells. This finding supports their postulated role in the catabolism of unwanted materials present in the lung. The activity of these lysosomes was, however, nowhere near as great as that of the free alveolar macrophages (Etherton and Conning 1971).

Finally, it should be noted that some progress has been made in isolating cell types from whole lung (Kikkawa and Yoneda 1974). When it is possible to analyze the enzyme profile of endothelial and interstitial cells separately, it should be possible to have more confidence about the fate of individual substances in the lung.

It is hoped that some of the above suggestions can be followed, because although enzyme and fluorescence histochemistry require a great deal of originality and careful work to test the validity of the conclusions drawn, they can provide some information unobtainable by other means. Enzyme histochemistry, in particular, can produce results quickly and more easily than almost any other technique.

References

Andersen, H. (1965). Sulphydryl "Nothing dehydrogenase" activity and lactic dehydrogenase-$NADH_2$ cytochrome C reductase reactions in tissues of the human foetus. *Acta Histochem.*, **21**:120–134.

Azzopardi, A. and Thurlbeck, W. M. (1969). The histochemistry of the nonciliated bronchiolar epithelial cell. *Am. Rev. Resp. Dis.*, **99**:516–525.

Barry, D. H. (1972). Quantitative enzyme histochemistry of acid phosphatase and its application to respiratory irritation. *Acta Histochem.*, **12**:121.

Barry, D. H. and Robinson, W. E. (1969a). Enzyme histochemical studies on rat lungs. I. An improved technique for the demonstration of enzyme activity in alveolar tissue. *Histochem. J.*, **1**:497–504.

Barry, D. H. and Robinson, W. E. (1969b). Enzyme histochemical studies on rat lungs. 2. Normal enzyme distribution in the alveolar tissue of the mature lung. *Histochem. J.*, **1**:505–515.

Barka, T. and Anderson, P. J. (1962). Histochemical methods for acid phosphatase using hexazonium pararosanilin as coupler. *J. Histochem. Cytochem.*, **10**:741–753.

Bowden, D. H. and Adamson, I. Y. R. (1972). The pulmonary interstitial cell as immediate precursor of the alveolar macrophage. *Am. J. Pathol.*, **63**:521–528.

Burton, J. F. and Pearse, A. G. E. (1952). A critical study of the methods for histochemical localization of beta-glucuronidase. *Br. J. Exp. Pathol.,* **33**: 87–97.

Caulet, T., Adnet, J. J., and Hopfner, C. (1968). Etude histo-chimique d'un type de cellules alveolaires du poumon: les cellules a inclusions lipidiques complexes. *Histochemie,* **15**:21–37.

Conning, D. M. and Etherton, J. E. (1971). The secretion of pulmonary surfactant in the mouse: an investigation using radioactive palmitic acid. *J. Pathol.,* **103**:IV–V.

Corrin, B. (1969). Phagocytic potential of pulmonary alveolar epithelium with particular reference to surfactant metabolism. *Thorax,* **24**:110–115.

Cross, S. A. M., Alabaster, V. A., Bakhle, Y. S., and Vane, J. R. (1974). Sites of uptake of ^{3}H-5-hydroxytryptamine in rat isolated lung. *Histochemistry,* **39**:83–91.

deDuve, C. (1963). In A. V. S. deReuck and M. P. Cameron (eds.): *Lysosomes.* Churchill, London.

Defendi, V. (1957). Observations on naphthol staining and the histochemical localization of enzymes by naphthol-azo dye technique. *J. Histochem. Cytochem.,* **5**:1–10.

Ellefsen, P. and Tos, M. (1972). Goblet cells in the human trachea. Quantitative studies of a pathological biopsy material. *Arch. Otolaryngol.,* **95**:547–555.

Esterly, J. R. (1972). Localization of trypsin-like activity in the lung. *J. Histochem. Cytochem.,* **20**:851–852.

Etherton, J. E. (1977). Pulmonary surfactant secretion and certain aspects of paraquat and tobacco smoke toxicity in small mammals. Ph.D. Thesis Submitted to Council for National Academic Awards, London.

Etherton, J. E. and Botham, C. M. (1970). Factors affecting lead capture methods for the fine localization of rat lung acid phosphatase. *Histochem. J.,* **2**:507–519.

Etherton, J. E. and Conning, D. M. (1971). A histochemical and ultrastructural examination of the irritant effects of tobacco smoke inhalation in mammalian lung. *Proc. R. Microsc. Soc.,* **6**:25.

Etherton, J. E., Conning, D. M., and Corrin, B. (1973a). Autoradiographical and morphological evidence for apocrine secretion of dipalmitoyl lecithin in the terminal bronchiole of mouse lung. *Am. J. Anat.,* **138**:11–36.

Etherton, J. E., Conning, D. M., and Jones, G. R. N. (1973b). The demonstration of mouse lung lactate-yellow tetrazolium reductase. *Histochemie,* **33**:287–290.

Etherton, J. E., Conning, D. M., and Purchase, I. F. H. (1974). A histochemical irritancy assay for the acute phase of tobacco smoke inhalation in rats. In Proceedings of the 128th Meeting of the Pathological Society of Great Britain and N. Ireland.

Fanchiotti, L. A. C. de, Jones, G. R. N., and Bradbury, S. (1971). The intramitochondrial localization of succinate-yellow tetrazolium reductase with the electron microscope. *Histochemie,* **27**:28–35.

Farber, E., Sternberg, W. H., and Dunlop, C. E. (1956). Histochemical localization of specific oxidative enzymes. I. Tetrazolium stains for diphosphopyridine nucleotide diaphorase and triphosphopyridine nucleotide diaphorase. *J. Histochem. Cytochem.*, **4**:254–265.

Fredricsson, B. (1956). The distribution of alkaline phosphatase in the rat lung. *Acta Anat.*, **26**:246–256.

Goldfischer, S., Kikkawa, Y., and Hoffman, L. (1968). The demonstration of acid hydrolase activities in the inclusion bodies of type II alveolar cells and other lysosomes in the rabbit lung. *J. Histochem. Cytochem.*, **16**:102–109.

Grasso, P., Williams, M., Hodgson, R., Wright, M. G., and Gangolli, S. D. (1971). The histochemical distribution of aniline hydroxylase in rat tissues. *Histochem. J.*, **3**:117–126.

Hanker, J. S., Kusyk, C. J., Bloom, F. E., and Pearse, A. G. E. (1973). The demonstration of dehydrogenases and monoamine oxidase by the formation of osmium blacks at the sites of Hatchett's brown. *Histochemie*, **33**: 205–230.

Hannibal, M. J. and Nachlas, M. M. (1959). Further studies on the lyo and desmo components of several hydrolytic enzymes and their histochemical significance. *J. Biophys. Biochem. Cytol.*, **5**:279–288.

Heppleston, A. G. and Young, A. E. (1973). Uptake of inert particulate matter by alveolar cells: an ultrastructural study. *J. Pathol.*, **111**:159–164.

Holt, S. J. and Hicks, R. M. (1961a). Studies on formalin fixation for electron microscopy and cytochemical staining purposes. *J. Biophys. Biochem. Cytol.*, **11**:31–45.

Holt, S. J. and Hicks, R. M. (1961b). The localization of acid phosphatase in rat liver cells as revealed by combined cytochemical staining and electron microscopy. *J. Biophys. Biochem. Cytol.*, **11**:47–66.

Jones, G. R. N. (1969a). The synthesis of yellow tetrazolium. *Histochemie*, **18**: 164–167.

Jones, G. R. N. (1969b). Yellow tetrazolium: a new reagent to serve a new concept. *Proc. R. Miscrosc. Soc.*, **4**:79–80.

Jones, R., Bolduc, P., and Reid, L. (1973). Goblet cell glycoprotein and tracheal gland hypertrophy in rat airways: the effect of tobacco smoke with or without the anti-inflammatory agent phenylmethyloxadiazole. *Br. J. Exp. Pathol.*, **54**:229–239.

Kalina, M., Graham, P. B., and Jones, G. R. N. (1965). An evaluation of the histochemical demonstration of certain pyridine nucleotide-linked dehydrogenases. *Nature*, **207**:647–648.

Kapanci, T., Assimacopoulos, A., Isle C., Zwahlen, A., and Gabbiani, G. (1974). "Contractile interstitial cells" in pulmonary alveolar septa: a possible regulator of ventilation/perfusion ratio. *J. Cell Biol.*, **60**:375–392.

Kawarai, Y. and Nakane, P. K. (1970). Localization of tissue antigens on the ultra-thin sections with peroxidase-labeled antibody method. *J. Histochem. Cytochem.*, **18**:161–166.

Kikkawa, Y. and Yoneda, K. (1974). The type II epithelial cell of the lung. I. Method of isolation. *Lab. Invest.*, **30**:76–84.

Klika, E. and Petrik, P. (1965). A study of the structure of the lung alveolus and bronchiolar epithelium. *Acta Histochem.*, **20**:331–342.

Lison, L. (1936). *Histochimie Animale.* Gauthier-Villars, Paris.

Meany, A., Gahan, P. B., and Maggi, V. (1967). Effects of Triton X-100 on acid phosphatases with different substrate specificities. *Histochemie,* 11:280–285.

Meban, C. (1972). Localization of phosphatidic acid phosphatase activity in granular pneumonocytes. *J. Cell Biol.,* 53:249–252.

Meyrick, B. and Reid, L. (1968). The alveolar brush cell in rat lung – a third pneumonocyte. *J. Ultrastruc. Res.,* 23:71–80.

Nachlas, M. M., Prinn, W., and Seligman, A. M. (1956). Quantitative estimation of lyo- and desmoenzymes in tissue sections with and without fixation. *J. Biophys. Biochem. Cytol.,* 2:487–502.

Nakane, P. K. (1968). Simultaneous localization of multiple tissue antigens using the peroxidase-labeled antibody method: a study on pituitary glands of the rat. *J. Histochem. Cytochem.,* 16:557–560.

Nairn, R. C. (1969). *Fluorescent Protein Tracing.* E & S Livingstone, Edinburgh and London.

Niden, A. H. (1967). Bronchiolar and large alveolar cell in pulmonary phospholipid metabolism. *Science,* 158:1323–1324.

Nissen, H. M. and Andersen, H. (1968). On the localization of a prostaglandin-dehydrogenase activity in the kidney. *Histochemie,* 14:189–200.

Pearse, A. G. E. (1957). Intracellular localization of dehydrogenase systems using monotetrazolium salts and metal chelation of their formazans. *J. Histochem. Cytochem.,* 5:515–527.

Pearse, A. G. E. (1960). *Histochemistry. Theoretical and Applied,* vol. 1, 2nd ed. J & A Churchill Ltd, London.

Pearse, A. G. E. (1968). *Histochemistry. Theoretical and Applied,* 3rd ed. J & A Churchill Ltd, London.

Pearse, A. G. E. and Rost, F. W. D. (1969). A microspectrofluorimeter with epi-illumination and photon counting. *J. Microsc.,* 89:321–328.

Pearse, A. G. E. (1972). *Histochemistry. Theoretical and Applied,* vol. 2, 3rd ed. Churchill Livingstone, Edinburgh and London.

Rost, F. W. D., Nägel, L. C. A., and Moss, D. W. (1970). Microfluorimetric investigations of enzyme kinetics in fixed and unfixed tissue sections. *Proc. R. Microsc. Soc.,* 5:76–77.

Ryan, J. W., Smith, U., and Niemeyer, R. S. (1972). Angiotensin I: metabolism by plasma membrane of lung. *Science,* 176:64–66.

Seligman, A. M., Ueno, H., Morizono, Y., Wasserkrug, H. L., Katzoff, L., and Hanker, J. S. (1967). Electron microscopic demonstration of dehydrogenase activity with a new osmiophilic ditetrazolium salt (TC-NBT). *J. Histochem. Cytochem.,* 15:1–13.

Smith, P. H., Heath, D., and Moosavi, H. (1974). The Clara cell. *Thorax,* 29:147–163.

Sorokin, S., Padykula, H. A., and Herman, E. (1959). Comparative histochemical patterns in developing mammalian lungs. *Develop. Biol.,* 1:125–151.

Stirling, W. (1875). On a new method of preparing the skin for histological examination. *J. Anat. Physiol.*, **10**:185–186.

Strum, J. M. and Junod, A. F. (1972). Radioautographic demonstration of 5-hydroxytryptamine-^{3}H uptake by pulmonary endothelial cells. *J. Cell Biol.*, **54**:456–457.

Tranzer, J-P., Thoenen, H., Snipes, R. L., and Richards, J. G. (1969). Recent developments on the ultrastructural aspect of adrenergic nerve endings in various experimental conditions. *Prog. Brain Res.*, **31**:33–46.

Tsou, K. C., Cheng, C. S., Nachlas, M. M., and Seligman, A. M. (1956). Synthesis of some *p*-nitrophenyl substituted tetrazolium salts as electron acceptors for the demonstration of dehydrogenases. *J. Am. Chem. Soc.*, **78**:6139–6144.

Tsou, K. C., Goodwin, C. W., Seamond, B., and Lynn, D. (1968). Intracristal localization of succinic dehydrogenase activity with a new osmium-containing tetra-tetrazolium salt. *J. Histochem. Cytochem.*, **16**:487–489.

Tyler, W. S. and Pearse, A. G. E. (1965). Oxidative enzymes of the interalveolar septum of the rat. *Thorax*, **20**:149–152.

Tyler, W. S., Pearse, A. G. E., and Rhatigan, P. (1965). Histochemistry of the equine lung: oxidative enzymes of the interalveolar septum. *Am. J. Vet. Res.*, **26**:960–964.

Vane, J. R. (1969). The release and fate of vaso-active hormones in the circulation. *Br. J. Pharmacol.*, **35**:209–242.

Wolfe, B. M. J., Rubinstein, D., and Beck, J. C. (1968). The metabolism of isolated pneumocytes from rabbit lung. *Can. J. Biochem. Physiol.*, **46**:151–154.

Part III

RELEASE OF BIOLOGICALLY ACTIVE MATERIALS FROM THE LUNG

9

Release Induced by Anaphylaxis

PRISCILLA J. PIPER

Institute of Basic Medical Sciences
Royal College of Surgeons of England
London, England

I. Introduction

The fact that the pulmonary circulation receives the entire cardiac output of
blood positions the lungs well to have important functions beside exchange of
gases in the alveoli. First, they are able to synthesize and store biologically
active substances. Second, in response to a variety of stimuli they are able
either to release stored materials or rapidly synthesize pharmacologically active
substances de novo, which may have a local action in the lung and/or enter
the pulmonary circulation. The stimuli, which cause the release of active
materials, may be immunologic, mechanical, or frankly pathologic (Piper and
Vane 1971). Since some mediators are released by all stimuli, their mechanism of release may be common to all stimuli. Third, there are enzyme systems in the pulmonary circulation, possibly in the vascular endothelium, which
may either activate substances present in the pulmonary circulation, for example, the conversion of angiotensin I to angiotensin II (Ng and Vane 1967)
or inactivate substances, such as bradykinin and prostaglandins, by converting

them to less active metabolites (Ferreira and Vane 1967a, Vane 1969, Piper et al. 1970).

This chapter will be confined to the discussion of the release of biologically active substances from the lung by anaphylaxis and its modification by drugs. Anaphylaxis is one of the conditions in which biologically active substances are released from the lungs of many, but not all, species. In man and guinea pig, the lung seems to be the major *shock* organ and source of mediators. In mouse, cat, monkey, rat, and calf, biologically active substances may be released from lung tissue, although the lung is not the main target organ of anaphylaxis. Release of mediators from guinea pig lung during anaphylactic shock and the effects of drugs on this release have been actively studied in the hope that the results will be relevant to man but there are important differences in the mechanism of anaphylaxis between species. One of these is that the antibody in guinea pig is IgG but is IgE in man. Another is that the relative sensitivity of bronchial smooth muscle to anaphylactic mediators differs between the two species. Although systemic anaphylaxis in man and bronchial asthma are both type I reactions (Gell and Coombs classification) with similar pathologic changes in the lungs, the main difference seems to be that asthma is usually a localized reaction in the lungs. Both conditions may be partly explained in terms of mediators released by antigen-antibody reactions, but it is important to realize that asthma is not synonymous with anaphylaxis in either man or animals, although there are similarities between the two conditions which merit consideration, including involvement of the same mediators.

Some of the mediators of anaphylaxis are also released by damage to lung tissue caused by overinflation, pulmonary embolism, or gentle agitation of chopped lung tissue. Biologically active substances are also released from the lung when various pharmacologic agents are injected or infused into the pulmonary circulation (Piper and Vane 1971, Palmer et al. 1973, Said, this volume).

II. Mediators Released from Lung During Anaphylaxis

A. Guinea Pig Lung

The signs of anaphylactic shock in the guinea pig are dyspnea, sneezing, coughing, acceleration of respiration and heart rate, collapse, and convulsions possibly followed by death. Guinea pigs have more airway smooth muscle than other species (Miller 1947) and the smooth muscle fibers of the trachea and bronchi are attached to the inner surface of the cartilage (Sanyal and West

1958). Contraction of these fibers in anaphylaxis may produce folding of the thick bronchial mucosa (Schultz and Jordan 1911), resulting in airway obstruction in such a way that air can be forced into the lungs but cannot be expelled again (Dale 1920). When the chest is opened postmortem, the lungs are bloodless, fully inflated, and do not collapse (Auer and Lewis 1910). A rise in blood pressure accompanies anaphylactic bronchoconstriction and may be the result of hypoxia caused by bronchoconstriction (Auer and Lewis 1910) and/or the action of one or more of the mediators released. These mediators are discussed in more detail below.

Histamine

Dale and Laidlaw (1910) noted, in the guinea pig, the similarity between anaphylaxis and the effects of injected histamine and Dale (1929) suggested that the release of histamine mediated effects of anaphylactic shock. The importance of histamine was confirmed when Watanabe (1931) showed that the histamine content of guinea pig lung was reduced after anaphylaxis, and Bartosch et al. (1933) demonstrated the release of histamine during anaphylaxis in isolated perfused lungs in vitro. An increase in histamine and a fall in histaminase levels in blood also occur during anaphylactic shock in the guinea pig in vivo (Code 1937, Eilbeck and Smith 1967). Guinea pig lung has numerous mast cells embedded between the smooth muscle cells of the bronchi, and during anaphylaxis histamine is released from the granules of these mast cells (Mota and Vugman 1956).

Following intravenous administration of antigen to a sensitized guinea pig in vivo or injection into the pulmonary artery of isolated lungs in vitro, the release of histamine is short-lasting and appears within 30 sec of antigen challenge, reaches a maximum in 2 min, and very little is released after 30 min (Brocklehurst 1960, Collier and James 1967).

Histamine is stored in the granules of mast cells in a complex with protein and heparin (Uvnäs 1974). So far the amine storage and release mechanism has only been studied in rat peritoneal mast cells, but mast cells from other species contain heparin and it seems possible that these cells store and release histamine in a similar way (Uvnäs 1974). Histamine release in response to antigen challenge is calcium dependent, requires an intact glycolytic pathway, and involves the action of a serine esterase which is sensitive to diisopropylfluorophosphate (DFP) (Schild 1936, 1968, Mongar and Schild 1958, Orange et al. 1971a).

Slow-Reacting Substance of Anaphylaxis

During anaphylaxis in guinea pig isolated perfused lungs, Kellaway and Trethewie (1940) observed the release of another mediator (in addition to histamine), which caused slow, long-lasting contraction of guinea pig ileum. This 'other' mediator they called slow-reacting substance of anaphylaxis (SRS-A). Brocklehurst (1960) described the actions of SRS-A and showed that in the presence of atropine and mepyramine it caused slow contraction of guinea pig ileum. SRS-A appears in the effluent from guinea pig isolated perfused lungs 30 sec after antigen challenge, reaches a maximum concentration after 4 min, but is still released in appreciable amounts after 30 min (Brocklehurst 1960, 1970). SRS-A is also released into the circulation during anaphylaxis in guinea pig in vivo caused by intravenous administration of antigen (Collier and James 1967, Stechschulte et al. 1973). The release of SRS-A from lungs depends on the antigen-antibody reaction and does not occur in response to any other stimulus that causes release of mediators from lungs (Said, this volume).

The exact structure of SRS-A has proved very difficult to elucidate and is still unknown. Brocklehurst (1963, 1968) described SRS-A as an acidic substance that is probably not a true lipid but which forms a loose association with lipid, protein, and other molecules, such as lecithin, and becomes very unstable when these are removed. SRS-A has been distinguished from bradykinin, prostaglandin $F_{2\alpha}$ ($PGF_{2\alpha}$), histamine, acetylcholine, 5-hydroxytryptamine, substance P, and angiotensin (Berry and Collier 1964) as well as from neuraminic acid (Änggård et al. 1963). Austen, Orange, and coworkers (for references see Austen 1974), using SRS-A from rat peritoneal cavity and human lung, which shows no demonstrable difference from guinea pig SRS-A, have obtained highly purified preparations and have used mass spectrometry in attempts to identify this substance. The release of SRS-A differs from that of histamine in that there are both biosynthetic and secretory stages involved in the release of SRS-A (Orange 1974), whereas histamine is released from a store of preformed material. SRS-A appears to be formed and released by enzymic processes activated by union of antigen and antibody (Brocklehurst 1970). SRS-A seems to be an unsaturated, acidic substance of low molecular weight (approx 400) (Orange et al. 1973). Its molecule contains both hydroxyl and carboxylic acid groups and it is biologically active at doses of less than a nanogram (Orange 1974). The activity of SRS-A is destroyed by the action of two preparations of arylsulfatase (Orange et al. 1974). These authors therefore concluded that SRS-A is a sulfate ester. The presence of a sulfate moiety in a substance reduces its volatility and prevents analysis by mass spectrometry, but analysis of a highly purified sample of SRS-A by spark-source mass spectrometry and electron probe confirmed the presence of sulfur in SRS-A molecules (Orange et al. 1974). Further confirmation of the presence of sulfur in SRS-A was obtained by Dawson et al. (1975) who administered radioactively labeled sulfur to sensitized guinea pigs and recovered the radioactivity in SRS-A prepared from their lungs after antigen challenge. The release of SRS-A from guinea pig and human lung is accompanied by an output of PGs of E and F series and their metabolites (Piper and Vane 1969a, Piper and Walker 1973, Mathé and Levine 1973, Liebig et al. 1974), but Dawson and Tomlinson (1974) have shown that SRS-A and PGs do not arise from a common precursor. The substrate for SRS-A is at present unknown.

Prostaglandins

When isolated lungs from sensitized guinea pigs are challenged in vitro, PGE_2 and $PGF_{2\alpha}$ are released and can be detected in the effluent from the lungs (Piper and Vane 1969a,b). Prostaglandin synthetase from sensitized guinea pig lungs is also capable of synthesizing PGD_2, but this has not yet been detected in lung effluent (Benzie et al. 1975). The release of the PG metabolites, 13,14-dihydro-15-keto PGE_2 and 13,14-dihydro $PGF_{2\alpha}$ has been detected in addition to that of their parent compounds during anaphylaxis in guinea pig perfused lungs (Mathé and Levine 1973, Dawson and Tomlinson 1974, Liebig et al. 1974). The release of PGs during anaphylaxis in vivo has been directly demonstrated by radioimmunoassay (Ruff et al. 1975), and with hindsight, Collier and James (1967) provided evidence for PG release by showing that aspirin-like drugs (inhibitors of PG synthetase, Vane (1971), partially antagonized anaphylactic bronchoconstriction in guinea pig in vivo and Strandberg and Hamberg (1974) have shown that, in guinea pigs, output of urinary metabolites of PGs almost doubled following anaphylactic shock.

The precursor of PGE_2 and $PGF_{2\alpha}$ is arachidonic acid and they are formed by the action of PG synthetase found in the lung (Änggård and Samuelsson 1965, Flower, this volume). Arachidonic acid is a component of phospholipids of the cell membrane and may be made available to PG synthetase by the action of phospholipase A_2 (Kunze and Vogt 1971). Prostaglandins are not stored in a preformed state in tissues and, therefore, their release from lungs represents their synthesis de novo by lung tissue (Piper and Vane 1971). Benzie et al. (1975) have shown that lungs taken from sensitized guinea pigs contain more PG synthetase than lungs from control animals.

Whether there is synthesis of PGs by a specific type of cell or all cells is not known. However, during challenge of peritoneal mast cells from sensitized rats, a small amount of PG-like material was released in addition to histamine (Piper, unpublished data). Since histamine is stored in lung mast cells, perhaps these cells may be a source of PGs released during anaphylaxis in the lung. Since PGs are released by distortion of cells (Piper and Vane 1971),

Piper and Walker (1973) suggested that, during anaphylaxis, PGs might be released from bronchial smooth muscle during contraction. Orehek et al. (1973) and Grodzinska et al. (1975) provided evidence for this by showing release of PGs during contraction of isolated trachea from guinea pig by anaphylaxis or by histamine or acetylcholine.

SRS-A also releases PGs from guinea pig lungs (Piper and Vane 1969b). All these results suggest that PGs are not primary mediators of anaphylaxis, for their release may be secondary to that of the primary mediators, histamine and SRS-A.

Rabbit Aorta Contracting
Substance (RCS)

The release of PGs during anaphylaxis in guinea pig isolated perfused lungs was detected by immediate continuous bioassay of the effluent (Piper and Vane 1969a). However, subsequent ethyl acetate extraction, identification, and quantitation of PGs by thin-layer chromatography showed a discrepancy between the amount of PG-like activity detected by the assay tissues and the quantity recovered by chemical extraction. The nonextractable activity was found to be due to an unstable substance with a half-life of 1 to 2 min in Krebs solution and characterized only by the fact that it strongly contracted isolated strips of rabbit aorta in the presence of antagonists to histamine, acetylcholine, 5-hydroxytryptamine, and catecholamines; this substance was named *rabbit aorta contracting substance* (RCS) (Piper and Vane 1969a,b, Palmer et al. 1973). The release of RCS has also been demonstrated during anaphylactic shock in anesthetized guinea pig in vivo (Palmer et al. 1973).

RCS is always released from lungs together with PGs, and nonsteroid antiinflammatory drugs such as aspirin or indomethacin block the release of these substances (Piper and Vane 1969b, Vane 1971). The inhibition of release by inhibitors of PG synthetase shows that RCS is a product of the PG synthetase system. Gryglewski and Vane (1972) produced RCS from dog spleen and showed that as the concentration of RCS declined, that of PG increased, suggesting that RCS might be a precursor of PGs. In fact, there are certain similarities between the biologic actions of PGG_2 and PGH_2 (the cyclic endoperoxide precursors of PGE_2 and $PGF_{2\alpha}$) and RCS, but their half-lives are different (Hamberg and Samuelsson 1973). The original observations that RCS might be converted to PGs have been substantiated by Hamberg et al. (1975) who have recently identified RCS formed during platelet aggregation as being a mixture of endoperoxide precursors of PGs and thromboxane A_2

Rabbit Aorta Contracting Substance Releasing Factor (RCS-RF)

In addition to RCS, a stable substance is released during anaphylactic shock in guinea pig isolated perfused lungs, which, when infused into unsensitized lungs causes a release of RCS and PGs but not histamine; this substance is known as rabbit aorta contracting substance releasing factor (RCS-RF). RCS-RF is stable to both freezing and boiling and at least part of its activity is nondialyzable (Piper and Vane 1969b). Since inhibitors of PG synthetase do not inhibit the release of RCS-RF, it seems unlikely to be a product of PG synthetase (Palmer et al. 1973).

Kinins

Brocklehurst and Lahiri (1962, 1963) showed that kininogen levels in the blood of sensitized guinea pigs decreased during anaphylaxis, thereby implying the release of bradykinin into the circulation during anaphylactic shock. Collier and James (1967) found that anaphylactic bronchoconstriction could be lessened by making sensitized guinea pigs tachphylactic to bradykinin before challenge and therefore indirectly confirmed the release of bradykinin during anaphylaxis. Jonasson and Becker (1966) showed the release of kallikrein from guinea pig isolated perfused lungs during anaphylaxis but, in isolated perfused lungs in the absence of blood and therefore substrate, no release of bradykinin was detected (Piper and Vane 1969b).

Eosinophil Chemotactic Factor in Anaphylaxis (ECF-A)

In addition to histamine and SRS-A, a factor specifically chemotactic for guinea pig eosinophil leukocytes (ECF-A) is released during anaphylactic shock in either guinea pig isolated perfused lungs or chopped lung tissue from actively or passively sensitized animals (Kay et al. 1971). The release of ECF-A follows a similar time-course to that of SRS-A appearing within 30 sec, reaching a peak in 4 min.

B. Human Lung

The signs of anaphylaxis in man include acute respiratory distress, asphyxia, angioneurotic edema, severe hypotension, and vascular collapse, which may cause death. The respiratory distress may result from upper airway obstruction caused by laryngeal edema and severe bronchospasm (Sheffer 1973). Postmortem examination of humans dying in anaphylactic shock shows changes in the lungs comparable with those seen in guinea pigs, i.e., hyperinflation with alternating areas of emphysema and collapse (Layton and Cameron 1971). Similar changes are seen in patients dying of status asthmaticus.

Histamine

The release of histamine from human asthmatic lung and bronchial tissue during challenge with specific antigen was demonstrated by Schild et al. (1951) and confirmed by Brocklehurst (1960), who perfused and challenged segments of lung from allergic patients and showed the release of both histamine and SRS-A. Sheard et al. (1967) passively sensitized human chopped lung tissue with reaginic serum and detected the release of histamine and SRS-A when this tissue was challenged.

SRS-A

The release of SRS-A from human lung was first demonstrated by Brocklehurst (1960) who obtained lung tissue from an allergic (actively sensitized) patient and challenged it with specific antigen. Since then several groups of workers have produced SRS-A by challenging fragments of human lung tissue, which have been passively sensitized with reaginic serum (Parish 1967, Sheard et al. 1967, Orange et al. 1971).

SRS-A appeared in the plasma of asthmatic children when the patients were provoked with specific antigen administered by aerosol. The maximum concentration of SRS-A occurred 20 min after provocation (Orange and Langer 1973). Since the antigen was administered by aerosol, the SRS-A detected in the circulation must have been formed in the lungs as a result of antigenantibody interaction on the surface of sensitized target cells.

Although SRS-A formed by human lung tissue has similar actions to guinea pig SRS-A, it has not yet been determined whether or not SRS-A from the two species is identical. However, Webster et al. (1975) have recently partially purified human SRS-A and suggest that it consists of four substances that differ from SRS-A of guinea pig or rat.

Prostaglandins

Piper and Walker (1973) detected the release of PGs E_1, E_2, and $F_{2\alpha}$ during antigen challenge of passively sensitized human lung tissue. The amount of

PGs released was not related to antigen dose, which is another indication that PG release is secondary to that of other mediators.

Recently, Green et al. (1974) found indirect evidence of the release of PGs from human lung in vivo by detecting an increase of up to eightfold in the PG metabolite, 13,14-dihydro-15-keto $PGF_{2\alpha}$ in peripheral venous blood soon after allergen-provoked attack of asthma. Since PGs of the E and F series are extensively metabolized (90% to 95%) in the pulmonary circulation of cat, dog, rabbit and guinea pig, both in vivo and in vitro, and also in man in vivo (Ferreira and Vane 1967b, Piper et al. 1970, Crutchley and Piper 1974, 1975a,b, Jose et al. 1976) this strongly suggests that at least $PGF_{2\alpha}$ is released from the lung during an asthmatic attack. However, Smith and Dunlop (1975) treated asthmatic patients with indomethacin before challenge and found no significant change in percentage fall of FEV during challenge, which indicates that PGs do not play an important role in the bronchoconstriction of asthma.

RCS

In contrast to anaphylaxis in the guinea pig, no detectable amount of RCS was released from passively sensitized human lung tissue when challenged (Piper and Walker 1973).

ECF-A

ECF-A is released in addition to histamine and SRS-A when human lung tissue which has been passively sensitized is challenged with specific antigen (Kay et al. 1971). ECF-A, like histamine, is stored preformed in human lung tissue, possibly in mast cell granules (Wasserman et al. 1974a). The molecular weight of ECF-A is approximately 500, and it appears to be an acidic peptide (Austen 1974). The release of ECF-A requires an intact glycolytic pathway, divalent cations and activation of DFP-sensitive esterase. Cyclic nucleotides modify the release of ECF-A in the same way as that of histamine and SRS-A (Wasserman et al. 1974b).

Kinins

Since most investigations of mediator release have been carried out on fragments of human lung tissue in vitro in the absence of substrate for kinin formation, there is little evidence available on the release of kinins during anaphylaxis in human lung. However, Abe et al. (1967) reported that the blood level of bradykinin is raised during severe bronchial asthma, which suggests that kinins might also be formed in anaphylaxis in vivo.

C.   Monkey Lung

The *shock* organ appears to vary with species of monkey but when Rhesus monkeys, which have been either passively sensitized with human reaginic sera or actively sensitized to *Ascaris* are challenged, the lungs are involved in the anaphylactic response (Patterson et al. 1965, 1970). The respiratory signs of anaphylaxis in this species are similar to those seen in asthma in man and include increase in respiratory frequency, decrease in tidal volume, edema of the bronchial mucosa, and bronchoconstriction and appear to be caused by antigen-antibody response in the bronchial tree (Patterson and Talbot 1969). Brocklehurst (1960) showed the release of histamine and SRS-A in perfused lungs from Rhesus monkeys sensitized to ovalbumen. Histamine and SRS-A are released by challenge of monkey lung tissue passively sensitized with human atopic serum (Ishizaka et al. 1970); these mediators are also released from lung mast cells during antigen challenge (Ishizaka et al. 1972). Patterson and associates (1965) detected increased blood levels of histamine during anaphylactic shock in vivo. Other mediators besides histamine and SRS-A may be involved in anaphylaxis in monkey lung but this has not been closely investigated. Since administration of bradykinin or $PGF_{2\alpha}$ by aerosol to monkeys did not cause bronchoconstriction, these mediators do not seem to be of prime importance in anaphylaxis in monkeys (Patterson and Talbot 1972, Patterson and Kelly 1973).

D.   Bovine Lung

Calves have been actively sensitized to horse serum (Eyre et al. 1973) and anaphylaxis elicited in either isolated perfused lungs in vitro or in the intact anesthetized animal in vivo. The lungs are involved in acute bovine anaphylaxis and calves suffer apnea or dyspnea. The respiratory changes are accompanied by initial bradycardia followed by tachycardia. The release of SRS-A has been detected from isolated perfused lungs of sensitized calves during antigen challenge (Burka and Eyre 1974). Plasma histamine levels rise during anaphylaxis in vivo and Eyre and associates (1973) suggested that the signs of anaphylaxis in vivo may be caused by interaction of histamine, SRS-A, and 5-hydroxytryptamine. Eyre et al. (1973) found that meclofenamate suppressed bovine anaphylactic shock by 80% and attributed this to antagonism of SRS-A. However, since meclofenamate is a potent inhibitor of PG synthetase

(Flower et al. 1972) this may be a strong indication that PGs are released in bovine anaphylaxis. Eyre and Lewis (1972) showed that blood levels of kinins increase greatly during anaphylaxis in calves, but Eyre and associates (1973) suggested that these substances did not play an important role in bovine anaphylaxis.

III. Release of Mediators by Components of Anaphylactic Release

The infusion of some of the mediators of anaphylaxis, or their precursors, or substances involved in anaphylaxis, into the pulmonary circulation of guinea pig isolated perfused lungs causes the release of prostaglandins and RCS and sometimes histamine from the lungs (Palmer et al. 1973, Piper 1974). These substances may be divided into two groups: those that cause a short-lasting release of biologically active substances, however long they are infused, and those that cause a maintained output which only terminates when the infusion is stopped (Table 1).

Bradykinin, partially purified SRS-A, histamine, and RCS-RF all cause the release of PGs and RCS from lungs. Although bradykinin, SRS-A, or RCS-RF may be infused for up to 15 min, the release of mediators is always short-lasting. Since RCS-RF is present in perfusate from challenged guinea pig lungs, it may have been contained in the partially purified SRS-A. It is not yet known whether highly purified SRS-A releases PGs and RCS from lungs.

TABLE 1   **Release of Histamine, PGs, and RCS from Guinea Pig Lung**

		Mediators released		
Duration of release	Substance	Hista-mine	PGs	RCS
Short-lasting release	Bradykinin 1–5 μg/ml	–	+	+
	Anaphylatoxin (C5a) 1–2 μg/ml	+	+	+
	RCS-RF	–	+	+
	SRS-A (charcoal purified)	–	+	+
	Histamine	–	+	+
Maintained output	Arachidonic acid 1–5 μg/ml	–	+	+
	Dihomo-γ-linolenic acid 5–10 μg/ml	–	+	+

The release of PGs by bradykinin is important, since there is increasing evidence that at least some of the actions of bradykinin are mediated by PGs (McGiff et al. 1975). Vargaftig and Dao Hai (1972) showed that the release of RCS by bradykinin is inhibited by mepacrine, whereas that caused by arachidonic acid is not, and suggested that bradykinin might be activating phospholipase A. Perhaps all short-lasting releases of RCS and PGs are initiated by phospholipase A, which may cleave the precursor fatty acids from the phospholipids of the cell membrane (Kunze and Vogt 1971, Flower, personal communication). Purified anaphylatoxin, the C5a fraction of complement, releases histamine in addition to PGs and RCS (Pavek and Piper, unpublished, Piper 1974).

The maintained output of PGs produced by the PG precursors arachidonic and dihomo-γ-linolenic acids is probably due to conversion of the precursors to PGs rather than to release of mediators.

IV.   Actions of Released Mediators

A.   Histamine

Histamine strongly contracts bronchial smooth muscle both in vivo and in vitro. The bronchoconstrictor action in vivo is due to a direct action of histamine on H_1 receptors in the smooth muscle of the bronchial tree (Black et al. 1972) and also to a nonvagal effect on lung compliance (Mills and Widdicombe 1970). The reduction in compliance is due to constriction of the terminal airways caused by histamine stimulation of 'lung irritant receptors' (Mills et al. 1969). However, histamine has also been reported to contract smooth muscle throughout the bronchial tree (Collier 1970). Histamine released by anaphylaxis or pulmonary damage in vivo will therefore cause constriction of the bronchi by direct and neuronal actions, but at the same time this substance paradoxically relaxes the trachea in guinea pig in vivo by stimulating adrenergic receptors (James 1969). When given intravenously to guinea pigs, histamine releases catecholamines by a direct action on the adrenal medulla and perhaps reflexly as a result of hypoxia (Piper et al. 1967). The catecholamines released by histamine will tend to reverse its bronchoconstrictor action.

Since there are both H_1 and H_2 receptors in pulmonary blood vessels, histamine has a dual mode of action in this vascular bed. When injected into the pulmonary artery of guinea pig isolated perfused lungs, histamine causes vasoconstriction and an increase in pulmonary arterial pressure. This action is inhibited by mepyramine and converted to vasodilatation, showing that it is caused by H_1 receptor stimulation. The vasodilatation is mediated by H_2 receptors, since it is blocked by burimamide (Okpako 1972, Goadby and Phillips 1973, Turker 1973).

Histamine may contribute to the pulmonary edema that occurs in anaphylaxis and following pulmonary embolism, since it increases vascular permeability and causes leaking venules. These changes are attributed to partial disconnection of the endothelial cells.

When histamine is injected into the pulmonary circulation of guinea pig isolated perfused lungs, prostaglandins are released into the effluent from the lungs (Palmer et al. 1973) so that histamine released during anaphylactic shock and pulmonary damage may in turn contribute to the release of PGs. However, whether PGs are released as a direct action of histamine or as a result of contraction of bronchial or perhaps vascular smooth muscle has yet to be determined.

B. Slow-Reacting Substance of Anaphylaxis (SRS-A)

The actions of SRS-A are difficult to describe accurately, because (a) SRS-A is not yet available in an absolutely pure form and (b) preparations of SRS-A vary between laboratories.

Berry and Collier (1964) showed that a charcoal-purified sample of SRS-A from guinea pig lung caused bronchoconstriction in the same species in vivo. However, more recent studies with highly purified SRS-A from rat peritoneal cavity showed that intravenous administration to an unanesthetized guinea pig decreased pulmonary compliance without appreciable change in pulmonary resistance (Drazen et al. 1973). Charcoal-purified SRS-A also contracts smooth muscle from the trachea and bronchioles of guinea pig and man, respectively (Berry and Collier 1964, Collier and Shorley 1963). Smooth muscle from human bronchioles is contracted by much lower concentrations of SRS-A than bronchial smooth muscle from any other species, suggesting that SRS-A is perhaps relatively more important in man than in other species (Brocklehurst 1970). Herxheimer and Streseman (1963) found that when SRS-A prepared from guinea pig was given by aerosol to human asthmatics, it caused bronchoconstriction. SRS-A caused prolonged contraction of isolated smooth muscle, especially after a long contact time. This indicates either that SRS-A causes changes in smooth muscle or becomes firmly attached to the tissue and is not easily destroyed (Brocklehurst 1970). When more highly purified preparations of SRS-A are used, the smooth muscle contractions last for a shorter time.

When SRS-A (charcoal-purified) is injected into the aorta of an anesthetized guinea pig, it causes slight lowering of blood pressure (Piper 1969).

However, when given intravenously, SRS-A has a pressor effect. SRS-A from bovine lung contracted bovine isolated pulmonary vein (Burka and Eyre 1974) and this may also occur in other species. The systemic vasoconstriction may be a reflex effect of the bronchoconstriction that occurs, since both the pressor and bronchoconstrictor effects are antagonized by treatment with aspirin-like drugs (Berry and Collier 1964, Piper 1969). Since these are inhibitors of PG synthetase, it strongly suggests that PGs play a part in the bronchoconstrictor and vasoconstrictor effects of SRS-A. Indeed Piper and Vane (1969b) showed that charcoal-purified SRS-A causes the release of PGs and RCS from guinea pig isolated perfused lungs but, as with histamine, this might be a result of contraction of bronchial smooth muscle. Stechschulte and associates (1973) showed that SRS-A caused increased vascular permeability in guinea pig skin. If SRS-A released during anaphylaxis caused a similar increase in vascular permeability in the pulmonary circulation, it would contribute to edema formation.

C. Prostaglandins

In the lungs the exact role of prostaglandins released from lung tissue by anaphylaxis seems hard to define, since both E and F-type PGs are released and they have directly opposing actions on some smooth muscles. Sweatman and Collier (1968) showed that PGE_2 relaxed, whereas $PGF_{2\alpha}$ contracted human isolated bronchial smooth muscle. Prostaglandin E_2 relaxed previously contracted bronchial smooth muscle of cat (Main 1964) and, when given by aerosol, produced bronchodilatation in guinea pig, dog, and monkey in vivo (Rosenthale et al. 1970). The bronchoconstrictor effects of $PGF_{2\alpha}$ in guinea pig were shown by Berry and Collier (1964). Smith and Cuthbert (1973) studied the effects of PG E_2 and $F_{2\alpha}$ in the lungs of both normal and asthmatic human subjects and found them basically the same as in guinea pig. Given by aerosol, PGE_2 increased forced expiratory ventilation (FEV_1) whereas $PGF_{2\alpha}$ decreased this function. However, when given intravenously PGE_2 had variable effects on the airways of asthmatic patients (Smith 1974), probably because of its rapid metabolism in the pulmonary circulation. Mathé and associates (1974) found asthmatic patients to be 8,000 times more sensitive to the bronchoconstrictor effects of $PGF_{2\alpha}$ given by aerosol than normal patients. Smith and Cuthbert confirmed an increased sensitivity to $PGF_{2\alpha}$ but found that the increase was only 161-fold (Smith, personal communication).

Prostaglandin E_2 is a vasodilator in a wide variety of vascular beds in a number of species (Horton 1969), whereas the actions of $PGF_{2\alpha}$ on the circulation are complex and vary between species. F-type PGs exert mild-to-moderate depressor actions in the cat and rabbit but are pressor in rat and dog

(Änggård and Bergstrom 1963, Horton and Main 1963, Du Charme et al. 1968) In cats, $PGF_{2\alpha}$ caused an increase in right ventricular pressure and increased pulmonary resistance (Änggård and Bergstrom 1963). In the guinea pig, anaphylaxis is accompanied by a marked rise in pulmonary arterial pressure, but PGs seem to play little part in this since indomethacin did not alter the pressor effect (Okpako 1972). Piper and Vane (1971) suggested that a function of PGs released in the lung by damage, anaphylaxis or the mediators released by these conditions might be to divert blood from underventilated areas of the lung to better ventilated areas. This would help to maintain the vitally important ventilation/perfusion ratios.

Pulmonary metabolites of PGs are released during anaphylaxis in guinea pig lung both in vitro and in vivo (Mathé and Levine 1973, Dawson and Tomlinson 1974, Liebig et al. 1974) and during asthmatic attacks in humans, so perhaps these compounds have important actions in the lung. Since metabolism in the pulmonary circulation is very rapid, PG metabolites may also be released by the other stimuli that release PGs from lung tissue (see Said, this volume). Dawson et al. (1974) have shown that 15-keto $PGF_{2\alpha}$ is more potent than the parent PG in contracting human isolated bronchial smooth muscle. Similarly 15-keto PGE_2 is more active in relaxing guinea pig isolated trachea than is PGE_2 (Crutchley and Piper 1975c). Prostaglandins are known to sensitize pain receptors in human skin to the actions of other agonists, such as histamine and bradykinin (Ferreira 1972) and to potentiate vascular permeability (Williams and Morley 1973 and Moncada et al. 1973). At least one of the pulmonary metabolites of PGE_2 sensitizes guinea pig bronchial smooth muscle to contraction by histamine, both in vitro and in vivo (Dawson, personal communication). Therefore, perhaps one of the actions of PGs and their metabolites released in the lung is to sensitize bronchial and vascular smooth muscle to the actions of other mediators.

Prostaglandins E_1, E_2, and $F_{2\alpha}$ increase levels of cyclic AMP in rat peritoneal mast cells and human lung fragments (Kaliner and Austen 1974a, Tauber et al. 1973, Walker 1973). In concentrations of 10^{-4} to 10^{-7} M, which raise the levels of cyclic AMP, exogenous PGs inhibit the release of histamine and SRS-A during challenge of passively sensitized human lung fragments and rat peritoneal mast cells. Walker (1973) found evidence that endogenous PGs modulate and tend to inhibit the release of SRS-A from human lung tissue but could find no evidence of modification of histamine release. The evidence described suggests that a feedback mechanism may exist in lung tissue whereby kinins, SRS-A, and histamine released in the lung by various stimuli subsequently release PGs in the lung tissue and these PGs then inhibit further mediator release.

D.　RCS

Although RCS is a vasoconstrictor in vitro (Piper and Vane 1969b, Palmer et al. 1973), it is not known what action RCS has on blood vessels in vivo. Similarly, RCS contracts human isolated bronchial muscle in vitro (Piper and Walker 1973), but its action on the bronchial tree in vivo is not known. However, RCS is now known to consist of a mixture of endoperoxide precursors of PGs and thromboxane A_2 (Hamberg et al. 1975) and the endoperoxides are bronchoconstrictor and vasoconstrictor in vivo.

E.　RCS-RF

RCS-RF appears to have little direct action on isolated smooth muscle but seems to act in the pulmonary circulation to release other mediators. If RCS-RF is released into the circulation during anaphylaxis in vivo, it might cause a prolonged release of PGs which could, in turn, affect the release and action of other mediators.

F.　Kinins

Bradykinin contracts isolated bronchial smooth muscle from man and guinea pig in vitro but is more potent as a bronchoconstrictor agent in guinea pig in vivo than in vitro. This led Collier and associates (1960) to suggest that part of its bronchoconstrictor action might be due to the release of an intermediate substance. Since the bronchoconstrictor action of bradykinin in vivo is antagonized by nonsteroid antiinflammatory drugs (Collier et al. 1960) and these drugs are potent inhibitors of PG synthetase (Vane 1971), this suggests that RCS and/or PGs may be involved in bronchoconstriction caused by bradykinin (Collier 1969, Palmer et al. 1973). To confirm this, bradykinin has been shown to release RCS and PGs from guinea pig isolated perfused lungs and to release RCS in vivo (Palmer et al. 1973).

In spontaneously breathing guinea pigs, bradykinin causes tachypnea (Gjuris and Westerman 1963), but when given to anesthetized or spinalized guinea pigs prepared for use in the Konzett-Rössler preparation, bradykinin, given intravenously, causes a marked increase in air overflow volume (Collier et al. 1959). This is mainly due to an increase in lung compliance (Widdicombe 1963) and may be explained by the fact that bradykinin selectively narrows the smaller airways and constricts respiratory bronchioles (Jänkälä and Virtame 1963). Bradykinin releases catecholamines from the adrenal medulla (Lecomte et al. 1964, Feldberg and Lewis 1964, Piper et al. 1967) and when given intravenously first causes bronchoconstriction and then releases catecholamines. The catecholamines consist mainly of adrenaline and tend to antagonize the bronchoconstriction (Piper et al. 1967). As with histamine, bradykinin paradoxically decreases intratracheal pressure, probably by stimulation of adrenergic receptors (James 1969). If bradykinin releases PGs of the E-type, they will also act to relax the trachea.

Bradykinin generally causes vasodilatation and lowers systemic blood pressure (Rocha e Silva et al. 1949, Elliot et al. 1960). In the guinea pig the duration of the hypotensive effect of bradykinin is shortened by antiinflammatory drugs (Collier et al. 1968a) and there is increasing evidence that hypotension caused by bradykinin is PG mediated. The PGs may be released by bradykinin from the walls of blood vessels. The hypotension caused by intravenous administration of bradykinin is sometimes followed by a rise in blood pressure (Collier and Shorley 1963, Lecomte et al. 1964). This rise in blood pressure is probably due to release by bradykinin of catecholamines from the adrenal medulla, which has been demonstrated in rabbit, rat, cat, dog, and guinea pig (Lecomte et al. 1961, Feldberg and Lewis 1964, Staszewska-Barczak and Vane 1967, Piper et al. 1967) and/or ganglionic stimulation by bradykinin (Trendelenberg 1966). Although bradykinin is hypotensive in the systemic circulation, it constricts the pulmonary vein in guinea pig and decreases perfusion of isolated lungs (Greef and Moog 1964); this could be due to release of F-type PGs in the blood vessel walls. Capillary permeability is increased by bradykinin, and although this was demonstrated in skin (Bhoola and Schachter 1959, Elliot et al. 1960), a similar increase in vascular permeability may also occur in the lungs.

G. ECF-A

Eosinophil chemotactic factor (ECF-A) is selectively chemotactic towards eosinophils, and it is interesting to note that ECF-A attracts cells that contain arylsulfatase and are therefore capable of inactivating SRS-A (Austen 1974). Thus the release of ECF-A may be another example of a feedback mechanism occurring in the lung during anaphylaxis.

V. Inhibition of Release of Mediators

Substances used to inhibit the release of mediators in anaphylaxis are shown in Table 2.

TABLE 2   Inhibition of Release of Mediators from Lung Tissue during Anaphylaxis

Species	State of lung	Mediators	Inhibitors	Reference
Guinea pig	Perfused	Histamine	Adrenaline	Schild 1936
			Hydrocortisone	Trethewie 1958 Goadby and Smith 1964
		SRS-A	Calcium lack and DFP	Brocklehurst 1960
		Prostaglandins and RCS	Indomethacin Aspirin Nonsteroid, anti- inflammatory drugs	Piper and Vane 1969b Palmer et al. 1973

Guinea pig	Chopped	Histamine	Calcium lack and
			  DFP
				Mongar and Schild 1958
				Austen and Brocklehurst
				  1960

			Catecholamines	Assem and Schild 1971
		SRS-A	Dinitrophenol	Stechschulte et al. 1967
		Prostaglandins and RCS	Indomethacin Aspirin	Piper (unpublished)
			Nonsteroid, anti- inflammatory drugs	Piper (unpublished)
Human	Chopped	Histamine	β-adrenergic drugs	Assem and Schild 1969 Orange et al. 1971
			Methylxanthines	Kaliner et al. 1973
			Prostaglandin E_1, E_2, $F_{2\alpha}$, A_1	Tauber et al. 1973
			Cholera toxin	Kaliner et al. 1973
			Disodium cromo- glycate	Sheard and Blair 1970
			Calcium lack	Orange 1974
			Colchicine	Orange 1974
			Cytochalasin B	Orange 1974
		SRS-A	β-adrenergic drugs	Assem and Schild 1969 Orange et al. 1971
			Methylxanthines	Kaliner et al. 1973
			Prostaglandins E_1, E_2, $F_{2\alpha}$, A_1	Tauber et al. 1973
			Cholera toxin	Kaliner et al. 1973
			Disodium cromo- glycate	Sheard and Blair 1970
			Calcium lack	Orange et al. 1974
			Colchicine	Orange 1974
			Cytochalasin A	Orange 1974
		ECF-A	β-adrenergic drugs Methylxanthines	Wasserman et al. 1974b
			DFP	Orange and Austen 1972
			Disodium cromo- glycate	Orange and Austen 1972
		Prostaglandins	Indomethacin Disodium cromo- glycate	Piper and Walker 1973

TABLE 2 (continued)

Species	State of lung	Mediators	Inhibitors	Reference
Monkey	Chopped	Histamine	Catecholamines Theophylline cAMP	Ishizaka et al. 1971
			Chlorophenesin	Malley and Baecher 1971
		SRS-A	Catecholamines Theophylline cAMP Diethycarbamazine	Ishizaka et al. 1971
			Chlorphenesin	Malley and Baecher 1971
Bovine	Chopped	Histamine	High molecular weight fractions PPP	Burka and Eyre 1974
		SRS-A	High molecular weight fractions PPP	Burka and Eyre 1974

A. Histamine and SRS-A

In 1936 Schild showed that not only was adrenaline a *physiologic antagonist* of anaphylaxis but it also suppressed the antigen-induced release of histamine from guinea pig lung. The mechanism of this inhibition became clearer when Sutherland and Robison (1966) showed that α-adrenergic agonists stimulated formation of cyclic 3'5'-adenosine monophosphate (cyclic AMP) from adenosine triphosphate (ATP) by activation of membrane-bound adenylate cyclase. Lichtenstein and Margolis (1968) showed that β-adrenoceptor stimulants and methylxanthines protect cyclic AMP from breakdown by phosphodiesterases and prevent the release of histamine during antigen challenge of human sensitized leukocytes. In 1969 Assem and Schild found that isoprenaline, adrenaline, salbutamol, dopamine, and orciprenaline (in descending order of potency) prevent the release of histamine from challenged human lung fragments. In human chopped lung tissue or nasal polyps, there is a direct correlation between the increase in cyclic AMP levels (caused by drugs other than β-adrenoceptor stimulants and methylxanthines) and inhibition of mediator release (Orange et al. 1971, Kaliner et al. 1973). Prostaglandins E_1, E_2, $F_{2\alpha}$, A_1 and cholera toxin all increase cyclic AMP and inhibit antigen-induced release of histamine and SRS-A, either by stimulating adenyl cyclase or inhibiting phosphodiesterase (Table 2) (Tauber et al. 1973, Kaliner et al. 1973).

Disodium cromoglycate inhibits the antigen-induced release of histamine and SRS-A from human lung tissue in a dose-dependent manner (Sheard and Blair 1970). In addition this drug inhibits the release of PGs from human lung, but only in doses that completely inhibit histamine and SRS-A output (Piper and Walker 1973). Disodium cromoglycate does not inhibit mediator release in guinea pig lung (Cox et al. 1970). The mechanism of action of disodium cromoglycate is not completely understood, but it is not acting either as a stimulator of adenyl cyclase or inhibitor of phosphodiesterase (Cox et al. 1970). The action of disodium cromoglycate is further discussed in the Section *Antagonism of Anaphylaxis*.

Since the release mechanisms for histamine, SRS-A, and ECF-A are calcium-dependent and require the activation of a DFP-sensitive serine esterase (Orange et al. 1971, Mongar and Schild 1958, Wasserman et al. 1974b, Orange and Austen 1974, Schild 1936, 1968), lack of calcium and the presence of DFP prevent antigen-induced release of these mediators from human and guinea pig lung. Release of both histamine and SRS-A is blocked by colchicine, which may act by inhibiting the release but not the intracellular formation of SRS-A (Orange 1974).

Chlorophenesin prevented the antigen-induced release of histamine and SRS-A from monkey lung fragments sensitized with human reagin (Malley and Baecher 1971). The action of chlorophenesin was thought to be due to activation of adenylcyclase.

Release of SRS-A from lungs is prevented by diethylcarbamazine (Orange and Austen 1969) and this drug also blocks release of PG induced by amines (Bakhle and Smith 1972). The release of histamine and SRS-A from sensitized rat and primate lung tissue inhibited by diethylcarbamazine (Orange et al. 1968, Ishizaka et al. 1971). Since the action of diethylcarbamazine is not prevented by propranolol, it cannot be attributable to β-adrenoceptor stimulation. Diethylcarbamazine relieves asthma and exercise-induced asthma (Salazar-Mallen 1965, Sly and Matzen 1974). Diethylcarbamazine also blocks the release of PGs from isolated, perfused, rat lung (Bakhle and Smith 1972) so that its therapeutic action in the lung may be to inhibit release of mediators by an unknown mechanism.

B.   ECF-A

The release of ECF-A from human lung is modified in the same way as the release of histamine and SRS-A by increased cyclic AMP and cyclic GMP levels and cholinergic stimulation (Wasserman et al. 1974b). Disodium cromoglycate probably also inhibits the release of ECF-A from human lung (Kaliner and Austen 1974b).

The high molecular weight fractions of polyphloretin phosphate inhibit release of histamine and SRS-A from rat peritoneal mast cells (Strandberg 1973) and bovine lung (Burka and Eyre 1974).

C. Prostaglandins and RCS

Whenever RCS and PGs are released from lungs or lung fragments by immuno-logic stimuli, their release is prevented by nonsteroid antiinflammatory drugs (Piper and Vane 1969b, 1971, Palmer et al. 1973, Piper and Walker 1973). These inhibitors of PG synthetase selectively prevent the release of PGs and RCS and do not reduce the output of histamine and SRS-A. Walker (1973) observed that the amount of SRS-A released on challenge of human lung was increased when the release of PGs had been inhibited by indomethacin. Similarly, Engineer, Piper, and Sirois (1976) found an increase in the amount of SRS-A released from guinea pig perfused lungs after treatment with indomethacin. However, indomethacin did not affect the reduction in FEV_1 during antigen challenge of asthmatic patients (Smith and Dunlop 1975). The release of RCS during anaphylaxis in guinea pig in vivo was prevented by treating the animal with aspirin (Palmer et al. 1973). This also abolished the release of RCS caused by bradykinin. Inhibition of the release of RCS (and possibly PGs) by nonsteroid antiinflammatory drugs, measured by direct bio-assay methods in vivo, explains the partial protection against anaphylaxis seen with these drugs in guinea pig in vivo (Collier et al. 1968b).

Aitken and Sanford (1972) and Eyre et al. (1973) found that meclo-fenamate protected calves against acute systemic anaphylaxis, whereas mepy-ramine or methysergide were either totally or partially ineffective. The authors interpreted these results as showing inhibition of the action of SRS-A and bradykinin, but an alternative conclusion would be that meclofenamate blocked the release of RCS and PGs, which might be important mediators in anaphylaxis in the calf (Bakhle and Vane 1974).

Vargaftig and Dao Hai (1972) observed that mepacrine selectively inhib-ited the bradykinin-induced release of RCS from guinea pig lungs but did not inhibit release caused by arachidonic acid.

Mathé and Levine (1972) found that adrenaline inhibited the release of PGs and their metabolites from challenged guinea pig perfused lungs.

The release of RCS-RF was not blocked by antiinflammatory drugs (Palmer et al. 1973) and no inhibitor of its release has yet been found.

VI. Pharmacologic Antagonism of Actions of Mediators

Pharmacologic antagonism of the actions of mediators released from the lung has been studied in terms of antagonism of the effects of anaphylaxis.

Collier and James (1967) treated sensitized anesthetized guinea pigs in vivo with a combination of aspirin or meclofenamate and mepyramine before challenge with antigen. This treatment suppressed most but not all of the anaphylactic bronchoconstriction. The authors concluded that the residual bronchoconstriction was due to the action of unknown bronchoconstrictor factor(s).

Disodium cromoglycate inhibits anaphylaxis in human lung fragments by preventing the release of histamine and SRS-A, presumably from mast cells (Sheard et al. 1967). This drug also prevents the release of PGs during anaphylaxis in human lung tissue but only at doses that almost completely inhibit the release of histamine and SRS-A (Piper and Walker 1973). During anaphylaxis in the rat, although the lung is not the *target* organ, bronchoconstriction can occur, and disodium cromoglycate inhibits this anaphylactic bronchoconstriction (Church et al. 1972). Disodium cromoglycate inhibits the release of histamine from rat peritoneal mast cells caused either by antigen challenge or phospholipase A (Cox et al. 1970) and may therefore exert a similar action on mast cells in the lung. However, disodium cromoglycate has no protective action during anaphylaxis in the guinea pig chopped lung during challenge (Cox et al. 1970, Assem and Mongar 1970). The exact mode of action of disodium cromoglycate is unknown, but the fact that it inhibited the release of mediators from mast cells by phospholipase A suggests that it may act on an enzyme or enzyme substrate(s) activated by the antigen-antibody reaction, thus preventing the release of mediators (Cox et al. 1970) and antagonizing the effects of anaphylaxis.

In dogs polyphloretin phosphate inhibited the bronchoconstrictor action of $PGF_{2\alpha}$ (Villaneuva et al. 1972) but the effects of this compound on the actions of PGs released in anaphylaxis is not known.

There is some evidence that the antiinflammatory steroids, such as hydrocortisone, reduce the amount of histamine and SRS-A released from guinea pig lung during anaphylaxis (Trethewie 1958, Goadby and Smith 1964). The animals used in these experiments had been sensitized with low doses of antigen. Cortisone and hydrocortisone suppressed the response of isolated, guinea pig intestinal smooth muscle to histamine and SRS-A (Trethewie 1958, Goadby and Smith 1964). Hydrocortisone suppresses the response of isolated assay tissues to the effects of PGs released during anaphylaxis in guinea pig isolated lungs (Palmer and Piper unpublished data). Church et al. (1972) inhibited anaphylactic bronchoconstriction in the rat with dexamethasone but gave no evidence whether this was due to inhibition of mediator release or to direct antagonism of bronchoconstriction.

VII. Discussion

Immunologic stimulation of lungs or lung fragments results in the release of a number of chemical substances that have potent biologic actions. The release may be from stores of preformed mediator, for example, histamine and ECF-A or, as is the case with SRS-A and prostaglandins, a result of synthesis de novo in response to the stimulus. Once released, the mediators may act locally in the lung or, if they are not metabolized in the pulmonary circulation, enter the systemic circulation to act on some other organ, perhaps to release further substances.

Certainly, in anaphylaxis in the guinea pig, when histamine, bradykinin, and SRS-A are released as a result of antigen-antibody union, they subsequently cause release of catecholamines from the adrenal medulla by direct or indirect action. This means that catecholamines are secondary mediators of anaphylaxis. The PGs and their metabolites are the latest additions to the list of mediators released from lungs and there is evidence that their release may be secondary to other factors, such as anaphylactic contraction of bronchial smooth muscle, hypoxia (Said 1974), and histamine or other bronchoconstrictive mediators entering the pulmonary circulation. The original detection of PGs released from lungs was by means of continuous bioassay and thin layer chromatography when PG metabolites were not available. It is impossible to distinguish biologically between high concentrations of metabolites and low concentrations of parent PGs (Crutchley and Piper 1975c). It appears that the PG metabolites detected in anaphylaxis are formed at extravascular sites and not in the pulmonary circulation (Piper 1974), and there is evidence that there is uptake of PGs prior to metabolism (Ryan et al. 1975).

In guinea pig lung, stimuli that release PGs also release RCS, but this substance is not released from either human or rat lung by anaphylaxis. However, it is released from human, rat, or cat lung by mechanical stimulation (Palmer et al. 1973, Piper and Walker 1973). This finding indicates that RCS is released from any species of lung tissue by damage but only by anaphylaxis involving IgG antibodies. RCS released during platelet aggregation has recently been identified as a mixture of thromboxane A_2 and endoperoxides, and certainly endoperoxides have been shown to be bronchoconstrictor in vivo (Hamberg and Samuelsson 1973). Thus RCS may be a contributing factor to the bronchoconstriction that accompanies pulmonary embolism.

Some mediators released from the lung have bronchoconstrictor actions, such as histamine, SRS-A, and bradykinin formed by lung kallikrein. All of these substances may also act on the pulmonary circulation. The actions of the PGs and their metabolites are harder to define. Since pretreatment of sensitized guinea pigs with aspirin alone does not greatly lessen anaphylaxis and PGs of the E and F series often have directly opposing actions, it is difficult to explain why these substances should be released in anaphylaxis. The release of PG metabolites also occurs from perfused lungs and suggests that the parent PGs have an action and are metabolized before entering the pulmonary circulation. Prostaglandin metabolites themselves may be important in anaphylaxis and certainly 15-keto PGE_2 and $F_{2\alpha}$ are more potent in relaxing or contracting bronchial smooth muscle than the parent prostaglandins. Prostaglandins are not circulating hormones, and their local action in the lung may be the maintenance of ventilation/perfusion ratios, an important function when damage to the lung has occurred. For instance, $PGF_{2\alpha}$ might be released in areas of bronchoconstriction and hypoxia and cause vasoconstriction in these areas, whereas PGE_2 may cause bronchodilatation and vasodilatation in areas of the lung that are better ventilated.

Prostaglandins have been shown to potentiate the actions of inflammatory mediators in human and guinea pig skin and increase passive cutaneous anaphylaxis in guinea pig (Ferreira 1972, Williams and Morley 1973, and Ferreira et al. 1973) and may therefore potentiate the action of other mediators in the lung. At least one metabolite potentiates the bronchoconstrictor action of histamine in vitro and in vivo (Dawson, personal communication).

Sensitization with antigen may modify the enzymes controlling both synthesis and metabolism of PGs, since an increased concentration of prostaglandin synthetase has been found in sensitized lungs, explaining the greater amounts of PGs released from sensitized lungs by pulmonary embolism (Palmer et al. 1973).

In describing the various functions of mediators released from the lung, it seems that several negative feedback mechanisms may exist, either in the whole animal in vivo or chopped lung tissue in vitro, or perhaps in both systems. Histamine, bradykinin, and SRS-A are bronchoconstrictor, and catecholamines released into the circulation during anaphylaxis act to reverse this bronchoconstriction. Also in chopped lung catecholamines inhibit the anaphylactic release of histamine, SRS-A and ECF-A, but whether catecholamines released as a result of anaphylaxis in vivo tend to cause similar inhibition is not known. Similarly, PGs inhibit mediator release in challenged, chopped and perfused lungs (Walker 1973, Engineer, Piper, Sirois, 1976) and may possibly do so in vivo. ECF-A may exert another negative feedback mechanism against the action of SRS-A. This substance is released together with SRS-A and is chemotactic towards eosinophils, which contain arylsulfatase, an enzyme that destroys the activity of SRS-A. It seems, therefore, that release of the primary mediators of anaphylaxis triggers a series of events that tend either to reverse the bronchoconstriction caused by anaphylactic mediators or to inhibit their release. Since some anaphylactic mediators are released by damage to the lung, they may also exert negative feedback control (Fig. 1).

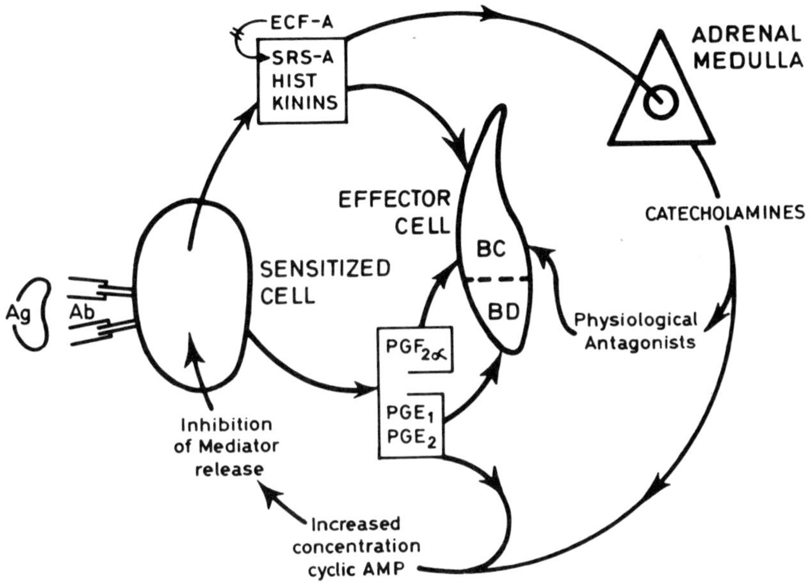

FIGURE 1 Negative feedback mechanisms that may exist in the lung during anaphylaxis. BC = bronchoconstriction, BD = bronchodilatation.

The release of substances in anaphylaxis may be modified as described previously. Sometimes inhibition of the release of one mediator(s) leads to an increase in the amount of others, which again emphasizes the interaction of biologically active mediators released from the lung.

References

Abe, K., Watanabe, N., Kumagai, N., Mouri, T., Seki, T., and Yoshinaga, K. (1967). Circulating plasma kinin in patients with bronchial asthma. *Experientia,* **23**:626–627.

Aitken, M. M. and Sanford, J. (1972). Modification of acute systemic anaphylaxis in cattle by drugs and by vagotomy. *J. Comp. Pathol.,* **82**:247–256.

Änggård, E., Bergqvist, U., Hogberg, B., Johansson, K., Thon, I. L., and Uvnas, B. (1963). Biologically active principles occurring on histamine release from cat paw, guinea pig lung and isolated rat mast cells. *Acta Physiol. Scand.,* **59**:97–110.

Änggård, E. and Bergstrom, S. (1963). Biological effects of an unsaturated trihydroxy acid (PGF$_{2\alpha}$) from normal swine lung. *Acta Physiol. Scand.,* **58**: 1–12.

Änggård, E. and Samuelsson, B. (1965). Biosynthesis of prostaglandins from arachidonic acid in guinea pig lung. *J. Biol. Chem.,* **240**:3518–3521.

Assem, E. S. K. and Mongar, J. L. (1970). Inhibition of allergic reactions in man and other species by cromoglycate. *Int. Arch Allergy Appl. Immunol.*, **38**: 68–77.

Assem, E. S. K. and Schild, H. O. (1969). Inhibition by sympathomimetic amines of histamine release induced by antigen in passively sensitized human lung. *Nature,* **224**:1026–1029.

Assem, E. S. K. and Schild, H. O. (1971). Antagonism of β-adrenoceptor blocking agents of the antianaphylactic effect of isoprenaline. *Br. J. Pharmacol.,* **42**:620–630.

Auer, J. and Lewis, P. A. (1910). The physiology of the immediate reaction of anaphylaxis in the guinea pig. *J. Exp. Med.,* **12**:151–175.

Austen, K. F. (1974). A review of immunological, biochemical and pharmacological factors in the release of chemical mediators from human lung. In K. F. Austen and M. Lichtenstein (eds.): *Asthma, Physiology, Immunopharmacology and Treatment.* Academic Press, London, pp. 109–122.

Austen, K. F. and Brocklehurst, W. E. (1960). Inhibition of the anaphylactic release of histamine from chopped guinea pig lung by chymotrypsin substrates and inhibitors. *Nature,* **186**:866–868.

Bakhle, Y. S. and Smith, T. W. (1972). Release of spasmogenic substances induced by vasoactive amines from isolated lungs. *Br. J. Pharmacol.,* **46**: 543–544P.

Bakhle, Y. S. and Vane, J. R. (1974). Pharmacokinetic function of the pulmonary circulation. *Physiol. Rev.,* **54**:1007–1045.

Bartosch, R., Feldberg, W., and Nagel, E. (1933). Weitere Versuche über das Freiwerden eines histaminähnlichen Stoffes aus der durchströmten Lunge sensibilisieter Meerschweinchen beim Auslösen einer anaphylaktischen Lungenstarre. *Arch. Physiol.,* **231**:616–629.

Benzie, R., Boot, J. R., and Dawson, W. (1975). A preliminary investigation of prostaglandin synthetase activity in normal, sensitized and challenged sensitized guinea pig lungs. *J. Physiol.,* **246**:80P.

Berry, P. A. and Collier, H. O. J. (1964). Bronchoconstrictor action and antagonism of a slow-reacting substance from anaphylaxis of guinea pig lung. Br. J. Pharmacol., **23**:201–216.

Bhoola, K. D. and Schachter, M. (1959). A comparison of serum kallikrein, bradykinin and histamine on capillary permeability in the guinea pig. *J. Physiol.,* **149**:80–81P.

Black, W., Duncan, W. A. M., Durant, C. J., Ganellin, R., and Parsons, E. M. (1972). Definition and antagonism of histamine receptors. *Nature,* **236**: 385–390.

Brocklehurst, W. E. (1960). The release of histamine and formation of a slow-reacting substance (SRS-A) during anaphylactic shock. *J. Physiol.,* **151**: 416–435.

Brocklehurst, W. E. (1963). Recent advances in the pharmacology of toxins. In H. W. Roudonat (ed.): Proceedings of the Second International Pharmacology Meeting, Prague, 1963, vol. 9. Pergamon, Oxford.

Brocklehurst, W. E. (1968). The probable role of known mediators in hypersensitivity reactions. In H. O. Schild (ed.): *Immunopharmacology*. Pergamon Press, Oxford, pp. 67–75.

Brocklehurst, W. E. (1970). The role of slow-reacting substance in asthma. In M. H. Harper and S. B. Simmonds (eds.): *Advances in Drug Research*, vol. 5. Academic Press, London, New York, pp. 109–113.

Brocklehurst, W. E. and Lahiri, S. C. (1962). The production of bradykinin in anaphylaxis. *J. Physiol.*, **160**:15–16P.

Brocklehurst, W. E. and Lahiri, S. C. (1963). Formation and destruction of bradykinin during anaphylaxis. *J. Physiol.*, **165**:39–40P.

Burka, J. F. and Eyre, P. (1974). The immunological release of slow-reacting substance of anaphylaxis from bovine lung. *Can. J. Physiol. Pharmacol.*, **52**:1201–1204.

Church, M. K., Collier, H. O. J., and James, G. W. L. (1972). The inhibition by dexamethasone and disodium cromoglycate of bronchoconstriction in the rat. *Br. J. Pharmacol.*, **46**:56–65.

Code, C. F. (1937). The quantitative estimation of histamine in the blood. *J. Physiol.*, **89**:257–268.

Collier, H. O. J. (1969). New light on how aspirin works. *Nature*, **223**:35–37.

Collier, H. O. J. (1970). Endogenous broncho-active substances and their antagonism. In M. H. Harper and S. B. Simmonds (eds.): *Advances in Drug Research*, vol. 5. Academic Press, London and New York, pp. 95–107.

Collier, H. O. J., Dineen, L. C., Perkins, A. C., and Piper, P. J. (1968a). Curtailment by aspirin and meclofenamate of hypotension induced by bradykinin in the guinea pig. *Naunyn-Schmiedebergs Arch. Exptl. Pathol. Pharmakol.*, **259**:159–160.

Collier, H. O. J., Holgate, J. A., Schachter, M., and Shorley, P. G. (1959). An apparent bronchoconstrictor action of bradykinin and its suppression by some anti-inflammatory drugs. *J. Physiol.*, **149**:54–55P.

Collier, H. O. J., Holgate, J. A., Schachter, M., and Shorley, P. G. (1960). The bronchoconstrictor action of bradykinin in the guinea pig. *Br. J. Pharmacol.*, **15**:290–297.

Collier, H. O. J. and James, G. W. L. (1967). Humoral factors affecting pulmonary inflation during acute anaphylaxis in the guinea pig in vivo. *Br. J. Pharmacol. Chemother.*, **30**:283–301.

Collier, H. O. J., James, G. W. L., and Piper, P. J. (1968b). Antagonism by fenamates and like-acting drugs of bronchoconstriction induced by bradykinin or antigen in the guinea pig. *Br. J. Pharmacol.*, **34**:76–87.

Collier, H. O. J. and Shorley, P. G. (1963). Antagonism by mefenamic and flufenamic acids of the bronchoconstrictor action of kinins in the guinea pig. *Br. J. Pharmacol.*, **20**:345–351.

Cox, J. S. G., Beach, J. E., Blair, A. M. J. N., Clarke, A. J., King, J., Lee, T. B., Loveday, D. E. E., Moss, G. F., Orr, T. S. G., Ritchie, J. T., and Sheard, P. (1970). Disodium cromoglycate (Intal). In M. H. Harper and A. B. Simmonds (eds.): Advances in Drug Research, vol. 5. Academic Press, London, New York, pp. 115–196.

Crutchley, D. J. and Piper, P. J. (1974). Prostaglandin inactivation in guinea pig lung and its inhibition. *Br. J. Pharmacol.,* **52**:197–203.

Crutchley, D. J. and Piper, P. J. (1975a). Inhibition of the pulmonary inactivation of prostaglandins in rabbit in vivo. *Br. J. Pharmacol.,* **53**:467P.

Crutchley, D. J. and Piper, P. J. (1975b). Inhibition of the pulmonary inactivation of prostaglandins in vivo by di-4-phloretin phosphate. *Br. J. Pharmacol.,* **54**:301–307.

Crutchley, D. J. and Piper, P. J. (1975c). Comparative bioassay of pulmonary metabolites of prostaglandin E_2. *Br. J. Pharmacol.,* **54**:397–399.

Dale, H. H. (1920). The biological significance of anaphylaxis. *Proc. R. Soc. (London) Ser. B.,* **91**:126–146.

Dale, H. H. (1929). Some chemical factors in the control of the circulation. *Lancet,* **1**:1179–1290.

Dale, H. H. and Laidlaw, P. P. (1910). The physiological action of β-iminazolyl-ethylamine. *J. Physiol.,* **41**:318–341.

Dawson, W., Lewis, R. L., McMahon, R. E., and Sweatman, W. J. F. (1974). Potent bronchoconstrictor activity of 15-keto prostaglandin $F_{2\alpha}$. *Nature,* **250**:331–332.

Dawson, W., Lewis, R. L., and Tomlinson, R. (1975). The release of ^{35}S-labelled material and SRS-A from immunologically challenged guinea pig lungs. *J. Physiol.,* **247**:37–38P.

Dawson, W. and Tomlinson, R. (1974). Effect of cromoglycate and eicosatetraynoic acid on the release of prostaglandins and SRS-A from immunologically challenged guinea pig lungs. *Br. J. Pharmacol.,* **52**:107–108P.

Drazen, J. M., Imming, D. J., Stechschulte, D. J., Amdur, M. O., Austen, K. F., and Mead, J. (1973). Effects of intravenous slow-reacting substance of anaphylaxis (SRS-A) on respiratory mechanics. *Federation Proc.,* **32**:402 (abstr.).

DuCharme, D. W., Weeks, J. R., and Montgomery, R. G. (1968). Studies on the mechanism of the hypertensive effect of prostaglandin $F_{2\alpha}$. *J. Pharmacol. Exp. Ther.,* **160**:1–10.

Eilbeck, J. F. and Smith, W. G. (1967). Histamine release from the mast cells of guinea pig lung. *J. Pharm. Pharmacol.,* **19**:374–382.

Elliott, D. F., Horton, E. W., and Lewis, G. P. (1960). Actions of pure bradykinin. *J. Physiol.,* **153**:473–480.

Eyre, P. and Lewis, A. J. (1972). Production of kinins in bovine anaphylactic shock. *Br. J. Pharmacol.,* **44**:311–313.

Eyre, P., Lewis, A. J., and Wells, P. W. (1973). Acute systemic anaphylaxis in the calf. *Br. J. Pharmacol.,* **47**:504–516.

Feldberg, W. and Lewis, G. P. (1964). The action of peptides on the adrenal medulla. Release of adrenaline by bradykinin and angiotensin. *J. Physiol.,* **171**:98–108.

Ferreira, S. H. (1972). Prostaglandins, aspirin-like drugs and analgesia. *Nature, New Biol.,* **240**:200–203.

Ferreira, S. H. and Vane, J. R. (1967a). The disappearance of bradykinin and eledoisin in the circulation and vascular beds of the cat. *Br. J. Pharmacol.,* **30**:417–424.

Ferreira, S. H. and Vane, J. R. (1967b). Prostaglandins: their disappearance from and release into the circulation. *Nature,* **216**:868–873.

Flower, R. J., Gryglewski, R., Herbaczynska-Cedro, K., and Vane, J. R. (1972). Effects of anti-inflammatory drugs on prostaglandin biosynthesis. *Nature, New Biol.,* **238**:104–106.

Flower, R. J. and Vane, J. R. (1974). Inhibition of prostaglandin biosynthesis. *Biochem. Pharmacol.,* **23**:1439–1450.

Gjuris, V. and Westermann, E. (1963). Zur Frage der bronchoconstrictorischen Wirkung des Bradykinins, Kallidins und Eledoisins. Naunyn-Schmiedebergs *Arch. Expth. Pathol Pharmakol.,* **246**:17–19.

Goadby, P. and Phillips, E. A. (1973). Some effects of burimamide on the isolated perfused pulmonary circulation of the guinea pig. *Br. J. Pharmacol.,* **49**:368–369.

Goadby, P. and Smith, W. G. (1964). Observations on the anti-anaphylactic activity of hydrocortisone and related steroids. *J. Pharm. Pharmacol.,* **16**: 108–114.

Greeff, K. and Moog, E. (1964). Vergleichende Untersuchunge über die broncho-constrictorische und gefüssconstrictorische Wirkung des Bradykinins, Histamins und Serotonins an isolierten Lungenprüparaten. *Naunyn-Schmiedebergs Arch. Exptl. Pathol. Pharmakol.,* **248**:204–215.

Gréen, K. Hedqvist, P., and Svanborg, N. (1974). Increased plasma levels of 15-keto-13, 14-dihydroprostaglandin $F_{2\alpha}$ after allergen-provoked asthma in man. *Lancet,* **2**:1419–1421.

Grodzinska, L., Panczenko, B., and Gryglewski, R. J. (1975). Generation of prostaglandin E-like material by the guinea pig trachea contracted by histamine. *J. Pharm. Pharmacol.,* **27**:88–91.

Gryglewski, R. J. and Vane, J. R. (1972). Generation from arachidonic acid of rabbit aorta contracting substance (RCS) by a microsomal enzyme preparation which also generates prostaglandins. *Br. J. Pharmacol.,* **46**:449–457.

Hamberg, M. and Samuelsson, B. (1973). Role of endoperoxides in the biosynthesis and actions of prostaglandins. In H. J. Robinson and J. R. Vane (eds.): *Prostaglandin Synthetase Inhibitors.* Raven Press, New York, pp. 107–119.

Hamberg, M., Svensson, J., and Samuelsson, B. (1975). Involvement of endoperoxides and thromboxanes in anaphylactic reactions. In *Prostaglandins and Thromboxanes.* Raven Press, New York, pp. 495–501.

Herxheimer, H. and Stresemann, E. (1963). The effect of slow reacting substance (SRS-A) in guinea pigs and asthmatic patients. *J. Physiol.,* **165**: 78–79P.

Horton, E. W. (1969). Hypotheses on physiological roles of prostaglandins. *Physiol. Rev.,* **49**:122–161.

Horton, E. W. and Main, I. H. M. (1963). A comparison of the biological activity of four prostaglandins. *Br. J. Pharmacol.,* **21**:182–189.

Ishizaka, T., Ishizaka, K., Orange, R. P., and Austen, K. F. (1970). The capacity of human immunoglobulin E to mediate the release of histamine and slow reacting substance of anaphylaxis (SRS-A) from monkey lung. *J. Immunol.,* **104**:335–343.

Ishizaka, T., Ishizaka, K., Orange, R. P., and Austen, K. F. (1971). Pharmacologic inhibition of the antigen-induced release of histamine and slow reacting substance of anaphylaxis (SRS-A) from monkey lung tissues mediated by human IgE. *J. Immunol.*, **106**:1267–1273.

Ishizaka, T., Ishizaka, K., and Tomioka, H. (1972). Release of histamine and slow reacting substance of anaphylaxis (SRS-A) by IgE-anti-IgE reactions on monkey mast cells. *J. Immunol.*, **108**:513–520.

James, G. W. L. (1969). The use of the in vivo trachea preparation of the guinea pig to assess drug action on lung. *J. Pharm. Pharmacol.*, **21**:379–386.

Jänkälä, E. O. and Virtama, P. (1963). Bronchographic demonstration of the bronchoconstrictor effect of bradykinin in the guinea pig. *Arch. Med. Exp. Fem.*, **41**:436–440.

Jonasson, O. and Becker, E. L. (1966). Release of kallikrein from guinea pig lung during anaphylaxis. *J. Exp. Med.*, **123**:509–522.

Jose, P., Niederhauser, U., Piper, P. J., Robinson, C., and Smith, A. P. (1976). Inactivation of prostaglandin $F_{2\alpha}$ in the pulmonary circulation. *Br. J. Clin. Pharmacol.*, **3**:342P.

Kaliner, M. and Austen, K. F. (1974a). Cyclic AMP, ATP and reversed anaphylactic histamine release from rat mast cells. *J. Immunol.*, **112**:664–674.

Kaliner, M. and Austen, K. F. (1974b). Cyclic nucleotides and modulation of effector systems of inflammation. *Biochem. Pharmacol.*, **23**:763–771.

Kaliner, M., Wasserman, S. I., and Austen, K. F. (1973). The immunologic release of chemical mediators from human nasal polyps. *N. Engl. J. Med.*, **289**:277–281.

Kay, A. B., Stechschulte, D. J., and Austen, K. F. (1971). An eosinophil leukocyte chemotactic factor of anaphylaxis. *J. Exp. Med.*, **133**:602–619.

Kellaway, C. H. and Trethewie, E. R. (1940). The liberation of a slow-reacting smooth muscle-stimulating substance in anaphylaxis. *Q. J. Exp. Physiol.*, **30**:121–145.

Kunze, H. and Vogt, W. (1971). Significance of phospholipase A for prostaglandin formation. *Ann. N. Y. Acad. Sci.*, **180**:123–125.

Layton, J. J. and Cameron, J. M. (1971). Post-mortem findings in anaphylactic shock. *The Practitioner*, **206**:383–385.

Lecomte, J., Troquet, J., and Cession-Fossion, A. (1964). Sur la nature de l'hypertension arterielle provoquée par la bradykinine et la kallidine. *Arch. Int. Pharmacodyn. Ther.*, **147**:518–524.

Lecomte, J., Troquet, J., and Dresse, A. (1961). Stimulation medullosurrenalienne par la bradykinine. *Arch. Int. Physiol.*, **69**:89–91.

Lichtenstein, L. M. and Margolis, S. (1968). Histamine release in vitro: inhibition by catecholamines and methylxanthines. *Science*, **161**:902–903.

Liebig, R., Bernauer, W., and Peskar, B. A. (1974). Release of prostaglandins, a prostaglandin metabolite, slow-reacting substance and histamine from anaphylactic lungs and its mofification by catecholamines. *Naunyn-Schmiedeberg's Arch. Pharmacol.*, **284**:279–293.

Main, I. H. M. (1964). The inhibitory actions of prostaglandins on respiratory smooth muscle. *Br. J. Pharmacol.*, **22**:511–519.

Malley, A. and Baecher, L. (1971). Inhibition of histamine and SRS-A from monkey lung tissue by chlorophenesin. *J. Immunol.*, **107**:586–588.

Mathé, A. A., Hedqvist, P., Holmgren, A., and Svanborg, N. (1974). Bronchial hyperactivity to $PGF_{2\alpha}$ and histamine in patients with asthma. *Br. Med. J.*, **1**:193–196.

Mathé, A. A. and Levine, L. (1973). Release of prostaglandins and metabolites from guinea pig lung: inhibition by catecholamines. *Prostaglandins*, **4**: 877–890.

McGiff, J. C., Itskovitz, H. D., and Terragno, N. A. (1975). The action of brady-kinin in the canine isolated kidney: relationships to prostaglandins. *Clin. Sci. Molec. Med.*, **39**:125–331.

Miller, W. S. (1947). *The Lung,* 2nd Ed. Blackwell, Oxford.

Mills, J. E., Sellick, H., and Widdicombe, J. G. (1969). The activity of lung ir-ritant receptors in pulmonary micro-embolism, anaphylaxis and drug-induced bronchoconstrictions. *J. Physiol. (Lond.)*, **203**:337–357.

Mills, J. E. and Widdicombe, J. G. (1970). Role of the vagus nerves in anaphy-laxis and histamine-induced bronchoconstrictions in guinea pigs. *Br. J. Pharmacol.*, **39**:724–731.

Moncada, S., Ferreira, S. H., and Vane, J. R. (1973). Prostaglandins, aspirin-like drugs and the oedema of inflammation. *Nature*, **246**:217–219.

Mongar, J. L. and Schild, H. O. (1958). The effect of calcium and pH on the ana-phylactic reaction. *J. Physiol. (Lond.)*, **140**:272–284.

Mota, I. and Vugman, I. (1956). Effects of anaphylactic shock and compound 48/80 on the mast cells of the guinea pig lung. *Nature*, **177**:427–429.

Ng, K. K. F. and Vane, J. R. (1967). The conversion of angiotensin I to angio-tensin II. *Nature*, **216**:762–766.

Okpako, D. T. (1972). A dual action of histamine on guinea pig lung vessels. *Br. J. Pharmacol.*, **44**:311–321.

Orange, R. P. (1974). Formation and release of slow reacting substance of ana-phylaxis in human lung tissues. In L. Brent and J. Holborow (eds.): *Pro-gress in Immunology II*, vol. 4, *Clinical Aspects I.* American Elsevier, New York, pp. 29–39.

Orange, R. P. and Austen, K. F. (1969). Slow reacting substance of anaphylaxis. *Adv. Immunol.*, **10**:105.

Orange, R. P. and Austen, K. F. (1972). Immunologic and pharmacologic re-ceptor control of the release of chemical mediators from human lung. In D. D. Dayton (ed.): *The Biological Role of the Immuno-globulin E Sys-tem.* U.S Government Printing Office, pp. 151–164.

Orange, R. P., Austen, W. G., and Austen, K. F. (1971). Immunological release of histamine and slow reacting substance of anaphylaxis from human lung. I. Modulation by agents influencing cellular levels of cyclic 3', 5'-adenosine monophosphate. *J. Exp. Med.*, **134**:136S.

Orange, R. P. and Langer, H. (1973). Bronchial asthma: hyperreactivity of air-ways and target cells. *Int. Congr. Ser.*, **323**, Allergology, pp. 325–333.

Orange, R. P., Murphy, R. C., and Austen, K. F. (1974). Inactivation of slow reacting substance of anaphylaxis (SRS-A) by arylsulfatases. *J. Immunol.*, **113**:316–322.

Orange, R. P., Murphy, R. C., Karnovsky, M. L., and Austen, K. F. (1973). The physiochemical characteristics and purification of slow-reacting substance of anaphylaxis. *J. Immunol.*, **110**:760–770.

Orange, R. P., Valentine, M. D., and Austen, K. F. (1968). Inhibition of the release of slow-reacting substance of anaphylaxis in the rat with diethylcarbamazine. *Proc. Soc. Exp. Biol. Med.*, **127**:127–132.

Orehek, J., Douglas, J. S., Lewis, A. J., and Bouhuys, A. (1973). Prostaglandin regulation of airway smooth muscle tone. *Nature, New Biol.*, **245**:84–85.

Palmer, M. A., Piper, P. J., and Vane, J. R. (1973). Release of rabbit aorta contracting substance (RCS) and prostaglandins induced by chemical or mechanical stimulation of guinea pig lungs. *Br. J. Pharmacol.*, **49**:226–242.

Parish, W. E. (1967). Release of histamine and slow reacting substance with mast cell changes after challenge of human lung sensitized passively with reagin in vitro. *Nature*, **215**:738–739.

Patterson, R., Fink, J. N., Nishimura, E. T., and Pruzansky, J. J. (1965). The passive transfer of immediate-type hypersensitivity from man to other primates. *J. Clin. Invest.*, **44**:140–148.

Patterson, R. and Kelly, J. F. (1973). Cellular and physiologic studies of immediate-type respiratory reactions. *Int. Arch. Allergy Appl. Immunol.*, **45**:98–109.

Patterson, R. and Talbot, C. H. (1969). Respiratory responses in subhuman primates with immediate-type hypersensitivity. *J. Lab. Clin. Med.*, **75**:924–933.

Patterson, R. and Talbot, C. H. (1972). A comparison of immediate-type respiratory reactions to immunologic and pharmacologic agents in rhesus monkeys. *J. Allergy Clin. Immunol.*, **49**:292–300.

Patterson, R., Talbot, C. H., and Booth, B. H. (1970). IgE mediated respiratory responses of subhuman primates. Reproducibility and effect of certain pharmacologic agents. *Am. Rev. Resp. Dis.*, **102**:412–421.

Piper, P. J. (1969). Release of catecholamines and other substances by antigen and mediators of the anaphylactic reaction. Ph.D. Thesis, University of London.

Piper, P. J. (1974). Release and metabolism of prostaglandins in lung tissue. *Pol. J. Pharmacol.*, **26**:61–72.

Piper, P. J., Collier, H. O. J., and Vane, J. R. (1967). Release of catecholamines in the guinea pig by substances involved in anaphylaxis. *Nature*, **213**:838–840.

Piper, P. J. and Vane, J. R. (1969a). The release of prostaglandins during anaphylaxis in guinea pig isolated lungs. In P. Mantegazza and E. W. Horton (eds.): *Prostaglandins, Peptides and Amines.* Academic Press, London, pp. 15–19.

Piper, P. J. and Vane, J. R. (1969b). Release of additional factors in anaphylaxis and its antagonism by anti-inflammatory drugs. *Nature*, **223**:29–35.

Piper, P. J. and Vane, J. R. (1971). The release of prostaglandins from lung and other tissues. *N. Y. Acad. Sci.*, **180**:363–385.

Piper, P. J., Vane, J. R., and Wyllie, J. H. (1970). Inactivation of prostaglandins by lungs. *Nature*, **225**:600–604.

Piper, P. J. and Walker, J. L. (1973). Release of spasmogenic substances from human chopped lung tissue and its inhibition. *Br. J. Pharmacol.*, **47**:291–304.

Rocha e Silva, M., Beraldo, W. T., and Rosenfeld, G. (1949). Bradykinin, a hypotensive and smooth muscle stimulating factor released from plasma globulin by snake venoms and by trypsin. *Am. J. Physiol.*, **156**:261–273.

Rosenthale, M. E., Dervinis, A., Begany, A. J., Lapidus, M., and Gluckman, M. I. (1970). Bronchodilator activity of prostaglandin E_2 when administered by aerosol to three species. *Experientia*, **26**:1119–1121.

Ruff, F., Dray, R., Santais, M.-C., Allouche, G., Foussard, C., Salem, A., and Parrot, J-L. (1975). Measurements of pulmonary prostaglandins, histamine and cyclic AMP during induced anaphylactic shock in guinea pig. In Proceedings of the Sixth International Congress of Pharmacology, Helsinki (Abstr 904).

Ryan, J. W., Niemeyer, R. S., and Ryan, U. (1975). Metabolism of prostaglandin $F_{1\alpha}$ in the pulmonary circulation. *Prostaglandins*, **10**:101–108.

Said, S. I., Yoshida, T., Kitamura, S., and Vreim, C. (1974). Pulmonary alveolar hypoxia: release of prostaglandins and other humoral mediators. *Science*, **185**:1181–1183.

Salazar-Mallen, M. (1965). Treatment of intractable asthma with diethylcarbamazine citrate. *Ann. Allergy*, **23**:534–537.

Sanyal, R. K. and West, G. B. (1958). The relationship of histamine and 5-hydroxytryptamine to anaphylactic shock in different species. *J. Physiol. (Lond.)*, **144**:525–531.

Schild, H. O. (1936). Histamine release and anaphylactic shock in isolated lungs of guinea pigs. *Q. J. Exp. Physiol.*, **26**:165–179.

Schild, H. O. (1968). Mechanism of anaphylactic histamine release. In K. F. Austen and E. L. Becker (eds.): Biochemistry of the acute allergic reaction. Blackwell, Oxford, pp. 99–118.

Schild, H. O., Hawkins, D. F., Mongar, J. L., and Herxheimer, H. (1951). Reactions of isolated human asthmatic lung and bronchial tissue to a specific antigen. Histamine release and muscular contraction. *Lancet*, **2**:376–382.

Schultz, W. H. and Jordan, H. E. (1911). Physiological studies in anaphylaxis — a microscopic study of the anaphylactic lungs of the guinea pig and mouse. *J. Pharmacol. Exp. Ther.*, **2**:375–389.

Sheard, P. and Blair, A. M. J. N. (1970). Disodium cromoglycate: activity in three in vitro models of the immediate hypersensitivity in lung. *Int. Arch. Allergy Appl. Immunol.*, **38**:217–224.

Sheard, P., Killingback, P. G., and Blair, A. M. J. N. (1967). Antigen induced release of histamine and SRS-A from human lung passively sensitized with reaginic serum. *Nature*, **216**:283–284.

Sheffer, A. L. (1973). Treatment of anaphylaxis. *Postgrad. Med.*, **53**:62–66.

Sly, R. M. and Matzen, K. (1974). Effect of diethylcarbamazine pamoate upon exercise-induced obstruction in asthmatic children. *Ann. Allergy*, **33**:138–144.

Smith, A. P. (1974). A comparison of the effects of prostaglandin E_2 and

salbutamol by intravenous infusion on the airways obstruction of patients
with asthma. *Br. J. Clin. Pharmacol.*, **1**:399–404.

Smith, A. P. and Cuthbert, M. F. (1973). Effects of inhaled prostaglandins on
bronchial tone in man. In S. Bergström and S. Bernhard (eds.): *Advances
in the Biosciences*, vol. 9. Pergamon Press Vieweg, Braunschweig, pp. 213–
217.

Smith, A. P. and Dunlop, L. (1975). Prostaglandins and asthma. *Lancet*, **1**:39.

Staszewska-Barczak, J. and Vane, J. R. (1967). The release of catecholamines
from the adrenal medulla by peptides. *Br. J. Pharmacol. Chemother.*, **30**:
655–667.

Stechschulte, D. J., Austen, K. F., and Block, K. J. (1967). Antibodies involved
in antigen-induced release of slow-reacting substance of anaphylaxis (SRS-
A) in the guinea pig and rat. *J. Exp. Med.*, **125**:127–147.

Stechschulte, D. J., Orange, R. P., and Austen, K. F. (1973). Detection of slow-
reacting substance of anaphylaxis (SRS-A) in plasma of guinea pigs during
anaphylaxis. *J. Immunol.*, **111**:1585–1589.

Strandberg, K. (1973). Inhibition of histamine release and formation of slow
reacting substance by poly-phloretin phosphate. *Acta Pharmacol. Toxicol.*,
32:33–45.

Strandberg, K. and Hamberg, M. (1974). Increased excretion of 5α, 7α-dihydroxy-
11-keto tetranor-prostanoic acid on anaphylaxis in the guinea pig. *Prostaglandins*, **6**:159–170.

Sutherland, E. W. and Robison, G. A. (1966). The role of cyclic 3', 5'-AMP in
response to catecholamines and other hormones. *Pharmacol. Rev.*, **18**:
145–161.

Sweatman, W. J. F. and Collier, H. O. J. (1968). Effects of PGs on human
bronchial muscle. *Nature*, **217**:69.

Tauber, A. I., Kaliner, M., Stechschulte, D. J., and Austen, K. F. (1973). Immunologic release of histamine and slow reacting substance of anaphylaxis
from human lung. V. Effects of prostaglandins on release of histamine.
J. Immunol., **111**:27–32.

Trendelenberg, U. (1966). Observations on the ganglion-stimulating action of
angiotensin and bradykinin. *J. Pharmacol. Exp. Ther.*, **154**:418–425.

Trethewie, E. R. (1958). Cortisone and anaphylaxis. *Austr. J. Exp. Biol.*, **36**:
275–284.

Turker, R. K. (1973). Presence of histamine H_2-receptors in the guinea pig pulmonary vascular bed. *Pharmacology*, **9**:306–311.

Uvnäs, B. (1974). The molecular basis for the storage and release of histamine
in rat mast cell granules. *Life Sci.*, **14**:2355–2365.

Vane, J. R. (1969). Release and fate of vasoactive hormones in the circulation.
Br. J. Pharmacol., **35**:209–243.

Vane, J. R. (1971). Inhibition of prostaglandin synthesis as a mechanism of
action for aspirin-like drugs. *Nature, New Biol.*, **231**:232–235.

Vargaftig, B. B. and Dao Hai, N. (1972). Interference of thiol derivatives with
the pharmacological effects of arachidonic acid and slow reacting substance and with the release of rabbit aorta contracting substances. *Eur. J.
Pharmacol.*, **18**:43–55.

Villanueva, R., Hinds, L., Katz, R. L., and Eakins, K. E. (1972). The effect of polyphloretin phosphate on some smooth muscle actions of prostaglandins in the cat. *J. Pharmacol. Exp. Ther.,* **180**:78–84.

Walker, J. L. (1973). The regulatory role of prostaglandins in the release of histamine and SRS-A from passively sensitized human lung tissue. In S. Bergstrom and S. Bernhard (eds.): Advances in the Biosciences, vol. 9. Pergamon Press, Vieweg, Braunschweig, pp. 235–239.

Wasserman, S. I., Goetzl, E. J., and Austen, K. F. (1974a). Preformed eosinophil chemotactic factor of anaphylaxis. *J. Immunol.,* **112**:351–378.

Wasserman, S. I., Goetzl, E. J., Kaliner, M., and Austen, K. F. (1974b). Modulation of the immunological release of the eosinophil chemotactic factor of anaphylaxis from human lung. *Immunology,* **26**:677–684.

Watanabe, K. (1931). Quantitative Untersuchungen über den Gehalt an darmkontrahierenden Stoffen von Lunge und Leber bei Meerschweinchen in Stadium der Eiweisssensibilisierung und in anaphylaktischen Schock. *Z. Immunol. Forsch. Exp. Ther.,* **72**:50–56.

Webster, Marion E., Takahashi, H., and Newball, H. H. (1975). SRS-A (slow reacting substance of anaphylaxis) from human lung: its purification and separation into four active fractions. Proceedings of the Sixth International Congress of Pharmacology, Helsinki, 1975 (abstr. 905).

Widdicombe, J. G. (1963). Regulation of tracheobronchial smooth muscle. *Physiol. Rev.,* **43**:1–37.

Williams, T. J. and Morley, J. (1973). Prostaglandins as potentiators of increased vascular permeability in inflammation. *Nature,* **246**:215–217.

10

Release Induced by Physical and Chemical Stimuli

SAMI I. SAID

University of Texas Southwestern Medical School
and Veterans Administration Hospital,
Dallas, Texas

I.   Introduction

It has been known for some time that the lung may, under certain conditions, release biologically active substances (Said 1968, Vane 1969). Except in anaphylaxis, however, this phenomenon, and its possible role in the pathogenesis of pulmonary or other disorders, has only recently been systematically investigated.

Evidence for the release of biologically active compounds from the lung has, in large measure, been derived from experiments on animals or in vitro and has been based on bioassay or on the use of pharmacologic antagonists and metabolic inhibitors. Confirmation of this release, therefore, and assessment of its importance in humans, is frequently lacking. Also, in many instances the identities and concentrations of released agents remain to be established by more specific and precise techniques.

Supported in part by a Lung Center Award (HL-14187) from the National Heart and Lung Institute, N.I.H.

It must be noted, further, that the release of active substances, as measured in many experiments, represents a balance between two sets of reactions: (a) de novo synthesis followed by discharge of these substances, and (b) their removal or inactivation by the lung.

II. Methods for Detection and Assay of Released Substances

Much of the data on the pulmonary release of biologically active substances has been acquired through bioassay techniques. In one such technique (Gaddum 1953, Vane 1964, 1968, 1969), which has proved especially valuable, a series of sensitive smooth muscle organs, attached to transducers, are superfused with physiologic salt solutions (Fig. 1). The addition of biologically

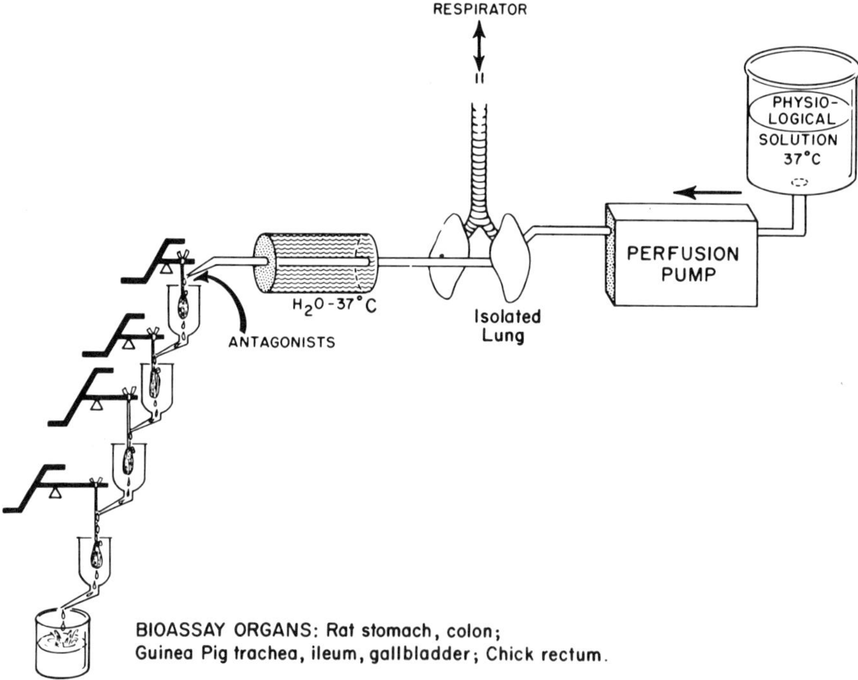

FIGURE 1   Schema for bioassay of lung perfusate, using the superfusion technique. Cat lung is isolated and perfused in situ, at constant flow, with physiologic solution at 37°C. Perfusate is rewarmed and pumped onto isolated smooth muscle organs, placed in series. Lung may be ventilated mechanically at different tidal volumes, using different gas mixtures.

active substances to the superfusing solution is detected by the responses of assay organs, and the approximate concentration of a given humoral agent is estimated by comparing the response it elicits with that elicited by standard reference solutions of known concentrations. Selection of assay organs depends on the substance being sought. The specificity of their responses may be enhanced by pretreating them with appropriate antagonists or inhibitors (Fig. 2; See also Vane 1969). This technique is equally applicable for the analysis of "spot" samples, as for the continuous assay of a perfusate from an isolated lung or a stream of blood from a living animal. Other advantages of this method are its relative simplicity, sensitivity, and the promptness with which results may be gathered and conclusions reached. Its main drawback is that it can permit only a tentative identification based on one type of biologic action, i.e., the contraction or relaxation of certain smooth muscles. Other limitations of this method are that it is semiquantitative and insensitive to released substances, if these are inactive on smooth muscle organs selected for the assay or mediators are released locally as *tissue hormones*, without being discharged into the perfusate or other external medium.

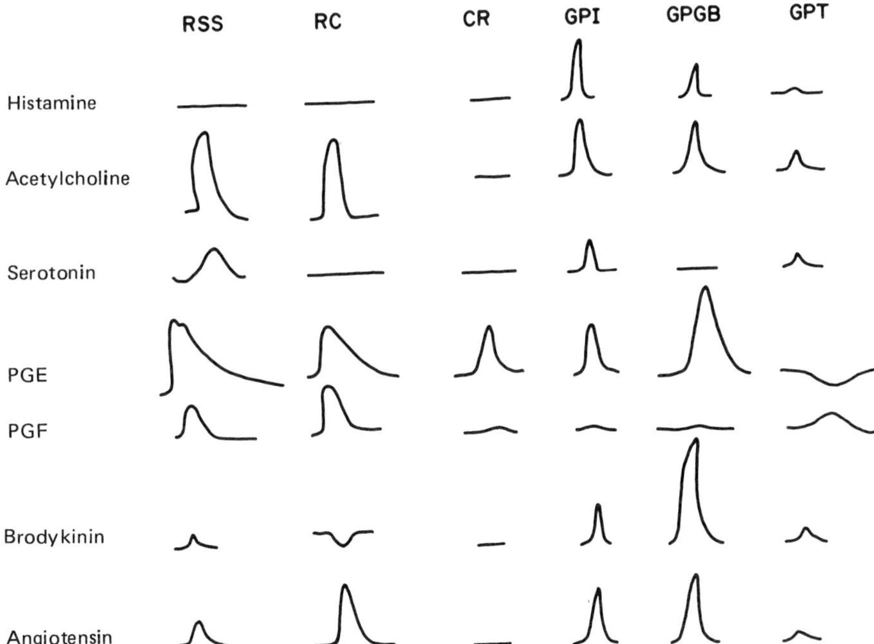

FIGURE 2 Characteristic responses of smooth muscle organs to various biologically active substances. RSS = rat stomach strip, RC = rat colon, CR = chick rectum, GPI = guinea pig ileum, GPGB = guinea pig gallbladder, GPT = guinea pig trachea. (Reprinted by permission from Said (1974). *Amer. J. Med.,* **57**:433–465).

Another important approach to the investigation of release of humoral agents from the lung has been the use of inhibitors of biosynthesis of these agents. This approach is based on the premise that, at least for the prostaglandins (PGs), their release from the lung follows stimulation of their biosynthesis, rather than their discharge from stores. Thus, if the biosynthesis of PGs is prevented, none could be released (Vane 1971). The discovery that aspirin and indomethacin can inhibit the biosynthesis of PGs in many systems (Vane 1971) has thus provided a valuable tool in exploring the occurrence, magnitude, and impact of PG synthesis and release (Robinson and Vane 1974).

III. Biologically Active Substances Released from Lung

It is possible that any substance the lung is capable of storing or synthesizing may, under certain conditions, be released into the bloodstream. Active substances whose release from the lung has been demonstrated or, at least, suspected include: biogenic amines, polypeptides, proteins, lipids, and other compounds that remain incompletely identified (Tables 1 and 2). Most of these substances are discussed in detail either elsewhere in this volume, or in recent publications, some of which are referred to in the tables. A few of the more newly identified or characterized substances are here briefly reviewed.

TABLE 1 Biologically Active Substances that may be Released from the Lung in Conditions other than Anaphylaxis

A. Biogenic Amines
 1. Histamine
 2. 5-hydroxytryptamine (serotonin)

B. Polypeptides
 1. ACTH, ADH and other polypeptide hormones (please refer to Table 2)
 2. Other, incompletely identified polypeptides, e.g., vasoactive lung peptides and renally active "lung substance" (LS)

C. Proteins
 1. Kallikrein and other proteolytic enzymes
 2. Other proteins, e.g., clotting and fibrinolytic factors

D. Lipids
 1. Prostaglandins (PGs), intermediate and PG-like compounds
 2. Rabbit aorta contracting substance (RCS)
 3. Slow reacting substance (SRS)

TABLE 2 Polypeptide Hormone Secretion in Pulmonary Disease: Resultant Syndromes and Commonly Associated Lesions*

Hormone	Syndrome	Lesion
ACTH	Hypokalemic alkalosis, edema, Cushing's syndrome	Oat cell carcinoma, adenoma
ADH (arginine vasopressin)	Hyponatremia (SIADH)	Oat cell carcinoma, adenoma, tuberculosis, pneumonia, aspergillosis
PTH or related peptide	Hypercalcemia	Squamous cell, adenocarcinoma and large-cell undifferentiated carcinoma
Gonadotropins	Gynecomastia (adults), precocious puberty (children)	Large cell anaplastic carcinoma
Calcitonin	No clinical findings	Adenocarcinoma, squamous and oat cell carcinoma
VIP or related peptide	Watery diarrhea or no symptoms	Squamous, large or oat cell carcinoma
? Growth hormone	Hypertrophic osteoarthropathy	Squamous cell carcinoma
Serotonin, kinins (and PGs, other)	"Carcinoid"	Bronchial adenoma, oat cell carcinoma
Insulin-like peptide	Hypoglycemia	Mesenchymal cell tumors
Glucagon or related peptide	Hyperglycemia	Fibrosarcoma
Prolactin	Galactorrhea (or no symptoms)	Anaplastic cell carcinoma
Combinations of above	Multiple syndromes	Anaplastic cell carcinoma

[a] Abbreviations: ACTH = adrenocorticotrophic hormone; SIADH = syndrome of inappropriate secretion of antidiuretic hormone; PTH = parathyroid hormone; PGs = prostaglandins; VIP = vasoactive intestinal polypeptide.
[b] For additional reading, please see: Lipsett 1968, Hall (Editor) 1974, References in Said 1974. More recent references: calcitonin (Becker et al. 1975), VIP (Said and Faloona 1975).

A.   Rabbit Aorta Contracting Substance (RCS)

Released from the lung by a variety of immunologic, mechanical, and chemical stimuli, this substance contracts not only rabbit aorta (Piper and Vane 1969) but also other vascular tissues, including pulmonary and systemic arteries and veins from several species (Palmer et al. 1973) and human bronchial smooth muscle (Piper and Walker 1973). The smooth muscle actions of RCS are not prevented by antagonists of histamine, 5-hydroxytryptamine, adrenergic or cholinergic stimulants, but its release may be prevented by aspirin or indomethacin. The latter finding led to the speculation that RCS may be a precursor or an intermediate in the biosynthesis of PGs (Gryglewski and Vane 1971, 1972), but recent evidence suggests that RCS is a nonprostaglandin product of the endoperoxide intermediates which is related to thromboxane A_2 (Samuelsson and Hamberg 1974, and Hamberg et al. 1975). RCS has a short ($<$2-min) biologic half-life (Palmer et al. 1973).

B.   Vasoactive Lung Polypeptides

Normal lung has been found to contain at least two vasoactive polypeptides, which are also active on extravascular smooth muscle (Said et al. 1975). Both peptides, which have been partially purified from hog lungs, dilate systemic vessels, but one contracts and the other relaxes various smooth muscles, including rat stomach strip, rat colon, guinea pig trachea, guinea pig gallbladder, and chick rectum. The chemical compositions of these peptides remain to be determined, but cross-immunoreactivity between lung peptide fractions and the vasoactive intestinal polypeptide (VIP) (Said and Mutt 1970), suggests a degree of structural similarity between the relaxant lung peptide and the recently isolated vasoactive intestinal peptide (Said and Mutt, unpublished observations).

C.   Renally Active Lung Substance

A lung substance (LS), believed to be a peptide, acts on the kidney to promote sodium and water retention, without affecting total renal blood flow (Lockett 1971). Thought to be formed through the action of lung on a plasma globulin, LS has been demonstrated in lung tissue and in arterial blood, but not in perfusate from isolated lung perfused with Tyrode solution (Lockett 1972).

IV. Experimental Conditions Associated with Pulmonary Release of Biologically Active Agents

A. Mechanical Stimulation

Stroking of Lung Surface and Stirring of Lung Fragments

Piper and Vane (1971) found that gentle stroking or massaging of the external surface of isolated, perfused guinea pig lungs (sensitized or unsensitized) led to the appearance, in the perfusate, of PGs, rabbit aorta contracting substance (RCS), and histamine. The force used to stroke the lung was equivalent to a weight of 30 to 40 g on a balance. This observation led these investigators to examine the release of spasmogens from chopped lung tissue. They found that when suspensions of chopped guinea pig lung (either sensitized or unsensitized) were stirred with a nylon rod for 5 to 6 min, a mixture of smooth muscle contracting substances, including histamine, PGs E_2, $F_{2\alpha}$, and RCS appeared in the medium. A similar release could be demonstrated when stirring was repeated once again, but the concentrations of released materials decreased with further attempts. In a later report, Piper and Walker (1973) described the release of a similar mixture of spasmogenic substances following mechanical agitation of chopped human lung tissue.

Hyperinflation of Isolated Lungs

The above observations provided the first suggestion that more physiologic forms of physical stimulation of the lung, such as stretching by hyperinflation, also may provoke the release of active agents. This possibility was tested in the isolated lung of dog and later in the intact animal. In the former preparation, dog lungs were mechanically ventilated with 5% CO_2 in O_2, and perfused at constant flow with Krebs solution (Said et al. 1972). The perfusate continually superfused strips of rat stomach and rat colon, which had been rendered insensitive to catecholamines, histamine, serotonin (5-hydroxytryptamine), and acetylcholine. During control ventilation, there was no evidence of spasmogenic activity in the perfusate. On increasing tidal volume by 50% to 100%, while maintaining the same minute ventilation and effluent pH, both smooth muscle strips contracted (Fig. 3). The contractions began within 2 min of increasing the tidal volume, correlated with breath size, and were consistent with the liberation of PGs E and F into the perfusate, in concentra-

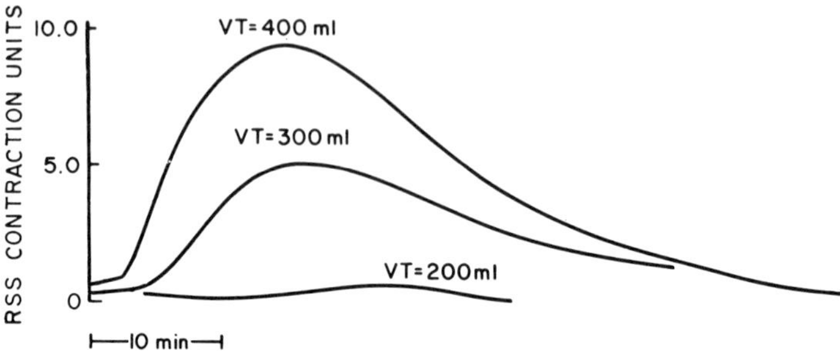

FIGURE 3   Contraction of rat stomach strip (RSS) in response to increasing tidal volume (VT) of isolated, perfused dog lung; evidence for release of PGs from lung during deeper breathing (Said et al. 1974a, reprinted from Ann. N.Y. Acad. Sci.).

tions of up to 150 ng/min (measured as PGE_1 equivalents) (Said et al. 1974a). Simultaneously, the perfusion pressure of the lung decreased, reflecting pulmonary vasodilation. After aspirin (1 mg) was infused into the pulmonary circulation, the hyperinflations no longer resulted in contraction of the smooth muscle organs (Fig. 4) or decrease in pulmonary perfusion pressure (Fig. 5). These findings suggested that stretching of the lung was capable of

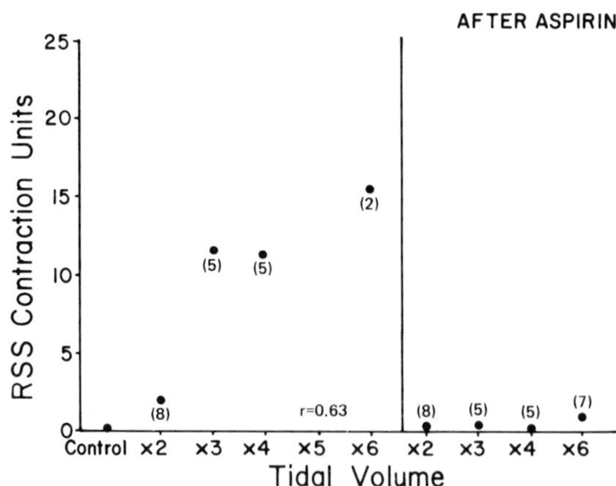

FIGURE 4   Release of PGs from lung and its prevention by aspirin. Contraction of rat stomach strip (RSS) in response to increasing tidal volume of isolated perfused dog lungs. Numbers in parentheses refer to the number of experiments. To right, same data after infusion of aspirin.

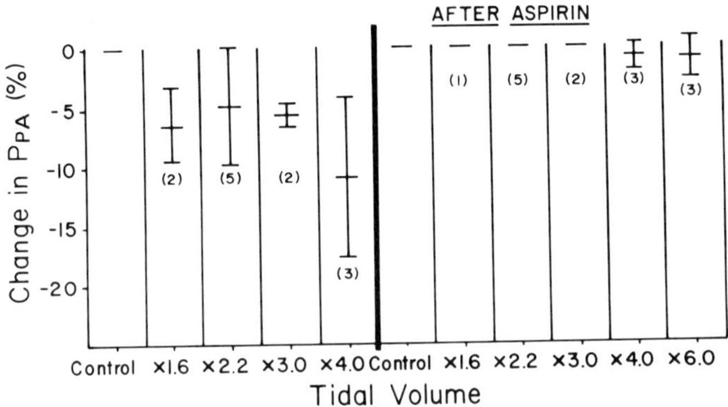

FIGURE 5   Fall in pulmonary arterial pressure P_{PA} (as percent of control values) with increasing tidal volume, before and after aspirin. Isolated dog lungs were perfused at constant flow. Numbers of experiments are given in parentheses.

provoking increased pulmonary synthesis of vasodilator PG-like compounds (and possibly other active substances), and their subsequent release into the circulation (Said et al. 1972). Similar conclusions were reached by Berry et al. (1971), in isolated guinea pig and rat lungs.

Hyperinflation and Hyperventilation In Vivo

Could a similar release of vasodilator PGs occur in the whole animal? If so, could it contribute to the systemic hypotension that frequently complicates mechanical ventilation at large tidal volumes? These questions were investigated in open-chested dogs, which were anesthetized with pentobarbital, paralyzed with succinylcholine, and mechanically ventilated (Said 1973, Kitamura et al. 1973). Following a control period of normal ventilation, tidal volume was increased fivefold and kept at that level for 5 min, without changing the frequency of respiration, before returning to normal ventilation. In order to separate the effects of hyperinflation alone from those of resultant respiratory alkalosis, the increased ventilation was carried out with two different inspired mixtures: air alone, and air to which was added 5% CO_2. Arterial blood pressure and cardiac output were monitored throughout these experiments. Hyperinflation with air was accompanied by severe hypocapnia (arterial blood P_{CO_2} fell from 41 to 15 mm Hg) and respiratory alkalosis (pH increased from 7.32 to 7.52). With the addition of CO_2 to the inspired air, however, arterial P_{CO_2} and pH remained unaltered during the increased ventilation. When hyperventilation was accompanied by respiratory alkalosis, mean arterial blood pressure fell by 32 (±18)% (Fig. 6). During hyperinflation alone, in the absence of respiratory alkalosis, the fall in blood pressure in the same animals was 13% (±12) of control value ($P < 0.001$). Simultaneously, cardiac output did not change significantly during hyperventilation, with or without supplemental CO_2. If these animals were pretreated with aspirin (30 mg/kg in saline, infused intravenously), the fall in blood pressure was reduced to 18% (±10) in the presence of respiratory alkalosis (reduction significant at $P < 0.02$), and to 8% (±5) without respiratory alkalosis. This group of experiments provided evidence that: (a) the systemic hypotension complicating mechanical hyperventilation is attributable in large measure to the release of vasodilator agents; (b) this release is greater in the presence of respiratory alkalosis than in its absence; and (c) the responsible vasodilator substances probably include PGs (possibly PGEs) or PG-like compounds (Kitamura et al. 1973, Said 1974).

Pulmonary Embolism

It has been suspected for some time that pulmonary embolism may be associated with the release of humoral mediators from the lung. This impression has been based largely on circumstantial and indirect evidence, such as: (a) the apparent inadequacy of mechanical obstruction and superimposed vagal re-

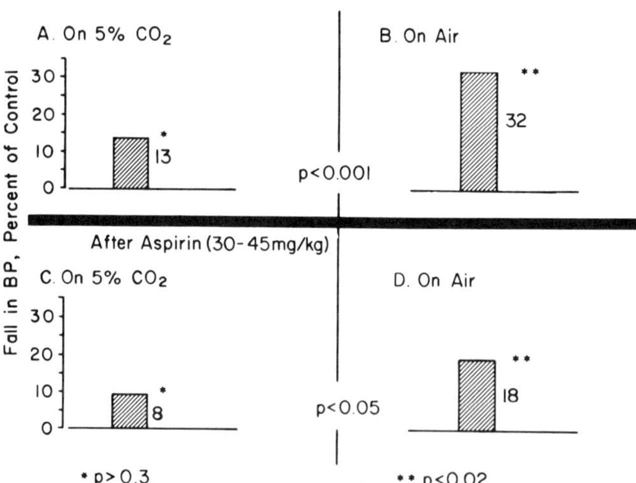

FIGURE 6   Fall in mean arterial blood pressure (BP) of anesthetized dogs during hyperinflation. Bars represent mean values in 7 dogs. Tidal volume was increased fivefold using 5% CO_2 in air (*upper left* (a) or air alone (*upper right* (b). Data after infusion of aspirin (30 to 45 mg/kg) are shown below.

flexes to account fully for pulmonary and systemic manifestations of pulmonary embolism (Smith and Smith 1955, Swedenborg 1971); (b) the capacity of certain humoral agents, including histamine and 5-HT, to mimic some of the vascular and airway changes seen in this condition (Comroe et al. 1953); (c) the reduction in the magnitude of these changes with pharmacologic agents that inhibit the actions of histamine and 5-HT, or deplete their tissue stores (Nadel et al. 1964, Gurewich et al. 1968); and (d) the transmission of cardio-respiratory effects of embolism in one animal to another by means of cross-circulation (Halmagyi et al. 1964). Despite evidence suggesting that both of these amines may be released following pulmonary embolism, their contributions to the pathogenesis of this condition remain uncertain (Stone and Nemir 1960, Marshall 1966, Puckett et al. 1973). The 5-HT released in this condition is probably derived largely from platelet aggregates acting as microemboli (Stein and Thomas 1967), though lung tissue of some animal species (e.g., rat, rabbit and mouse) contains relatively high concentrations of this biogenic amine (Weissbach et al. 1957).

More recently, the superfusion technique for bioassay has enabled investigators to obtain more direct evidence for the release of vasoactive substances after embolization of pulmonary vessels with a variety of particulate matter. Lindsey and Wyllie (1970), embolizing isolated lungs of guinea pigs and rats with particles ranging in size from 1 to 120 mμ in diameter, including fat emulsions, microspheres, and colloidal substances, found evidence for the release of PGE_2, even when the lungs were perfused with platelet-free solutions. Palmer et al. (1973), using the same experimental preparation, detected the release, not only of PGs but also of RCS and, possibly in some instances, histamine. An increase in lung weight accompanied the release of PGs, suggesting the concomitant development of pulmonary edema. In the latter experiments, the lungs had been previously sensitized to ovalbumin, so that the magnitude of the release of humoral agents could be compared with that induced by anaphylaxis. The release recurred when the embolization was repeated at least twice, but was always less intense than antigen-induced release (Piper and Vane 1971).

Additional, indirect evidence that PGs or related compounds may contribute to the mediation of the effects of pulmonary embolism has come from the use of inhibitors of PG synthesis. Rådegran and his colleagues (Rådegran 1972, Rådegran et al. 1971, 1972) found that pretreating anesthetized dogs with aspirin prevented the rise in pulmonary vascular and airway pressures that otherwise followed thrombin- or protamine-induced platelet aggregation in pulmonary vessels, without preventing the platelets from aggregating. Similarly, aspirin abolished the pulmonary hypertension caused by endotoxin-induced microembolization (Greenway and Murthy 1971), and the increase in airway pressure following barium sulfate microembolism (Nakano and McCloy 1973).

Pulmonary Edema

Pulmonary edema is a serious complication that may occur during the course
of a large variety of clinical disorders. Several vasoactive substances (e.g.,
histamine, bradykinin, epinephrine) are capable of causing pulmonary edema,
but the release of such active agents from the lung during, or as a result of,
this condition has been inadequately examined. Said and Yoshida (1974)
showed that following the induction of edema in isolated, perfused cat lungs,
perfusates and foam exhibited spasmogenic activity consistent with the presence of PGE_2 and $PGF_{2\alpha}$, and other unidentified materials. In more recent
experiments airway fluid and foam were extracted for PGs; thin layer chromatography of these extracts and bioassay of portions corresponding to PGE_2
and $PGF_{2\alpha}$ confirmed the presence of these compounds in concentrations of
up to 14 ng/ml of foam (Chijimatsu et al., unpublished observations). Using a
radioimmunoassay in which antibodies to VIP cross-react with one of the newly identified vasoactive lung peptides, Hara et al. (unpublished observations),
have found evidence for the presence of the spasmogenic lung peptide in foam
and perfusates from edematous cat lungs.

B.   Chemical Stimulation

Alveolar Hypoxia

Students of pulmonary physiology have long known that alveolar hypoxia induces pulmonary vasoconstriction, but the mechanism of this response has remained incompletely understood. In recent years several lines of evidence
have pointed to the likelihood that hypoxic pulmonary vasoconstriction depends on a metabolic reaction in the lung, which may include the release of
vasoactive mediators. This evidence includes (a) the failure of hypoxia to con-
strict pulmonary vessels in vitro when these vessels are stripped of all lung
tissue (Lloyd 1968); (b) the attenuation of the hypoxic pressor response with
cooling of the lung to $27°C$ (Hauge 1970); and (c) the degranulation during
hypoxic ventilation of pulmonary mast cells (Haas and Bergofsky 1972) and
neuroepithelial bodies (Lauweryns and Cokelaere 1973; Fig. 7), cellular elements that store a variety of vasoactive substances, especially histamine and
5-hydroxytryptamine (serotonin), respectively.

More direct evidence for the release of biologically active compounds
from the lung during hypoxia was derived from the assay of lung perfusates by
the superfused smooth muscle organ technique. In these experiments isolated
cat lungs were ventilated with either 21% O_2 − 5% CO_2 or 2% O_2 − 5% CO_2,
and were perfused with physiologic solutions, with or without blood. The
perfusate was continually assayed on a series of isolated, superfused smooth

muscle organs. Ventilation with the hypoxic gas mixture was followed by a rise in pulmonary vascular resistance, and the appearance in the perfusates, in 20 of 24 experiments, of biologically active substances (Fig. 8; Said et al. 1974b). These substances caused the contraction of one or more of these organs: guinea pig trachea, guinea pig gallbladder, rat stomach strip, rat colon, guinea pig ileum, and chick rectum. The contractions occurred even if the assay tissues had been pretreated with antagonists of histamine, 5-HT, and adrenergic and cholinergic agonists. These findings were consistent with the possibility that the vasoactive agents released during hypoxia may include PGs or PG-like substances (Said et al. 1974b).

In another group of 26 experiments in 6 anesthetized cats, infusions of aspirin ($>$ 50 mg/kg) were found to reduce by 52% the rise in pulmonary vascular resistance associated with breathing 8.7% O_2 (Said et al. 1975b; Fig. 9). The protection afforded by aspirin was dose related (Fig. 10). Though incomplete, it supported the conclusion that PGs, or related compounds (possibly including RCS), are among the mediators of the pulmonary pressor response to hypoxia, at least in the cat.

The role of PGs in the mediation of hypoxic pulmonary hypertension remains, nevertheless, unsettled. For example, indomethacin, another and usually more potent inhibitor of PG synthesis, did not have the protective effect of aspirin against hypoxic pulmonary vasoconstriction in cats or dogs, though it reduced the pulmonary arterial pressure both during air and hypoxic ventilation (Fig. 11; Said 1975b). Precise measurement of the concentrations of PGs in blood entering and leaving the lung has been limited by imperfections in the radioimmunoassay and the complexity of the chemical assay. Further, intermediate compounds in the biosynthesis of PGs, e.g., the cyclic endoperoxides, and other products that may be formed, for instance, thromboxanes are not measurable by some assays but have considerable biologic activity, often surpassing that of the PGs themselves (Samuelsson and Hamberg 1974).

Regardless of the final verdict on the role of PGs in the mediation of hypoxic pulmonary hypertension, it seems likely that additional vasoactive substances may participate in this response. Besides 5-HT, histamine, and PG-like compounds, newly identified vasoactive lung peptides are possibly among these mediators. One of these, the spasmogenic peptide, has smooth muscle contracting activity closely resembling that of the PGs, and its presence in lung perfusates could be mistaken for PGs on bioassay (Said et al. 1975a).

*Biogenic Amines, Peptides
and Other Chemical Influences*

There are several reports of one vasoactive substance provoking the release of another, during passage through the pulmonary circulation. For example,

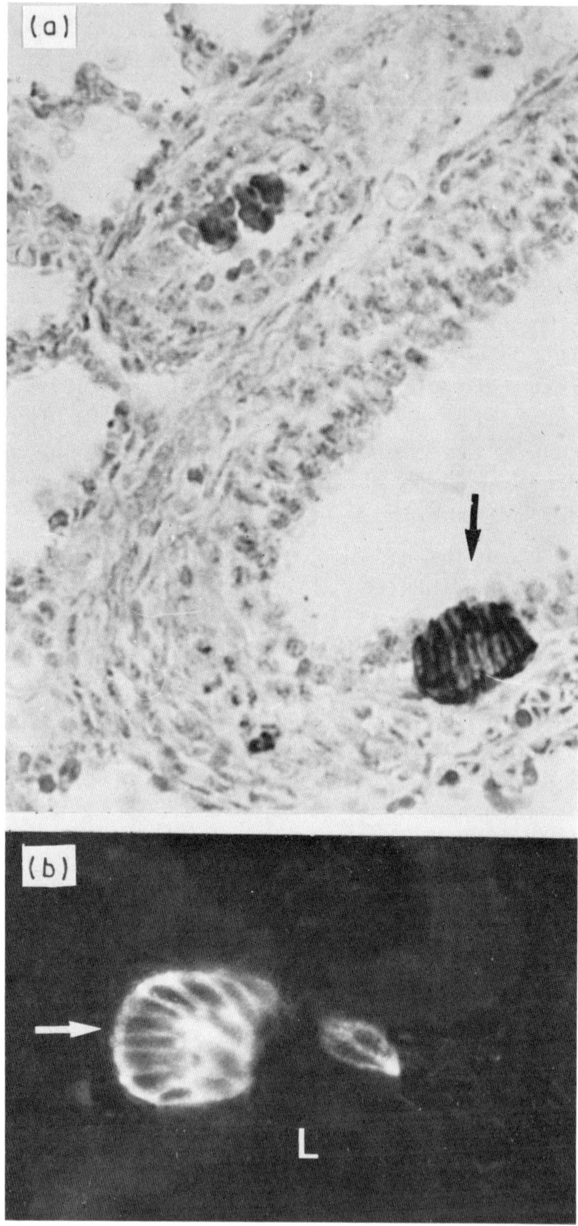

FIGURE 7 (a) Neuroepithelial body (arrow), exhibiting distinct argyrophilia, located within the bronchial mucosa. Neonatal rabbit lung; Van Campenhout's modification of Bodian's technique (magnification ×557). Besides this promi-

5-HT infused in relatively large concentrations (0.05 to 1 μg/ml) into the pulmonary artery of isolated lung from rats or dogs, stimulated the release from the lung of PG-like materials, a *slow-reacting substance* (causing contraction of guinea pig ileum, that is not blocked by mepyramine or atropine) and other active substances (Alabaster and Bakhle 1970, 1976). Infusions of tryptamine (0.5 to 2 μg/ml) had a similar releasing effect. This release by the tryptamines could be antagonized by methysergide, but was not dose-related once a threshold had been reached (Bakhle and Smith 1974). Tyramine and β-phenylethylamine, decarboxylation products of the amino acids l-tyrosine and l-phenylalanine, respectively, given in higher concentrations (10 to 100 μg/ml), also released PG-like substances and a slow-reacting substance from isolated, cat and dog lungs (Bakhle and Smith 1972).

Acetylcholine (0.5 to 1 μg/ml) also has been reported to induce the release of PG-like materials and a slow-reacting substance (Alabaster and Bakhle 1976). Bradykinin, in large doses (10 μg), was found to cause the release of RCS (Piper and Vane 1969, Vargaftig and Dao Hai 1972). Other examples of biologically active substances released by other active agents are RCS and PGE by dihomo-γ-linolenic and arachidonic acids (Palmer et al. 1973), and of RCS by *slow-reacting substance C* and arachidonic acid (Vargaftig and Dao Hai 1971) and by a releasing factor (RCS-RF) found in the effluent from shocked lungs (Piper and Vane 1969).

An additional chemical stimulus to PG release from the lung is respiratory alkalosis, discussed earlier in conjunction with hyperventilation. No data are available on the possible influence of other disturbances in acid-base balance and pH.

Norepinephrine and angiotensin I and II have been shown to release PGs from the kidney. Whether such release is specific to the kidney or may also

---

FIGURE 7 (continued)
nent cytoplasmic argyrophilia, the corpuscular cells display a less pronounced argentaffinity and react positively with α-glycerophosphate dehydrogenase, acetylcholinesterase and Solcia's lead hematoxylin stain for endocrine cells producing polypeptides and amines. (b) Cytoplasmic fluorescence (arrow) of a neuroepithelial body, showing also a small cut on the opposite side of the bronchus (B); L = bronchial lumen. Neonatal rabbit lung; specimen treated with Falck's freeze-drying and fluorescent amine technique, section studied with uv light alone (magnification ×747). Examined with this technique, fluorescence is yellow; microspectrographically, the fluorescence is maximal at 530 nm, corresponding to emission spectrum of serotonin and of colonic enterochromaffin cells. (Both figures courtesy of Professor Joseph M. Lauweryns, University of Leuven, Belgium. Reprinted from Said, S. I. (1974). *Am. J. Med,* 57:433–465.)

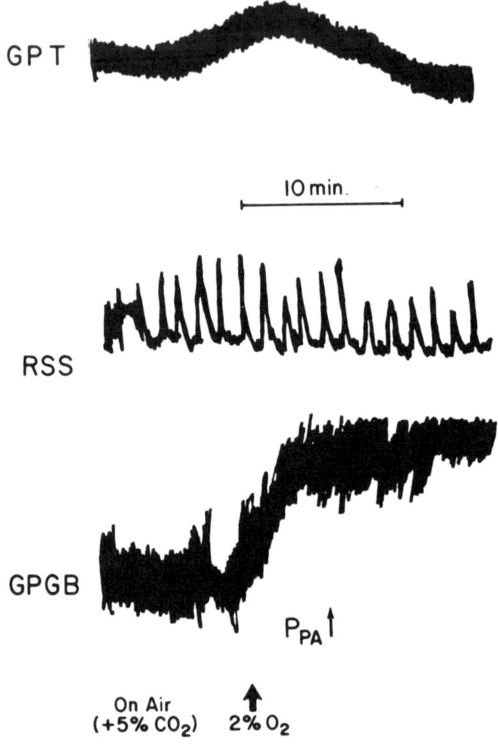

FIGURE 8   Release of biologically active substances from cat perfused lung during hypoxia. Contraction of guinea pig trachea (GPT) and guinea pig gallbladder (GPGB), superfused with lung effluent, on switching inspired gas from air plus 5% CO_2 to 2% O_2 plus 5% CO_2. These tissues were not treated with antagonists. Arrow labeled P_{PA} indicates point when pulmonary arterial pressure rose. RSS is rat stomach strip.

occur in the lung, is at present unknown. On the other hand, catecholamines may inhibit the release of PGs and their metabolites from the lung (Mathé and Levine 1973).

Stoner and associates (1973) have recently suggested that the stimulant action of bradykinin, acetylcholine, histamine, and, perhaps, other agents, on PG synthesis and release by the lung may be achieved through an increase in cellular levels of 3':5'-guanosine monophosphate (cyclic GMP). The authors reason that the enhanced PG production could serve an adaptive role similar to a compensatory increase in 3':5'-adenosine monophosphate (cyclic AMP).

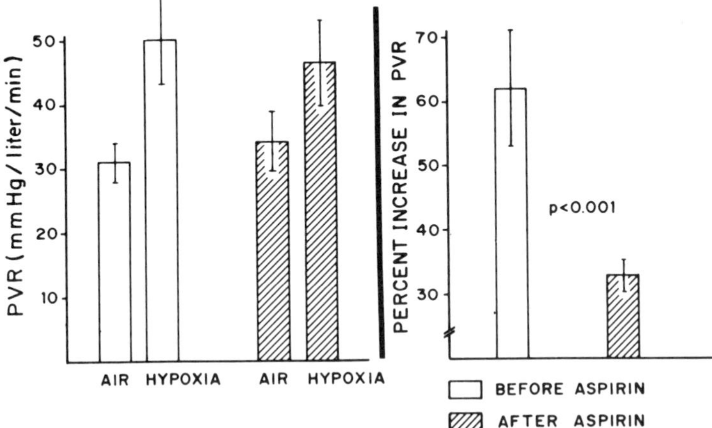

FIGURE 9　Rise in pulmonary vascular resistance (PVR) during hypoxic ventilation before (blank) and after aspirin (shaded). Figure shows means and ± SE of data from 17 cats. Percent increase in PVR is shown to right.

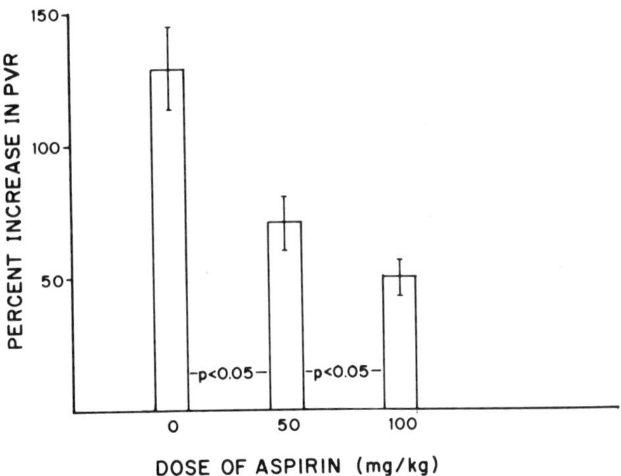

FIGURE 10　Dose-related inhibition by aspirin of hypoxic pulmonary pressor response (PPR) in cats. Plot shows percent increase in pulmonary vascular resistance (PVR) with hypoxic breathing. These tissues were not treated with antagonists.

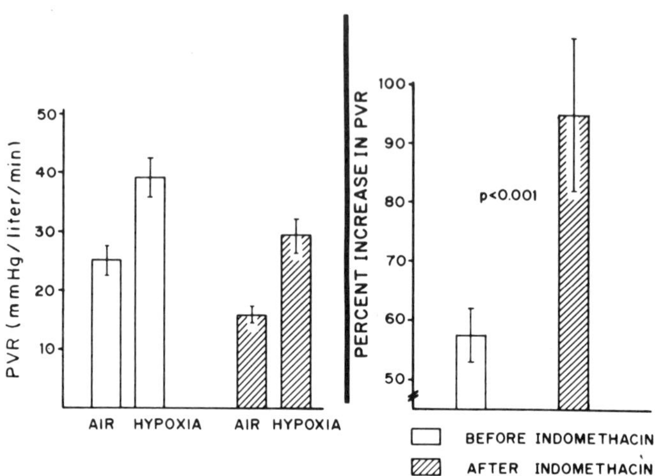

FIGURE 11   Rise in pulmonary vascular resistance (PVR) during hypoxic ventilation before (blank) and after indomethacin (shaded). Figure shows means and ± SE of data from 11 cats. Percent increase in PVR shown to right.

V.   Physiologic and Clinical Perspectives

It is still difficult to assess the full physiologic and clinical implications of the observations cited here. In several instances, however, such implications already seem likely, or at least possible.

1. The increased synthesis and release of bronchodilator and vasodilator PGE compounds during hyperventilation and increased ventilation, should promote the desired increase in air and blood flow, as during muscular exercise. The release of bronchodilator PGEs should at least moderate the bronchoconstrictor effect of hypocapnia (Said 1974).

2. The local release of bronchoconstrictor and vasoconstrictor agents, including PG-like compounds and the spasmogenic lung peptide, during alveolar hypoxia could be an adaptive response, serving to redirect ventilation and blood flow to better oxygenated parts of the lung. This response would protect arterial blood oxygen tension from falling excessively.

3. On the other hand, the liberation of vasodilator PGs (or other compounds) into the circulation could predispose, or contribute, to systemic hypotension. The importance of this factor has been demonstrated in experimental animals during mechanical ventilation

at increased tidal volumes, hyperventilation, and respiratory alkalosis. These observations have special clinical relevance to the management of patients in respiratory failure who are given respiratory assistance, often at larger tidal volumes and coupled with end-expiratory positive pressure (Petty and Ashbaugh 1971).

4. Pulmonary release of vasoactive materials is likely to be a major factor in the constriction of pulmonary vessels associated with hypoxic ventilation, pulmonary edema, and pulmonary embolism. These effects may be produced either by the same compounds that cause systemic vasodilation (e.g., PGE_2, spasmogenic lung peptide) or by other compounds that may be released simultaneously (e.g., $PGF_{2\alpha}$).

5. Similarly, the constriction of airway smooth muscle and other contractile elements in the lung (Kapanci et al. 1974), which often complicates these same conditions, appears to be mediated in large measure by active substances produced within the lung. In pulmonary embolism and in pulmonary edema, airway constriction could be a prominent clinical feature (Stein et al. 1973, Meth et al. 1975).

6. The aggravation of bronchial asthma by exercise (Chan-Yeung et al. 1971) may possibly be related to the excessive release of bronchoconstrictor substances, provoked by the hyperinflation of the lungs. However, since hyperinflation of dog lung stimulated the predominant release of bronchodilator PGE compounds, a hypothesis invoking PG release as a factor in exercise-induced asthma must also postulate an imbalance in the pulmonary synthesis or degradation of PGE and PGF compounds.

7. Some cases of severe lung *injury*, e.g., extensive pneumonia, are complicated by a process of disseminated intravascular coagulation. This grave complication, characterized by abnormal clot formation and lysis, may be precipitated in these patients by the discharge from the lung of *tissue factors* promoting the activation of prothrombin (thromboplastin, leading to fibrin formation) and of plasminogen (resulting in fibrinolysis).

8. A polypeptide with the immunoreactivity of the vasoactive intestinal peptide (VIP), and possibly one of the vasoactive lung peptides, is demonstrable in the plasma of some patients with bronchogenic carcinoma, who present no endocrine manifestations (Said, unpublished observations). This conclusion was reached through the use of a radioimmunoassay originally developed for the vasoactive intestinal polypeptide (VIP), and later found to detect certain lung peptides as well. Such an assay could serve as a useful test for the detection and follow-up of lung cancer.

9. Another polypeptide frequently present in neoplastic and even in normal lung tissue is adrenocorticotrophin (ACTH) (Holdaway et al. 1974). Elevated levels of this peptide hormone also are measurable in the plasma of most patients with bronchogenic carcinoma (Gewirtz and Yalow 1974) even in the absence of clinical signs of ACTH overproduction.

10. A great variety of endocrine syndromes may be associated with certain lung diseases, especially bronchogenic carcinoma. With few exceptions (e.g., hypercalcemia, osteoarthropathy, gonadotrophin secretion), most of these tumors are of the oat-cell variety. The subject of ectopic hormonal secretion by tumors (paraneoplastic syndromes) has been recently reviewed (Lipsett 1968, Hall 1974); some of these syndromes, which relate especially to pulmonary disorders, are listed in Table 2.

VI. Conclusions

The evidence that the lung may synthesize and release many biologically active materials is now overwhelming. This evidence is still largely based on animal experimentation, much of it on isolated lungs or fragments thereof. In many cases, the released materials have been described merely in terms of their biologic characteristics rather than their precise chemical identities. In the coming years, these gaps will no doubt be filled. Improved techniques will permit separation, isolation, and structure determination of released agents, as well as sensitive, specific means for assaying each of them. These advances should yield a better understanding of the normal regulation of pulmonary functions and improved methods for detecting, diagnosing, and treating lung disease.

Recent Developments

Recent work has shown that synthetic pathways beginning with arachidonic acid (and leading to prostaglandin formation) may also result in the production of other, even more potent, substances. These transformations of arachidonic acid include: (a) prostaglandin endoperoxides, precursors of PGs, and several times as active on smooth-muscle organs and platelets; (b) thromboxanes, nonprostaglandin, oxane derivatives of endoperoxides, including an extremely potent platelet aggregator, but unstable compound (thromboxane A_2), and another that is relatively inactive but more stable (thromboxane B_2). Thromboxane A_2 may be the major component of rabbit aorta contracting substance (RCS). In the lung and platelets, most arachidonic acid is transformed into thromboxanes rather than PGs. (M. Hamberg, J. Svensson and B. Samuelsson. Thromboxanes: A new group of biologically active compounds derived from prostaglandin endoperoxides. *Proc. Natl. Acad. Sci, USA,* **72**:2994–2998, 1975).

References

Alabaster, V. A. and Bakhle, Y. S. (1970). The release of biologically active substances from isolated lungs by 5-hydroxytryptamine and tryptamine. *Br. J. Pharmacol.,* **40**:582P–583P.

Alabaster, V. A. and Bakhle, Y. S. (1976). Release of smooth muscle contracting substances from isolated perfused lungs. *Eur. J. Pharmacol.,* **35**:349–360.

Bakhle, Y. S. and Smith, T. W. (1972). Release of spasmogenic substances induced by vasoactive amines from isolated lungs. *Br. J. Pharmacol.,* **46**: 543P–544P.

Bakhle, Y. S. and Smith, T. W. (1974). The nature of the tryptamine receptor mediating spasmogen release from rat isolated lungs. *Br. J. Pharmacol.,* **50**:463P.

Bakhle, Y. S. and Vane, J. R. (1974). Pharmacokinetic function of the pulmonary circulation. *Physiol. Rev.,* **54**:1007–1045.

Becker, K. L., Silva, O. L., Doppman, J., Primack, A., and Snider, R. H. (1975). Elevated serum calcitonin levels in nonthryoid cancer. *Clin. Res.,* **23**:41A.

Berry, E. M., Edmonds, J. F., and Wyllie, J. H. (1971). Release of prostaglandin E_2 and unidentified factors from ventilated lungs. *Br. J. Surg.,* **58**:189–192.

Chan-Yeung, M. M. W., Vyas, M. N., and Grzybowski, S. (1971). Exercise-induced asthma. *Am. Rev. Respir. Dis.,* **104**:915–923.

Comroe, Jr., J. H., Van Lingen, B., Stroud, R. C., and Roncoroni, A. (1953). Reflex and direct cardiopulmonary effects of 5-OH-tryptamine (serotonin). Their possible role in pulmonary embolism and coronary thrombosis. *Am. J. Physiol.,* **173**:379–386.

Gaddum, J. H. (1953). Technique of superfusion. *Br. J. Pharmacol. Chemother.,* **8**:321–326.

Gewirtz, G. and Yalow, R. S. (1974). Ectopic ACTH production in carcinoma of the lung. *J. Clin. Invest.,* **53**:1022–1032.

Greenway, C. V. and Murthy, V. S. (1971). Mesenteric vasoconstriction after endotoxin administration in cats pretreated with aspirin. *Br. J. Pharmacol.,* **43**:259–269.

Gryglewski, R. and Vane, J. R. (1971). Rabbit aorta contracting substance (RCS) may be a prostaglandin precursor. *Br. J. Pharmacol.,* **43**:420P.

Gryglewski, R. and Vane, J. R. (1972). The generation from arachidonic acid of rabbit aorta contracting substance (RCS) by a microsomal enzyme preparation which also generates prostaglandins. *Br. J. Pharmacol.,* **46**:449–457.

Gurewich, V., Cohen, M. D., and Thomas, D. P. (1968). Humoral factors in massive pulmonary embolism: an experimental study. *Am. Heart J.,* **76**: 784–794.

Haas, F. and Bergofsky, E. H. (1972). Role of the mast cell in the pulmonary pressor response to hypoxia. *J. Clin. Invest.,* **51**:3154–3162.

Hall, T. C. (ed.) (1974). Paraneoplastic syndromes. *Ann. N.Y. Acad. Sci.,* **230**: 1–577.

Halmagyi, D. F. J., Starzecki, B., and Horner, G. J. (1964). Humoral transmission of cardiorespiratory changes in experimental lung embolism. *Circ. Res.,* **14**:546–554.

Hamberg, M., Svensson, J., and Samuelsson, B. (1975). Thromboxanes. A new group of biologically active compounds derived from prostaglandin endoperoxides. *Proc. Natl. Acad. Sci. USA,* **72**:2994–2998.

Hauge, A. (1970). The pulmonary vasoconstrictor response to acute hypoxia. Studies on mechanism and site of action. *Progr. Respir. Res.,* **5**:145–155.

Holdaway, I. M., Bloomfield, G. A., Ratcliffe, J. G., Hinson, K. W. F., Rees, G. M., and Rees, L. H. (1974). Adrenocorticotrophin levels in normal and neoplastic lung tissue. In *Endocrinology 1973*: Proceedings of the Fourth International Symposium, London. William Heinemann Medical Books Ltd., London, pp. 309–315.

Kapanci, Y., Assimacopoulos, A., Irle, C., Zwahlen, A., and Gabbiani, G. (1974). "Contactile interstitial cells" in pulmonary alveolar septa: a possible regulator of ventilation/perfusion ratio? *J. Cell. Biol.,* **60**:375–392.

Kitamura, S., Preskitt, J., Yoshida, T., and Said, S. I. (1973). Prostaglandin release, respiratory alkalosis, and systemic hypotension during mechanical ventilation. *Fed. Proc.,* **32**:341.

Lauweryns, J. M. and Cokelaere, M. (1973). Intrapulmonary neuro-epithelial bodies: hypoxia-sensitive neuro (chemo-) receptors. *Experientia,* **29**: 1384–1386.

Lindsey, H. E. and Wyllie, J. H. (1970). Release of prostaglandins from embolized lungs. *Br. J. Surg.,* **57**:738–741.

Lipsett, M. B. (1968). Hormonal syndromes associated with neoplasia. *Adv. Metab. Disorders,* **3**:111–152.

Lloyd, Jr., T. C. (1968). Hypoxic pulmonary vasoconstriction: role of perivascular tissue. *J. Appl. Physiol.,* **25**:560–565.

Lockett, M. F. (1971). The separation of renal activity from lung and from venous effluent from perfused lung. *J. Physiol., Lond.,* **212**:719–731.

Lockett, M. F. (1972). The formation of a renally active peptide by cat lungs from γ-globulin in vitro and the plasma concentrations of this peptide in vivo. *J. Physiol., Lond.,* **224**:187–194.

Marshall, R. (1966). Serotonin and embolization by small blood clots in dogs. *Thorax,* **21**:266–271.

Mathé, A. A. and Levine, L. (1973). Release of prostaglandins and metabolites from guinea pig lung: inhibition by catecholamines. *Prostaglandins,* **4**: 877–890.

Meth, R. F., Tashkin, D. P., Hansen, K. S., and Simmons, D. H. (1975). Pulmonary edema and wheezing after pulmonary embolism. *Am. Rev. Respirat. Diseases,* **111**:693–698.

Nadel, J. A., Colebatch, J. H., and Olsen, C. R. (1964). Location and mechanism of airway constriction after barium sulfate microembolism. *J. Appl. Physiol.,* **19**:387–394.

Nakano, J. and McCloy, R. B. Jr. (1973). Effects of indomethacin on the pulmonary vascular and airway resistance responses to pulmonary microembolization. *Proc. Soc. Exp. Biol. Med.,* **143**:218–221.

Palmer, M. A., Piper, P. J., and Vane, J. R. (1973). Release of rabbit aorta contracting substance (RCS) and prostaglandins induced by chemical or mechanical stimulation of guinea pig lungs. *Br. J. Pharmacol.*, **49**:226–242.

Petty, T. L. and Ashbaugh, D. G. (1971). The adult respiratory distress syndrome. Clinical features, factors influencing prognosis and principles of management. *Chest*, **60**:233–239.

Piper, P. J. and Vane, J. R. (1969). Release of additional factors in anaphylaxis and its antagonism by anti-inflammatory drugs. *Nature*, **223**:29–35.

Piper, P. J. and Vane, J. R. (1971). The release of prostaglandins from the lung and other tissues. *Ann. N.Y. Acad. Sci.*, **180**:363–385.

Piper, P. J. and Walker, J. L. (1973). The release of spasmogenic substances from human chopped lung tissue and its inhibition. *Br. J. Pharmacol.*, **47**:291–304.

Puckett, C. L., Gervin, A. S., Rhodes, G. R., and Silver, D. (1973). Role of platelets and serotonin in acute massive pulmonary embolism. *Surg. Gynecol. Obstet.*, **137**:618–622.

Rådegran, K. (1972). The effect of acetylsalicylic acid on the peripheral and pulmonary vascular responses to thrombin. *Acta Anaesthesiol. Scand.*, **16**:140–146.

Rådegran, K., Bergentz, S. E., Lewis, D. H., Ljungqvist, U., and Olsson, P. (1971). Pulmonary effects of induced platelet aggregation. Intravascular obstruction or vasoconstriction? *Scand. J. Clin. Lab. Invest.*, **28**:423–427.

Rådegran, K., Swedenborg, J., and Olsson, P. (1972). Effect of defibrinogenation and acetylsalicylic acid on the circulatory response to thrombin. *Acta Chir. Scand.*, **138**:441–444.

Robinson, H. J. and Vane, J. R., eds. (1974). *Prostaglandin Synthetase Inhibitors – Their Effects on Physiological Functions and Pathological States.* Raven Press Books, Ltd., New York.

Said, S. I. (1968). The lung as a metabolic organ. *N. Eng. J. Med.*, **279**:1330–1334.

Said, S. I. (1973). The lung in relation to vasoactive hormones. *Fed. Proc.*, **32**:1972–1975.

Said, S. I. (1974). Endocrine role of the lung in disease. *Am. J. Med.*, **57**:433–465.

Said, S. I. and Faloona, G. R. (1975). Elevated plasma and tissue levels of vasoactive intestinal polypeptide in the watery diarrhea syndrome due to pancreatic, bronchogenic and other tumors. *N. Engl. J. Med.*, **293**:155–160.

Said, S. I., Hara, N., and Yoshida, T. (1975b). Hypoxic pulmonary vasoconstriction in cats: Modification by aspirin and by indomethacin. *Fed. Proc.*, **34**:438.

Said, S. I., Kitamura, S., and Vreim, C. (1972). Prostaglandins: Release from the lung during mechanical ventilation at large tidal volumes. *J. Clin. Invest.*, **51**:83A.

Said, S. I., Kitamura, S., Yoshida, T., Preskitt, J., and Holden, L. D. (1974a). Humoral control of airways. *Ann. N.Y. Acad. Sci.*, **221**:103–114.

Said, S. I. and Mutt, V. (1970). Polypeptide with broad biological activity: Isolation from small intestine. *Science*, **169**:1217–1218.

Said, S. I. and Yoshida, T. (1974). Release of prostaglandins and other humoral mediators during hypoxic breathing and pulmonary edema. *Chest,* **66**:12S.

Said, S. I., Mutt, V., Yoshida, T., and Hara, N. (1975a). Biologically active polypeptides from normal lung. *Clin. Res.,* **23**:351A.

Said, S. I., Yoshida, T., Kitamura, S., and Vreim, C. (1974b). Pulmonary alveolar hypoxia: release of prostaglandins and other humoral mediators. *Science,* **185**:1181.

Samuelsson, B. and Hamberg, M. (1974). Role of endoperoxides in the biosynthesis and action of prostaglandins. In H. J. Robinson and J. R. Vane (eds.): *Prostaglandin synthetase inhibitors.* Raven Press, New York, pp. 107–119.

Smith, G. and Smith, A. N. (1955). The role of serotonin in experimental pulmonary embolism. *Surg. Gynecol. Obstet.,* **101**:691–700.

Stein, M. and Thomas, D. P. (1967). Role of platelets in the acute pulmonary responses to endotoxin. *J. Appl. Physiol.,* **23**:47–52.

Stein, M., Hirose, T., Yasutake, T., and Tarabeih, A. (1973). Airway responses to pulmonary embolism – pharmacologic aspects. In K. M. Moser and M. Stein (eds.): *Pulmonary thromboembolism.* Yearbook Medical Publishers, Chicago, pp. 166–177.

Stone, H. H. and Nemir, P., Jr. (1960). Study of role of 5-hydroxytryptamine (serotonin) and histamine in the pathogenesis of pulmonary embolism in man. *Ann. Surg.,* **152**:890–900.

Stoner, J., Manganiello, V. C., and Vaughan, M. (1973). Effects of bradykinin and indomethacin on cyclic GMP and cyclic AMP in lung slices. *Proc. Natl. Acad. Sci. USA,* **70**:3830–3833.

Swedenborg, J. (1971). On the role of vasoactive substances in hemodynamic changes induced by thrombin. *Acta Chir, Scand.,* Suppl. **413**:1–20.

Vane, J. R. (1964). The use of isolated organs for detecting active substances in the circulating blood. *Br. J. Pharmacol. Chemother.,* **23**:360–373.

Vane, J. R. (1968). The release and assay of hormones in the circulation. In *The Scientific Basis of Medicine Annual Reviews,* pp. 336–358.

Vane, J. R. (1969). The release and fate of vasoactive hormones in the circulation. *Br. J. Pharmacol.,* **35**:209–242.

Vane, J. R. (1971). Inhibition of prostaglandin synthesis as a mechanism of action for aspirin-like drugs. *Nature New Biol.,* **231**:232–235.

Vargaftig, B. B. and Dao Hai, N. (1971). Release of vasoactive substances from guinea pig lungs by slow-reacting substance C and arachidonic acid. *Pharmacology,* **6**:99–108.

Vargaftig, B. B. and Dao Hai, N. (1972). Selective inhibition by mepacrine of the release of rabbit aorta contracting substance evoked by the administration of bradykinin. *J. Pharm. Pharmacol.,* **24**:159–161.

Weisbach, H., Waalkes, T. P., and Udenfriend, S. (1957). Presence of serotonin in lung and its implication in the anaphylactic reaction. *Science,* **125**:235–236.

Epilogue

Y. S. BAKHLE

Institute of Basic Medical Sciences
Royal College of Surgeons of England
London, England

Our contributors have provided ten excellent chapters for this monograph
and I have to provide an epilogue. The epilogue I would like to provide is
one which might also serve as a prologue to the next monograph on this subject. A summary of ten chapters would be both tedious and repetitive. What
I propose to do is to pick out some facets of these ten chapters which have
appealed to me and which I think may prove to be areas of advance.

First, a problem that underlies much of the work, the access of substrate
to enzyme. Time after time we have seen how enzymic activities present in
homogenates of lung are not exhibited by the whole lung either in vivo or in
isolated perfused preparations. Is this a discrepancy due to a lack of transport
mechanism, as seems to be the case with the catecholamines, or is it due to a
more gross separation of enzymic activity from substrate in the pulmonary circulation? If, for instance, all the acetylcholine esterase in lung homogenates
derived from cells perfused by the *bronchial* circulation, it would not be surprising that acetylcholine passes through the *pulmonary* circulation without
change. It is this localization of enzymic activity in lung that I hope will

become more apparent through ultrastructural, histochemical, and immuno-chemical techniques, such as the Ryans and Etherton and Conning have described. Histochemistry has so far largely concentrated on the enzymes of intermediate metabolism, but there is now a need for techniques related to enzymes of pharmacologic interest. I hope that a future monograph will be able to provide an atlas of enzymic activities in the lung.

In many other fields, the prostaglandins are giving fresh impetus to research and we shall, as the prostaglandin story unfolds, have to reassess their place in lung. We have considered the metabolism of PGs by the dehydrogenase and reductase enzymes as inactivation. However, even now there is evidence that PG derivatives inactive on one smooth muscle may be highly active on another so that what we have, up till now, called inactivation may in fact be activation but for a specific target organ. Another recent development in prostaglandin research, the identification and characterization of the thromboxanes derived from arachidonic acid, will cast its shadow (or its light, depending on one's own view of these discoveries) on what has been considered so far as prostaglandin synthesis in lung. If, as it seems at present, thromboxane A_2 is more potent as a spasmogen on smooth muscle and more active on platelets than the prostaglandins, in the next 5 years we shall probably be studying thromboxane synthesis and perhaps considering prostaglandins more as waste or alternative products, not in the main stream of arachidonic acid transformation. The ephemeral nature of thromboxane A_2 will inspire innumerable hypotheses as to its place in lung in health and disease, all sharing one essential component; that the short life of thromboxane A_2 makes critical testing of such hypotheses a very difficult task.

To turn towards the investigation and application of lung metabolism in man, I am encouraged by the results that have already been obtained, particularly by the group at Yale. It makes it all the more likely that in man, as in all other laboratory animals, the pulmonary circulation exerts an important control over biologically active substances in blood apart from its respiratory and filtering functions. We proposed some time ago (Bakhle and Vane 1974) that the postperfusion syndrome might be related to the absence of biochemical properties of lung, even though the gas exchange properties could be adequately substituted by heart-lung machines. Now we know amine uptake in human lungs after bypass is affected by the duration of bypass. So is the severity of postperfusion syndrome. This investigation should be pursued, and the extent to which the metabolic functions of lung are disturbed by heart-lung bypass clearly established. One way of correcting the biochemical deficiencies of present heart-lung machines would be to include column-coupled enzymes. The blood could then be scrubbed for the various substrates, just as effluents from industry are scrubbed to remove undesirable chemicals. Converting enzyme coupled to Sepharose has already been described, and I am sure that further progress will be made in this direction.

The metabolic properties of the pulmonary circulation also have significance for drug design. One of us has already pointed out (Vane 1970) that the inefficacy in vivo of a drug efficacious in vitro may be due to metabolism, and particularly to metabolism in the pulmonary circulation. As recent experience has shown for bradykinin (Ondetti and Engel 1975), it is possible to design analogs, which, although less active in vitro, are, because of their resistance to lung enzymes, much more potent in vivo.

Instead of considering lung metabolism as an obstacle to overcome, it could be turned to therapeutic advantage, particularly for drugs, acting on the lung, given by inhalation. The incentive to discover amines which are specifically bronchodilator derived from the unacceptable systemic effects of inhaled isoprenaline. An alternative approach to an isoprenaline substitute would be to look for an amine not *specifically* bronchodilator but which was susceptible to metabolism by lung. Such an amine could then be given by inhalation and its possible systemic effects eliminated through its inactivation in the lung. This approach has not yet been adopted or at least has not yet been successful. However, this principle may be operating in the case of beclamethasone, a synthetic steroid given by inhalation for the treatment of asthma. This steroid has potent antiasthmatic effects without the systemic effects that accompany treatment with other steroids. As the lung has significant steroid metabolizing capacity and can take up and transform native steroids, it is possible that the selective effect of beclamethasone inhalation is due, at least in part, to its metabolism in the lung. If this possibility is supported by experimental results, then clearly there will be a new approach to selectivity of drug action.

We have set out to provide, in this volume, a summary of what is known of the pharmacologically relevant metabolic functions of the pulmonary circulation. This summary is intended not as a definitive and final statement but as an incentive to further research. Whether this further research arises from a fascination with a problem of metabolism in lung or from a despairing vexation with the insufficiency of the work already described, it does not matter; this volume will have served its purpose. Three years ago John Vane and I wrote a review to bring to general notice the pharmacokinetic functions of the pulmonary circulation (Bakhle and Vane 1974). In 1975 there was an international symposium on lung pharmacokinetics, which demonstrated a widespread interest in this field (Bakhle and Hartiala 1976). Now there is this volume, which will soon be out of date (if it were not, that would be a sign of stagnation). In 5 years time each of our chapter headings will need a monograph of its own. All that we, the contributors and the readers, have to do now is to provide the experimental results to fill those monographs.

References

Bakhle, Y. S. and Hartiala, J. (eds.) (1976). Proceedings of Symposium on pharmacokinetic functions of lung, *Agents and Actions,* **6**:493–559.

Bakhle, Y. S. and Vane, J. R. (1974). Pharmacokinetic function of the pulmonary circulation. *Physiol. Rev.,* **54**:1007–1045.

Ondetti, M. A. and Engel, S. L. (1975). Bradykinin analogs containing β-homo-amino acids. *J. Med. Chem.,* **18**:761–763.

Vane, J. R. (1970). The alteration or removal of vasoactive substances by the pulmonary circulation. In D. H. Tedeschi and R. E. Tedeschi (eds.): *Importance of Fundamental Principles in Drug Evaluation.* Raven Press, New York, pp. 217–236.

AUTHOR INDEX

Italic numbers give the page on which the complete reference is listed.

T

SUBJECT INDEX